ADVANCED YANG STYLE TAI CHI CHUAN

Volume One
Tai Chi Theory and Tai Chi Jing

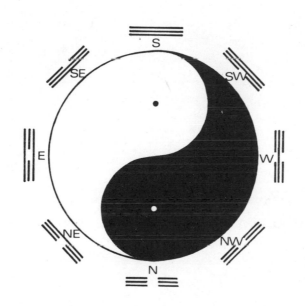

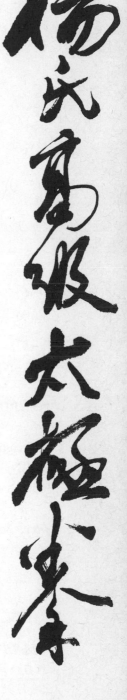

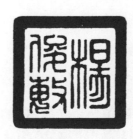

By Dr. Yang Jwing-Ming

DISCLAIMER

The author(s) and publisher of this material are **NOT RESPONSIBLE** in any manner whatsoever for any injury which may occur through reading or following the instructions in this material.

The activities, physical and otherwise, described in this material may be too strenuous or dangerous for some people, and the reader(s) should consult a physician before engaging in them.

YMAA PUBLICATION CENTER
A DIVISION OF YOAA, INC.
38 HYDE PARK AVENUE
JAMAICA PLAIN, MASSACHUSETTS 02130

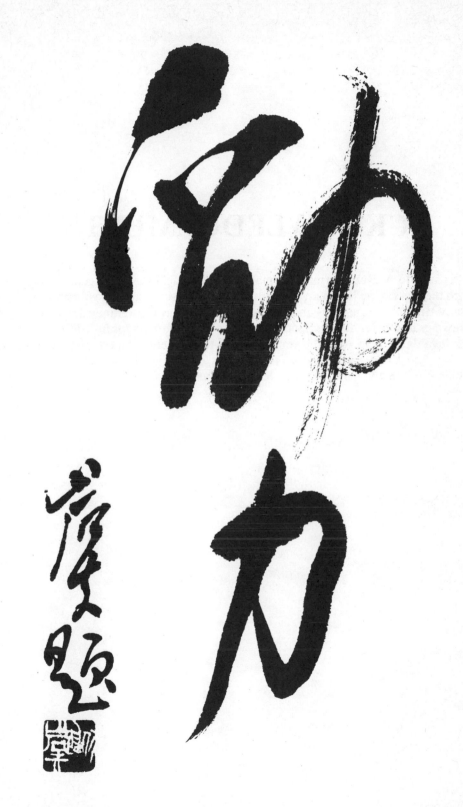

ACKNOWLEDGEMENTS

Thanks to A. Reza Farman-Farmaian and Michael Fioretti for general help with the work, Eric Hoffman for proofing the manuscript and for contributing many valuable suggestions and discussions, and John Casagrande Jr. for the drawings and cover design. Special thanks to Alan Dougall for his editing and his invaluable help with the translation of the ancient Chinese poetry and songs. And a very special thanks to the artist Zong Nian-Fu for his beautiful calligraphy on the front pages of both volumes.

ABOUT THE AUTHOR

DR. YANG JWING-MING

Dr. Yang Jwing-Ming was born in Taiwan, Republic of China, in 1946. He started his Wushu (Kung Fu) training at the age of fifteen under the Shaolin White Crane (Pai Huo) Master Cheng Gin-Gsao. In thirteen years of study (1961-1974) under Master Cheng, Dr. Yang became an expert in White Crane defense and attack, which includes both the use of barehands and of various weapons such as saber, staff, spear, trident, and two short rods. With the same master he also studied White Crane Chin Na, massage, and herbal treatment. At the age of sixteen Dr. Yang began the study of Tai Chi Chuan (Yang Style) under Master Kao Tao. After learning from Master Kao, Dr. Yang continued his study and research of Tai Chi Chuan with several masters in Taipei. In Taipei he became qualified to teach Tai Chi. He has mastered the Tai Chi barehand sequence, pushing hands, the two-man fighting sequence, Tai Chi sword, Tai Chi saber, and internal power development.

When Dr. Yang was eighteen years old he entered Tamkang College in Taipei Hsien to study Physics. In college, he began the study of Shaolin Long Fist (Chang Chuan) with Master Li Mao-Ching at the Tamkang College Kuoshu Club (1964-1968), and eventually became an assistant instructor under Master Li. In 1971 he completed his M.S. degree in Physics at the National Taiwan University, and then served in the Chinese Air Force from 1971-1972. In the service, Dr. Yang taught Physics at the Junior Academy of the Chinese Air Force while also teaching Wushu. After being honorably discharged in 1972, he returned to Tamkang College to teach Physics and resume study under Master Li Mao-Ching. From Master Li, Dr. Yang learned Northern style Wushu, which includes both barehand (especially kicking) techniques and numerous weapons.

In 1974, Dr. Yang came to the United States to study Mechanical Engineering at Purdue University. At the request of a few students, Dr. Yang began to teach Kung Fu which resulted in the foundation of the Purdue University Chinese Kung Fu Research Club in the spring of 1975. While at Purdue, Dr. Yang also taught college-credited courses in Tai Chi Chuan. In May of 1978, he was awarded a Ph.D. in Mechanical Engineering from Purdue.

Currently, Dr. Yang and his family reside in Massachusetts. In January of 1984, he gave up his engineering career to devote more time to research, writing, and teaching at Yang's Martial Arts Academy in Boston.

In summary, Dr. Yang has been involved in Chinese Wushu (Kung Fu) for more than twenty years. During this time, he has spent thirteen years learning Shaolin White Crane (Pai Huo), Shaolin Long Fist (Chang Chuan), and Tai Chi Chuan. Dr. Yang has seventeen years of instructional experience: seven years in Taiwan, five years at Purdue University, two years in Houston, Texas, and three years in Boston, Massachusetts.

Dr. Yang has published six other volumes on martial arts:
1. *Shaolin Chin Na;* Unique Publications, Inc., 1980.
2. *Shaolin Long Fist Kung Fu;* Unique Publications, Inc., 1981.
3. *Yang Style Tai Chi Chuan;* Unique Publications, Inc., 1981.
4. *Introduction to Ancient Chinese Weapons;* Unique Publications, Inc., 1985.
5. *Chi Kung - Health and Martial Arts;* Yang's Martial Arts Academy (YMAA), 1985.
6. *Northern Shaolin Sword;* Yang's Martial Arts Academy (YMAA), 1985.

In addition, Dr. Yang has published the videotape "Yang Style Tai Chi Chuan and Its Applications", Yang's Martial Arts Academy (YMAA), 1984.

Dr. Yang plans to publish a number of additional books including:
1. *Advanced Yang Style Tai Chi Chuan, Vol.2, Martial Applications*
2. *Analysis of Shaolin Chin Na - Instructor's Manual*
3. *Northern Shaolin Staff*
4. *Northern Shaolin Saber*
5. *Northern Shaolin Spear*

Several videotapes have also been scheduled for publication:
1. *"Shaolin Long Fist Kung Fu - Lien Bu Chuan"*
2. *"Shaolin Long Fist Kung Fu - Gung Li Chuan"*
3. *"Shaolin Long Fist Kung Fu - Yi Lu Mei Fu"*
4. *"Shaolin Long Fist Kung Fu - Shaw Fu Ien"*
5. *"Shaolin Long Fist Kung Fu - Shih Tzu Tan"*
6. *"Yang Style Tai Chi Sword and Its Applications"*

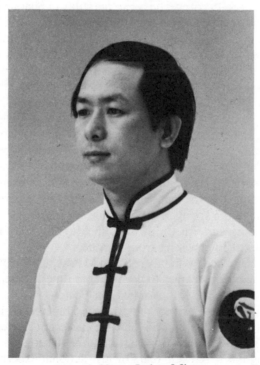

Master Yang Jwing-Ming.

FOREWORD

BY JOU, TSUNG HWA

It is with great pleasure that I introduce the reader to Dr. Yang, Jwing-Ming's new book on Tai Chi Chuan. In truth, I had come to know Dr. Yang first through his excellent books on the Chinese Martial Arts. Although we had corresponded, it was not until June of 1985 that I first met with Dr. Yang in person. I first met him at the National Chang, San Feng Festival held at the Tai Chi Foundation's training grounds in Warwick, New York. Dr. Yang had graciously accepted my invitation to teach a workshop for the numerous Tai Chi practitioners who had gathered together for the festival. It was at that time that I had the opportunity to see for myself that Dr. Yang's ability was of the same high caliber as his written treatises.

Many practitioners today are satisfied to merely run through the choreography of their particular Tai Chi form without putting any content or effort into their practice. While a routine run-through of Tai Chi may be enjoyable, it will not lead to progress. A hollow form will produce neither health nor martial benefits.

The practitioner who wishes to achieve progress in Tai Chi must be willing to put forth great efforts to master the necessary principles, and to practice diligently and with a sense of purpose, in order to get results. Tai Chi must be a blend of both Yin and Yang. Empty form alone will produce nothing. In Dr. Yang's first book the external, martial aspects of Tai Chi Chuan were clearly presented. In Dr. Yang's present work, he has made a clear and detailed presentation of the more "inner" mechanics of Tai Chi Chuan.

If the Tai Chi practitioner is willing to invest effort into developing his internal power and awareness, his Tai Chi form and applications will improve. Not everyone today has personal access to accomplished masters of Tai Chi Chuan. Furthermore, availiable written materials related to the development of internal energy and force have often been difficult to understand.

For these reasons I urge the reader to pay careful attention to this book. However, as Dr. Yang points out, reading alone will accomplish little. It is up to the individual practitioner to put these concepts into practice. In this regard, the reader is very fortunate to have Dr. Yang for a guide.

Jou, Tsung Hwa
Warwick, New York, June 9, 1985

PREFACE

Tai Chi Chuan has become a popular exercise, not only in China but even in many other countries around the world. Throughout most of its history the art was kept secret, and only taught to family members and trusted students. Since the beginning of this century, when the art was first opened up to the public, many people have taken advantage of Tai Chi's ability to improve health and cure a number of illnesses. In our present hectic society, people are looking for a way to release daily pressures, calm down their minds, and relax their bodies. Tai Chi has been shown to be an excellent way to achieve this.

In spite of the popularity of Tai Chi Chuan, whether in China, Taiwan, or other parts of the world, the art is gradually becoming incomplete. Because most Tai Chi practitioners are more interested in health than in self-defense, the deeper aspects of the art have been gradually ignored. Many people who have practiced Tai Chi Chuan for quite a few years still do not understand its theory and principles. They may not know how to coordinate their breathing with the forms, and many do not understand the relationship of Tai Chi and Chi Kung. Some even do not know what Chi is, or how to generate it through Tai Chi practice and still meditation. Because of this their art remains superficial. Furthermore, the original, major part of Tai Chi Chuan—the martial application—is dying out. The reader should understand that Tai Chi was created as a martial Chi Kung art. The self-defense applications remain a necessary part of the wholeness of Tai Chi Chuan. Its principles and techniques are unique in martial society.

The author hopes through this volume on theory and a subsequent volume on applications to fill in some of the gaps in the general knowledge, and to encourage Tai Chi practitioners to research the deeper aspects of the art. Because Tai Chi is so profound and covers so much, it is not possible for one book, or for that matter one person, to cover the art fully. The author hopes that more Tai Chi masters will share their research experience and knowledge with the public through publications, seminars, and classes. Only in this way can Tai Chi again become a living, vital, complete art.

In these two volumes, the author will discuss the deeper aspects of barehand Tai Chi Chuan based upon his personal experience and understanding, and the teachings of his masters. The theory and techniques of Tai Chi weapons will be published later. Also, these volumes will not discuss fundamental Tai Chi theory and training, the solo sequence, fundamental pushing hands, or the matching set, since they have already been covered in the author's first Tai Chi book: *Yang Style Tai Chi Chuan*, Unique Publications, Inc., 1982. The Tai Chi beginner should also study the author's book *Chi Kung–Health and Martial Arts*, YMAA, 1985, which explains general Chi Kung theory, methods of training, and the relationship of Chi Kung to health and the martial arts.

This first volume will discuss theory and principles. Chapter 1 will introduce the history of Yang Style Tai Chi Chuan, the definition of Tai Chi, its content and training procedures. Chapter 2 will discuss the deeper aspects of Tai Chi principles and theory. This chapter will be very important to both beginners and advanced students, and will help to build a comprehensive foundation for later discussion. The third chapter will discuss Tai Chi power—known by the Chinese word "Jing". Jing theory and training methods have been kept secret since the beginning of the art. To the author's knowledge, there is no extensive discussion published in English on this subject, and very little is available even in Chinese. The first volume will conclude with fifteen ancient Tai Chi poems and songs written by famous masters. Translations will be given as well as commentary by the author.

After the reader has studied and built up a foundation of knowledge from the first volume, the second chapter of the second volume will analyze the martial applications of each form in the solo sequence. All the postures in the sequence have a martial purpose—they are not done just for relaxation and the beauty of the exercise. Every posture has multiple levels of martial application. Tai Chi Chuan specializes in the techniques of Downing the Enemy, Chin Na Control, and Cavity Press. After the reader understands the applications of the Tai Chi forms, the third chapter will guide him through pushing hands training theory, methods, and applications. Only after the reader has practiced pushing hands extensively should he learn the Tai Chi fighting set in Chapter 4. This set was created to resemble real fighting, and will gradually lead the Tai Chi practitioner to an understanding of the techniques and the ability to use them in a real fight. Chapter 5 will discuss Tai Chi fighting strategy, which is very different from that of most of the external martial styles. Chapter 6 will conclude this volume with some guidelines to help the reader select a qualified instructor.

Throughout these two volumes are quotations from various Chinese sources. The author has chosen not to make the translations polished English, but rather to make them as accurate as possible. Wherever feasible the Chinese idioms, and even the Chinese sentence structure, have been used. It is hoped that this contributes enough in flavor and clarity to compensate for the distraction that this approach can cause.

VOLUME 1

TAI CHI THEORY AND TAI CHI JING

TABLE OF CONTENTS

VOLUME 2

MARTIAL APPLICATIONS

TABLE OF CONTENTS

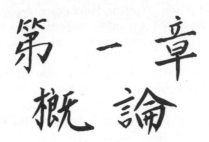

CHAPTER 1
GENERAL INTRODUCTION

1-1. Introduction

Chi Kung is a training system which helps to generate a strong flow of Chi (Internal Energy) inside the body and then circulate it through the entire body. Many martial and non-martial styles of Chi Kung training have been created in the last four thousand years. The most famous martial styles are Tai Chi Chuan, Ba Kua, Hsing Yi, and Liu Ho Ba Fa. These are considered "internal" styles (Nei Kung or Nei Jar in Chinese), as opposed to "external" styles like Shaolin, because they emphasize working with Chi. The best known non-martial styles, which emphasize the enhancement of Chi circulation to improve health, are Wu Chin Si (Five Animal Sport), Ba Tuan Gin (Eight Pieces of Brocade), Da Mo's Yi Gin Ching (Muscle Change Classic), and Shih Er Chuang (Twelve Postures).

Tai Chi Chuan, which is said to have been created by Chang San-Feng in the twelfth century, is now the most popular Chi Kung style in the world, even though it was shrouded in secrecy until the beginning of this century. At present it is widely practiced not only in China and the East but also in the Western world.

There are several reasons for the rapid spread of this art. The most important, perhaps, is that the practice of Tai Chi can help to calm down the mind and relax the body, which are becoming survival skills in today's hectic and stress-filled world. Secondly, since guns are so effective and easy to acquire, Tai Chi has been considered less vital for personal self-defense than it used to be. For this reason, more Tai Chi masters are willing to share their knowledge with the public. Thirdly, ever since Tai Chi was created, it has been proven not only effective for defense, but also useful for improving health and curing a number of illnesses.

Unfortunately, because of this healthful aspect the deeper theory and practice of Tai Chi Chuan, especially the martial applications, are being widely ignored. Most people today think that Tai Chi is not practical for self-defense. To approach the deeper aspects requires much time and patience, and there are very few people willing to make the necessary sacrifices. In addition, some Tai Chi experts are still withholding the secrets of the deeper aspects of the training, and not passing down the complete art.

Anyone who practices this art correctly for a number of years will soon realize that Tai Chi is not just an exercise for calmness and relaxation—it is a complex and highly developed art. It gives the practitioner a feeling of enjoyment and satisfaction which seems to go beyond that of any other art. This is because Tai Chi is smooth, refined, and elegant internally as well as externally. The practitioner can sense the Chi (energy) circulating within his body, and can achieve the peaceful mind of meditation. Chi circulation can bring good health and may even help you to reach enlightenment. Furthermore, when a Tai Chi practitioner has achieved Grand Circulation, he can use this Chi in self-defense. The principles that Tai Chi uses for fighting are quite different from most other martial styles, which rely on muscular force. Tai Chi uses the soft to defend against the hard, and weakness to defeat strength. The more you practice, the better you will become, and this defensive capability will grow with age instead of weaken. However, because the martial theory of Tai Chi Chuan is much deeper and more profound than that of most other systems, it is much harder to learn and takes a longer time to approach a high level of martial capability. A knowledgeable instructor is very important, for guidance from an experienced master can save many years of wandering and useless practice.

Today, there are still a number of interested practitioners who are researching and practicing the deeper aspects of Tai Chi Chuan with the help of the very few qualified experts and/or the limited number of in-depth publications. Many questions have arisen: Which is a good style of Tai Chi Chuan? How can I tell who is a qualified Tai Chi instructor? What is the historical background of the different styles? Which styles can be applied effectively? How do I generate Chi? How do I coordinate my breathing with the Chi circulation? How do I use Chi in self-defense? What is Jing (power) and is there more than one kind? How do I train my Jing correctly? How does the fighting strategy of Tai Chi differ from other styles? All these questions puzzle people even in China.

This volume will describe the deeper aspects of Tai Chi training and is written mainly for the reader who has practiced Tai Chi for a few years. The beginning Tai Chi practitioner should also refer to the author's books: *Yang Style Tai Chi Chuan* and *Chi Kung–Health and Martial Arts.*

1-2. General History of Tai Chi Chuan

Many people have learned Yang style Tai Chi Chuan, but few really understand the history, background, and variations of the style. Often a person who has learned Yang style Tai Chi Chuan will see forms which claim to be Yang style, but which look different from what he has learned. This sometimes causes consternation and doubt about which form, if any, is the correct "Yang style". A knowledge of the history can help to explain this discrepancy.

It is said that Tai Chi Chuan was created by Chang San-Feng in the Sung Wei Dsung era (c. 1101 A.D.). It is also said that techniques and forms with the same basic principles as Tai Chi were already in existence during the Liang Dynasty (502-557 A.D.), and were being taught by Han Goong-Yueh, Chen Ling-Shih, and Chen Bi. Later, in the Tang Dynasty (713-905), it was found that Sheu Hsuan-Pin, Li Tao-Tzu, and Ien Li-Hen were teaching similar martial techniques. They were called Thirty-Seven Postures (San Shih Chi Shih), Post-Heaven Techniques (Hou Tien Far), or Small Nine Heaven (Shao Jeou Tien) which had seventeen postures. The accuracy of these accounts is sometimes questionable, so it is not really known when and by whom Tai Chi Chuan was created. Because there is more formal history recorded about Chang San-Feng he has received most of the credit.

According to the historical record *Nan Lei Gi Wang Jeng Nan Moo Tzu Min:* "Chang San-Feng, in the Sung Dynasty, was a Wu Dan Taoist. Wei Dsung (a Sung Emperor) summoned him, but the road was blocked and he couldn't come. At night, (Wei Dsung) dreamed Emperor Yuen (the first Gin emperor) taught him martial techniques. At dawn, he killed a hundred enemies by himself". Also recorded in the Ming history *Ming Shih Fan Gi Chwan:* "Chang San-Feng, from Lieu Dong Yi county. Named Chuan-Yi. Also named Jiun-Bao. San-Feng was his nickname. Because he did not keep himself neat and clean, also called Chang Lar-Tar (Sloppy Chang). He was tall and big, shaped like a turtle, and had a crane's back. Large ears and round eyes. Beard long like a spear tassel. Wears only a priest's robe winter or summer. Will eat a bushel of food, or won't eat for several days or a few months. Can travel a thousand miles. Likes to have fun with people. Behaves as if nobody is around. Used to travel to Wu Dan (mountain) with his disciples. Built a simple cottage and lived inside. In the 24th year of Hung Wu (around 1392), Ming Tai Tzu (the first Ming emperor) heard of his name, and sent a messenger to look for him but he couldn't be found". It was also recorded in the Ming Dynasty in *Ming Lan Yin Chi Shou Lei Kou:* "Chang the Immortal, named Jiun-Bao, also named Chuan-Yi, nicknamed Shuan-Shuan, also called Chang Lar-Tar. In the third year of Tien Suen (1460) he visited Emperor Ming Ying Dsung. A picture was drawn. The beard and mustache were straight, the back of the head had a tuft. Purple face and big stomach, with a bamboo hat in his hand. On the top of the picture was an inscription from the emperor honoring Chang as 'Ton Wei Sien Far Jinn Zen' (a genuine Taoist who finely discriminates and clearly understands much" (Figure 1-1). This record is suspect, because if it were true, Chang San-Feng would have been at least 500 years old at that time. Other records state that Chang San-Feng's techniques were learned from the Taoist Fon Yi-Yuen. Another story tells that Chang San-Feng was an ancient hermit meditator. He saw a magpie fighting against a snake, had a sudden understanding, and created Tai Chi Chuan.

After Chang San-Feng, there were Wang Dsung in Sanshi province, Chen Ton-Jou in Wen County, Chang Soun-Shi in Hai Yen, Yeh Gi-Mei in Shyh Ming, Wang Dsung-Yueh in San You, and Chiang Fa in Hebei. The Tai Chi techniques were passed down and divided into two major styles, southern and northern. Later, Chiang Fa passed his art to the Chen family at Chen Jar Gou in Hwai Ching County, Henan. Tai Chi was then passed down for fourteen generations and divided into Old and New Styles. The Old Style was carried on by Chen Chang-Shen and the New Style was created by Chen You-Ban.

The Old Style successor Chen Chang-Shen then passed the art down to his son, Ken-Yun, and his Chen relatives, Chen Hwai-Yuen and Chen Hwa-Mei. He also passed his Tai Chi outside of his family to Yang Lu-Shann and Li Bao-Kuai, both of Hebei province. This Old Style is called Thirteen Postures Old Form (Shih San Shih Lao Jiah). Later, Yang Lu-Shann passed it down to his two sons, Yang Ban-Huo and Yang Chien-Huo. Then, Chien-Huo passed the art to his two sons, Yang Shao-Huo and Yang Chen-Fu. This branch of Tai Chi Chuan is popularly called Yang Style. Also, Wu Chun-Yu learned from Yang Ban-Huo and started a well known Wu style.

Also, Chen You-Ban passed his New Style to Chen Ching-Pin who created Tsao Bao Style Tai Chi Chuan. Wuu Yu-Larn learned the Old Style from Yang Lu-Shann and New Style from Chen Ching-Pin, and created Wuu Style Tai Chi Chuan. Li Yi-Yu learned the Wuu Style and created Li Style Tai Chi Chuan. Heh Wei-Jinn obtained his art from Li Style and created Heh Style Tai Chi Chuan.

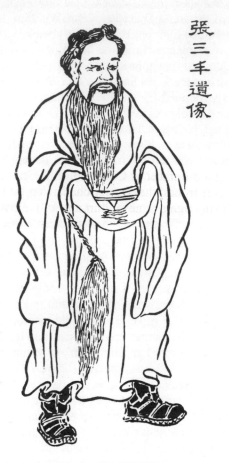

張三丰遺像

Figure 1-1. Chang San-Feng

Sun Lu-Tan learned from Heh Style and created Sun Style.

All the above mentioned styles are popular in China and Southeast Asia. Among them, Yang style has become the most popular. In the next section we will discuss the history of the Yang style.

1-3. History of Yang Style Tai Chi Chuan

Yang Style history starts with Yang Lu-Shann (1799-1872), also known as Fu-Kuai or Lu-Chan. He was born at Youn Nien Hsien, Kuan Pin County, Hebei Province. When he was young he went to Chen Jar Gou in Henan province to learn Tai Chi Chuan from Chen Chang-Shen. When Chen Chang-Shen stood he was centered and upright with no leaning or tilting, like a wooden signpost, and so people called him Mr. Tablet. At that time, there were very few students outside of the Chen family who learned from Chen Chang-Shen. Because Yang was an outside student, he was treated unfairly, but he still stayed and persevered in his practice.

One night, he was awakened by the sounds of "Hen" and "Ha" in the distance. He got up and traced the sound to an old building. Peeking through the broken wall, he saw his master Chen Chang-Shen teaching the techniques of grasp, control, and emitting Jing in coordination with the sounds Hen and Ha. He was amazed by the techniques and from that time on, unknown to master Chen, he continued to watch this secret practice session every night. He would then return to his room to ponder and study. Because of this, his martial ability advanced rapidly. One day, Chen ordered him to spar with the other disciples. To his surprise, none of the other students could defeat him. Chen realized that Yang had great potential and after that taught him the secrets sincerely.

After Yang Lu-Shann finished his study, he returned to his home town and taught Tai Chi Chuan for a while. People called his style Yang Chuan (Yang Style), Mei Chuan (Soft Style), or Far Chuan (Neutralizing Style), because his motions were soft and able to neutralize the opponent's power. He later went to Peking and taught a number of Ching officers. He used to carry a spear and a small bag and travel around the country challenging well known martial artists. Although he had many fights he never hurt anybody. Because his art was so high, nobody could defeat him. Therefore, he was called "Yang Wu Di", which means "Unbeatable Yang". He had three sons, Yang Chyi, Yang Yuh (Ban-Huo), and Yang Jiann (Chien-Huo). Yang Chyi died when he was young. Therefore, only the last two sons succeeded their father in the art.

There are a few stories about Yang Lu-Shann

1.   One time, when Yang was at Kuan Pin, he was fighting a martial artist on the city wall. The opponent was not able to defeat him and kept retreating to the edge of the wall. Suddenly he lost his balance and was about to fall. At that moment, Yang suddenly approached him from several yards distance, grasped his foot and saved his life.

2.   Yang was good at using the spear. He could pick up light objects by using his spear to adhere to the object, then tossing it up into his hand. He was also good at throwing arrows with his bare hand--he could hit the target accurately while on horse back without using a bow.

3.   One rainy day, while Yang was sitting in his living room, his daughter entered from outside holding a basin of water. When she opened the screen, she suddenly slipped on the wet step. Yang saw this and jumped up, held the screen with one hand, and caught his daughter's arm with the other. Not a drop of water splashed from the basin. From this anecdote one can see how quick his reactions were.

4.   One day, Yang was fishing at a lake. Two other martial artists were passing by and saw him. They had heard of Yang's reputation and were afraid to challenge him, so they decided to take the opportunity to push Yang into the lake and make him lose face. To their surprise, when their hands touched his back, Yang arched his back and bounced both of them into the lake.

5.   When Yang was in Peking, a famous martial artist was jealous of Yang's reputation and challenged him. Yang politely refused. However, the man insisted. Yang said, if you want to fight me, you can hit me three times first. The man was delighted and hit Yang's stomach. Yang suddenly uttered the "Ha" sound with a laugh. Before the laugh was finished, the challenger was already on the ground, bounced many yards away.

Yang's second son was Yang Yuh (1837-1890), also named Ban-Huo. People used to call him "Mr. The Second". He studied Tai Chi Chuan with his father since he was small. Even though he practiced very hard and continuously, he was still scolded and whipped by his father. He was good at free fighting. One day he was challenged by a strong martial artist. When the challenger grasped his wrist and would not let him escape, Yang Ban-Huo suddenly used his Jing to bounce the challenger away and defeat him. He was so proud he went home and told his father. Instead of praise, his father laughed at him, because his sleeve was torn. After that, he trained harder and harder and finally became a superlative Tai Chi artist. Unfortunately, he didn't like to teach very much and had few students, so his art did not spread far after he died. One of his students called Wu Chun-Yu later taught his son Wu Chien-Chun, whose art became the Wu Style Tai Chi Chuan. Yang Ban-Huo also had a son, called Jaw-Peng, who passed on the art.

The third son of Yang Lu-Shann was Yang Jiann (1842-1917), also named Chien-Huo and nicknamed Gien-Fu. People used to call him "Mr. The Third". He also learned Tai Chi from his father since he was young. His personality was softer and more gentle than his brother's and he had many followers. He taught three postures—large, medium, and small—although he specialized in the medium posture. He was also expert in using and coordinating both hard and soft power. He used to spar with his disciples who were good at sword and saber while using only a dust brush. Every time his brush touched the student's wrist, the student could not do anything but bounce out. He was also good at using the staff and spear. When his long weapon touched an opponent's weapon, the opponent could not approach him, but instead bounced away. When he emitted Jing it happened at the instant of laughing the "Ha" sound. He could also throw the small metal balls called "bullets". When he had a few balls in his hand, he could shoot three or four birds at the same time. The most impressive demonstration he performed was to put a sparrow on his hand. The bird could not fly away because when a bird takes off, it must push down first and use the reaction force to lift itself. Yang Chien-Huo could sense the bird's power and neutralize this slight push, leaving the bird unable to take off. From this demonstration, one can understand that his Listening Jing and Neutralizing Jing (see Chapter 3) must have been superb. He had three sons, Jaw-Shyong, Jaw-Yuen, and Jaw-Ching. The second son, Jaw-Yuen died at an early age.

Yang Chien-Huo's first son was Yang Jaw-Shyong (1862-1929), also named Mum-Shiang and later called Shao-Huo. People used to call him "Mr. Oldest". He practiced Tai Chi Chuan since he was six years old. He had a strong and persevering personality. He was expert in free fighting and very good at using various Jings like his uncle Yang Ban-Huo. He reached the highest level of Tai Chi Kung Fu. Specializing in small postures, his movements were fast and sunken. Because of his personality, he didn't have too many followers. He had a son called Yang Jen-Shen.

Yang Chien-Huo's second son, Jaw-Yuan, died at a young age. The third son was Yang Jaw-Ching (1883-1935), also named Chen-Fu. People called him "Mr. The Third". His personality was mild and gentle. When he was young, he did not care for martial arts. It was not until his teens that he started studying Tai Chi with his father. While his father was still alive Yang Chen-Fu did not really understand the key secrets of Tai Chi Chuan. It was not until his father died (1917) that he started to practice hard. His father had helped him to build a good foundation, and after several years of practice and research he was finally able to approach the level of his father and grandfather. Because of his experiences, he modified his father's Tai Chi Chuan and specialized in large postures. This emphasis was just completely reversed from that of his father and brother. He was the first Tai Chi master willing to share the family secrets with the public, and because of his gentle nature he had countless students. When Nanking Central Kuoshu Institute was founded in 1926 he was invited to be the head Tai Chi teacher, and his name became known throughout the country. He had four sons, Jeng-Min, Jeng-Gi, Jeng-Zer, and Jeng-Kuo.

Yang Style Tai Chi Chuan can be classified into three major postures: large, medium, and small. It is also divided into three stances: high, medium, and low. Large postures were emphasized by Yang Chen-Fu. He taught that the stances can be either high, medium, or low, but the postures are extended, opened, and relaxed. Large postures are especially suitable for improving health. The medium posture style requires that all the forms be neither too extended nor too restricted, and the internal Jing neither totally emitted nor too conserved. Therefore, the form and Jing are smoother and more continuous than the other two styles. The medium posture style was taught by Yang Chien-Huo. The small posture style, in which the forms are more compact and the movements light, agile, and quick, was passed down by Yang Shao-Huo. This style specializes in the martial application of the art. In conclusion, for martial application the small postures are generally the best, although they are the most difficult, and the large posture style is best for health purposes.

To summarize:

1. Chen Style Tai Chi Chuan was derived from Chiang Style. Before Chiang, the history is vague and unclear.
2. Chen Style was divided into two styles: Old and New. Chen Chang-Shen learned Old Style and later passed it down to Yang Lu-Shann. New Style was created by Chen You-Ban.
3. Yang Style was derived from Chen Style fourteen generations after the Chen family learned from Chiang.
4. Chen You-Ban passed his art to Chen Ching-Pin who created Tsao Bao Style.
5. Wuu Yu-Larn obtained the New style from Chen Ching-Pin and the Old Style from Yang Lu-Shann and created Wuu Style Tai Chi Chuan.
6. Li Yi-Yu learned Wuu Style and created Li Style.
7. Heh Wei-Jinn obtained his art from Li Style and started Heh Style Tai Chi Chuan.
8. Sun Lu-Tan learned from Heh Style and began Sun Style.
9. Wu Style was started by Wu Chun-Yu who learned from Yang Lu-Shann's second son Yang Ban-Huo.
10. Yang Style Tai Chi Chuan has been famous since its creation by Yang Lu-Shann in the early part of the last century.
11. Yang Chen-Fu's Tai Chi Chuan is not the same as his father's, uncle's, or brother's. He modified it and emphasized large postures and improving the health

The reader should now understand why there are so many variations within the art, even within a style such as the Yang style. After so many years and so many generations, countless students have learned the art. Many went on to modify the style in light of their own experiences and research. It is understandable that a student nowadays might learn Tai Chi Chuan and find that his style is different from another claiming to be from the same source. No one can really tell which is the original style or which is more effective than the others.

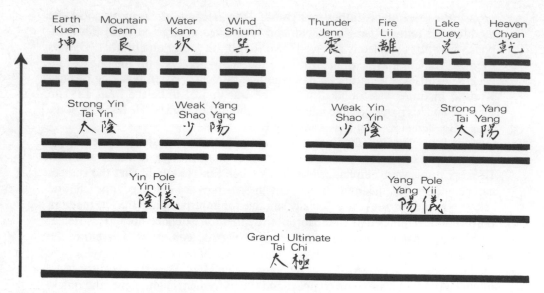

| Earth Kuen 坤 | Mountain Genn 艮 | Water Kann 坎 | Wind Shiunn 巽 | | Thunder Jenn 震 | Fire Lii 離 | Lake Duey 兌 | Heaven Chyan 乾 |

Strong Yin Tai Yin 太陰 　　Weak Yang Shao Yang 少陽 　　　Weak Yin Shao Yin 少陰 　　Strong Yang Tai Yang 太陽

Yin Pole Yin Yii 陰儀 　　　　Yang Pole Yang Yii 陽儀

Grand Ultimate Tai Chi 太極

Figure 1-2. The Eight Trigrams are derived from Tai Chi.

1-4. What is Tai Chi Chuan?

In Wang Dsung-Yueh's Tai Chi Classic he states "What is Tai Chi? It is generated from Wu Chi. It is the mother of Yin and Yang. When it moves, it divides. At rest it reunites" (see Appendix A-2). According to Chinese Taoist scripture, the universe was initially without life. The world had just cooled down from its fiery creation and all was foggy and blurry, without differentiation or separation, with no extremities or ends. This state was called "Wu Chi" (literally "no extremity"). Later, the existing natural energy divided into two extremities, known as Yin and Yang. This polarity is called Tai Chi, which means "Grand Ultimate" or "Grand Extremity", and also means "Very Ultimate" or "Very Extreme". It is this initial separation which allows and causes all other separations and changes.

When you are standing still before you start the sequence, you are in a state of Wu Chi. Your body is relaxed, with no intentions; your weight is evenly distributed on both legs. When you start the sequence, you are in a state of Tai Chi—you shift from side to side, foot to foot, and each part of your body becomes alternately substantial and insubstantial.

Once you start a motion it is possible to modify or redirect it, but this modification is only possible after the motion has been started. If one change is made, others can be made, and each change opens up other possibilities for variation. Each factor in the situation introduces other factors as possible influences. The initial motion made all other motions possible, and in a sense "created" the other motions. The Chinese express this by saying that Tai Chi is the mother of Yin and Yang. "Tai Chi begets two poles, two poles produce four phases, four phases generate eight trigrams (gates), and eight trigrams initiate sixty-four hexagrams". (Figure 1-2).

The Yin and Yang theory is used to classify everything, whether ideas, spirit, strategy, or force. For example, female is Yin and male is Yang, night is Yin and day is Yang, weak is Yin and strong is Yang. It is from the interaction of all the

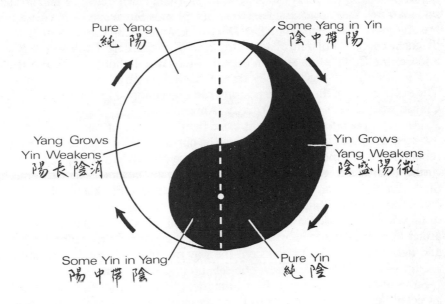

Figure 1-3. The Tai Chi diagram

Yin and Yang that life was created and grew. Tai Chi Chuan is based on this theory and applies it to form, motion, force, and fighting strategy. In the thousands of years since the Tai Chi theory was first stated, many Tai Chi symbols have been designed. The best one for both theory and application is a circle which contains Yin and Yang (Figure 1-3). In this figure, the circle and the curved dividing line between Yin and Yang imply that both Yin and Yang are generated and contained in roundness. The smooth dividing line between Yin and Yang means that they interact smoothly and efficiently. Extreme Yang weakens and evolves into Yin, first weak and then extreme Yin. Extreme Yin, in turn, evolves into Yang. One evolves into the other and back again, continuously and without stopping. The diagram also shows a small dot of Yin in the center of the greatest concentration of Yang, and a little bit of Yang inside the greatest concentration of Yin. This means that there is no absolute Yin or Yang. Yang always reserves some Yin and vise versa. This also implies that there is a seed or source of Yin in Yang and of Yang in Yin.

Tai Chi Chuan is based on this theory, and therefore it is smooth, continuous, and round. When it is necessary to be soft, the art is soft, and when it is necessary to be hard, the art can be hard enough to defeat any opponent. Yin-Yang theory also determines Tai Chi fighting strategy and has led to thirteen concepts which guide practice and fighting. Thus, Tai Chi Chuan is also called "Thirteen Postures". Chang San-Feng's Tai Chi Chuan Treatise states "What are the thirteen postures? Peng (Wardoff), Lu (Rollback), Ghi (Press), An (Push), Chai (Pluck), Lie (Split), Zou (Elbow-Stroke), Kau (Shoulder-Stroke), these are the eight trigrams. Jinn Bu (Forward), Twe Bu (Backward), Dsao Gu (Beware of the Left), Yu Pan (Look to the Right), Dsung Dien (Central Equilibrium), these are the five elements. Wardoff, Rollback, Press, and Push are Chyan (Heaven), Kuen (Earth), Kann (Water), and Lii (Fire), the four main sides. Pluck, Split, Elbow-Stroke, and Shoulder-Stroke are Shiunn (Wind), Jenn (Thunder), Duey (Lake), and Genn (Mountain), the four diagonal corners. Forward, Backward, Beware of the Left, Look to the Right, and Central Equilibrium are Gin (Metal), Moo (Wood), Sui (Water), For (Fire), and Tu (Earth). All together they are the thirteen postures" (see Appendix A-1). The explanation of the thirteen postures can also be found in the Tai Chi Chuan Classic written in the Ching Dynasty (Appendix A-13).

The eight postures are the eight basic fighting moves of the art, and can be assigned directions according to where the opponent's force is moved. Wardoff rebounds the opponent back in the direction he came from. Rollback leads him further than he intended to go in the direction he was attacking. Split and Shoulder-Stroke lead him forward and deflect him slightly sideward. Pluck and Elbow-Stroke can be done so as to catch the opponent just as he is starting forward, and strike or unbalance him diagonally to his rear. Push and Press deflect the opponent and attack at right angles to his motion. The five directions refer to stance, footwork, and fighting strategy. They concern the way one moves around in response to the opponent's attack, and how one sets up one's own attacks.

Since ancient times, many Tai Chi masters have tried to explain the deeper aspect of these thirteen postures by using the eight trigrams and the five elements. In order to find a satisfactory explanation, various correspondences between the eight basic techniques and the eight trigrams, and also between the five directions and the five elements, have been devised. Unfortunately, none of the explanations are completely reasonable and without discrepancy. The author will not attempt to find another explanation which might be just as unsatisfactory. However, in order to help the interested reader in pondering this mystery, we will include some of the available diagrams and an explanation considered the most accurate. We hope that someday someone who is a master of Yi Ching and Ba Kua theory and also an experienced Tai Chi researcher can untie this knot of mystery.

First, the relationship of the eight basic techniques (Wardoff, Rollback, Press, Push, Pluck, Split, Elbow-Stroke, and Shoulder-Stroke) with the eight trigrams and the Tai Chi symbol is shown in Figure 1-4. This diagram is drawn following Chang San-Feng's Tai Chi Chuan classic. Two alternatives are found in some of the available Tai Chi books and are shown in Figures 1-5 and 1-6. None of the above three diagrams give a satisfactory explanation of the connection between the Ba Kua eight "gates" and the eight techniques. However, from the viewpoint of Yin and Yang one can obtain a more or less satisfactory explanation. Here, we will discuss the diagram as described in Chang San-Feng's classic. In a trigram, a straight line expresses Yang and a broken line implies Yin. Therefore, when two straight lines are put together it means strong Yang, and when three straight lines are put together it means very strong Yang. The same can be applied to Yin. The Chinese have used the trigrams to analyze the seasons, the weather, and even the destiny of a person or a country. Initially three lines were used, but when understanding of the relationships grew, trigrams were used in pairs, allowing things to be divided and analyzed in 64 different ways. These 64 hexagrams are the basis of the Yi Ching (Book of Changes), which has exerted an enormous influence on Chinese culture.

From Figure 1-4, one can see several things. Wardoff is expressed by three straight lines, which means very strong Yang. This means power, aggression and

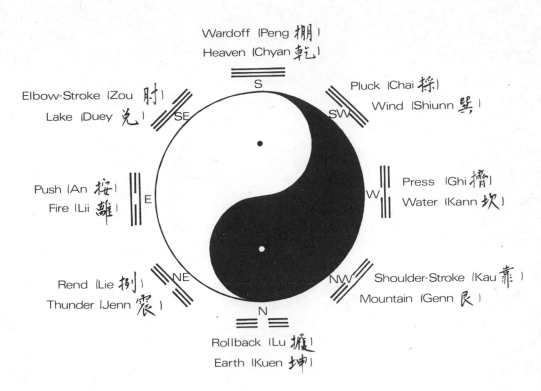

Figure 1-4. The directions of the eight basic techniques according to Chang San-Feng.

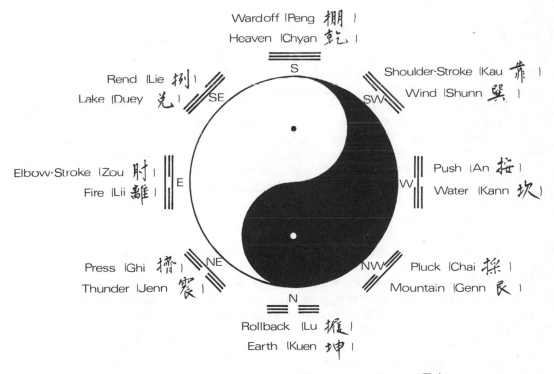

Figure 1-5. The directions of the eight basic techniques according to "Tai Chi Touchstones" (See Bibliography).

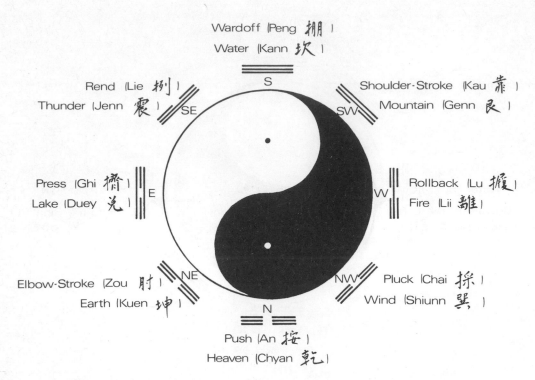

Figure 1-6. The directions of the eight basic techniques according to J. J.
Soong (See Bibliography).

offense. The opponent's attack is bounced back in the direction it came from.
Rollback is expressed by three broken lines, which implies defense, withdrawal,
or retreat. The opponent's attack is diffused by taking away its target. Pluck, Elbow-
Stroke, and Push are constructed of one Yin and two Yang lines, which shows
that there is offense with some defense. Split, Shoulder-Stroke, and Press are
characterized by two Yin lines and one Yang line, which shows that defense is
more important than offense in their fighting strategy.

As is the case with the eight trigrams and the eight techniques, the various
documents show different ways of matching the five elements with the five directions (Forward, Backward, Beware of the Left, Look to the Right, and Central
Equilibrium). Similarly, none of the explanations are completely satisfactory. Figure
1-7 shows the correspondence according to Chang San-Feng's classic. Figures 1-8
and 1-9 show two other published interpretations.

Before going further, the reader should first know the general rules and relationships of the five elements. This is shown in Figure 1-10. There are two main
cycles of relationships—production and destruction. One can see from the figures
that Metal generates Water, Water produces Wood, Wood produces Fire, Fire
leads to Earth, and the Earth gives Metal. In the Yi Ching, Metal belongs to
Heaven and generates water and rain, Rain will make wood grow, Wood can
generate Fire, Fire generates ashes (earth), and Earth includes and produces Metal.
It can also be seen from the figure that Water conquers Fire, Fire conquers Metal,
Metal subdues Wood, Wood defeats Earth, and finally Earth defeats Water. In
the real world water can extinguish fire, fire can melt metal, metal can cut wood,
wood (roots) can break up earth (rock), and finally dirt can dam the flow of water.

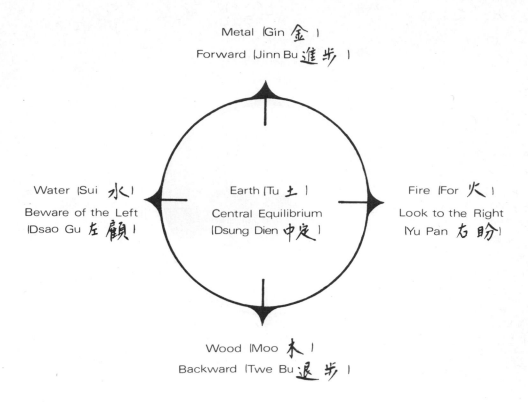

Metal (Gin 金)
Forward (Jinn Bu 進步)

Water (Sui 水)
Beware of the Left
(Dsao Gu 左顧)

Earth (Tu 土)
Central Equilibrium
(Dsung Dien 中定)

Fire (For 火)
Look to the Right
(Yu Pan 右盼)

Wood (Moo 木)
Backward (Twe Bu 退步)

Figure 1-7. The directions of the Five Elements according to Chang San-
Feng.

As with the eight trigrams and techniques, we will only discuss the five elements and directions as they are delineated in the Classic of Chang San-Feng. This is shown in Figure 1-7. Water conquering Fire corresponds to Beware of the Left defeating Look to the Right. This means that if the opponent attacks from your right, you go to the left to avoid his attack and at the same time you can attack his right from your left. Fire conquering Metal matches Look to the Right defending against an attack from the front. That means if your opponent attacks from your front, you can defend against him by sticking to his hand and pulling to the right to immobilize him. Metal conquering Wood matches Forward defeating Backward. This means that when your opponent withdraws, you want to move forward and use Adhere-Connect and Stick-Follow to follow his retreat and immobilize him aggressively. Wood subduing Earth corresponds to using Backward to defeat Central Equilibrium. This refers to using backward pulling power to destroy the opponent's stability and root. Finally, Earth conquering Water matches Central Equilibrium defeating Beware of the Left. This means that in order to defend against force from the left, you have to find your center and stability.

As one can see, trying to fit the five directions into the pattern of the five elements can be even more frustrating and unsatisfactory than is the case with the eight trigrams. It may very well be that the masters of old did not ever intend these philosophical explanations to be taken literally. If you train yourself to always

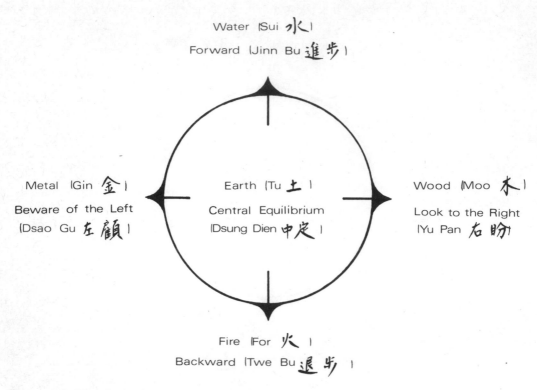

Figure 1-8. The directions of the Five Elements according to "Tai Chi Touchstones" (See Bibliography).

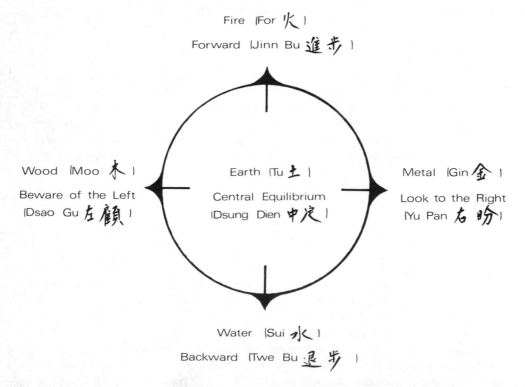

Figure 1-9. The directions of the Five Elements according to J.J. Soong (See Bibliography).

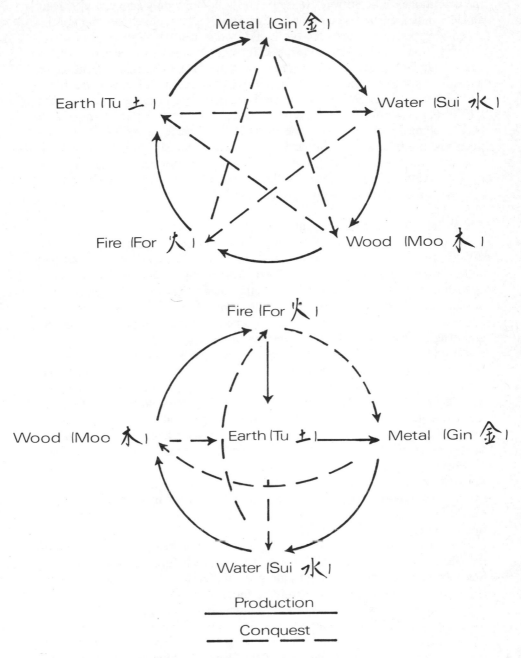

Figure 1-10. The Five Elements and the cycles of production and conquest.

respond a certain way to a certain attack, you are depriving yourself of flexibility and perhaps setting yourself up to be countered. The key point which this philosophy teaches is probably that one must always remain mobile and flexible in both hands and footwork. There are many ways to respond to each and every attack, and the more thinking and research you do, the better off you are. The various interpretations of the philosophy reflect different points of view and give the practitioner different ways to train. The philosophy may give you ideas, but all ideas must be tested out. In the final analysis, it is not the philosophy but the practical experiences which are the foundation of Tai Chi Chuan.

In addition to the Thirteen Postures, Tai Chi Chuan is also commonly called Mei Chuan (Soft Sequence). This is because when Tai Chi is practiced, the forms are soft and smooth, the mind is calm, the Chi is round, and Jing is fluid. Tai Chi Chuan is also called Chang Chuan (Long Sequence). Chang San-Feng's Tai Chi Treatise states "What is the long sequence? It is like a long river and a large ocean, rolling ceaselessly" (see Appendix A-1). That means, when Tai Chi is practiced, the forms flow smoothly and continuously. The Chi flow is also smooth and continuous, and the Jing is unbroken. There is another martial style also called Chang Chuan. However, this Shaolin style should be translated as "Long Fist" because it specializes in long range fighting.

1-5. What does Tai Chi Training Include?

Tai Chi has been evolving for more than seven hundred years, and it is very difficult to state just exactly what makes up the art. The content of the art has varied from one generation to the next. For example, one generation might specialize in the Tai Chi spear, and gradually come to ignore other aspects of the art such as the sword or saber. The contents of the system can also vary from one teacher to another. One might have learned only the sword from his master, and so naturally the sword would be the only weapon he could teach. Some masters will emphasize a particular principle or training method because of their experience, temperament or research, or perhaps create a new training style for a new weapon.

Since the beginning of this century, Tai Chi weapons practice has been increasingly ignored. Frequently only the barehand solo sequence is taught. In some cases the solo sequence has been modified to make it simpler and shorter, and therefore more accessible to a greater number of people. Although a number of techniques have been eliminated, the sequence still serves the purpose of improving health. However, a simplified sequence may not be enough if one is interested in deeper research and practice. Additionally, the coordination of breath and Chi circulation is often ignored. Most people these days learn Tai Chi without ever being exposed to the martial applications of the postures, the concept of Jing, barehand fighting sets, or Tai Chi sparring.

Tai Chi sword and saber sequences, because of their beauty, are practiced in the United States, although the applications of the techniques are seldom taught. Chi enhancement and extension training seems almost to have disappeared. Tai Chi spear, staff, and ruler can hardly be found in this country.

The reason for this is nothing new. The practitioners today are usually looking for a relatively quick and easy way to improve and maintain their health. Very few are willing to sacrifice their time for the long, hard training required to develop the other aspects of the art. Because of this, both in China and the rest of the world, even if a master is qualified to teach the whole art, he may be reluctant to pass it down to an unappreciative, if not actually doubting, generation. It seems very possible that the deeper aspects of Tai Chi Chuan will die out in the near future.

The various aspects of Tai Chi Chuan that are still available are listed below for reference:
1. Barehand:
    a. Tai Chi Solo Sequence
    b. Applications from the Solo Sequence

    c. Fast Tai Chi Training
    d. Still Meditation
    e. Chi Circulation Training
    f. Jing Training
    g. Pushing Hands and its Applications
    h. Tai Chi Fighting Set and Deeper Martial Applications
    i. Tai Chi Free Pushing Hands and Sparring
2. Tai Chi Sword:
    a. Tai Chi Sword Solo Sequence
    b. Chi Enhancement and Extension Training
    c. Martial Applications
    d. Tai Chi Sword Matching Forms
    e. Tai Chi Sword Sparring
3. Tai Chi Saber:
    a. Tai Chi Saber Solo Sequence
    b. Martial Applications
    c. Tai Chi Saber Matching Forms
    d. Tai Chi Saber Sparring
4. Tai Chi Spear and Staff:
    a. Individual Spear and Staff Martial Techniques
    b. Spear and Staff Sticking-Matching Practice
    c. Long Weapons Sparring
5. Tai Chi Ball:
    a. Listening and Understanding Jing Training
    b. Adhere-Stick Jing Training
    c. Two-person Tai Chi Ball Training
6. Tai Chi Ruler:
    Unknown to author

It can be seen that some of the training areas are already incomplete. For example, there is no longer a complete traditional staff or spear sequence, although a few individual techniques are still taught by some masters. In mainland China, complete sequences are being practiced for a number of weapons, but these sequences have been developed only in the last few years. There are very few masters anywhere who still know and train with the Tai Chi ruler or ball. However, even with the abridged list of Tai Chi activities available today, it would still take about twenty years to learn the art.

1-6. The Proper Approach to Learning Tai Chi, and the Sequence of Training
The Proper Approach to Learning Tai Chi:
   Whether or not a person learns something depends upon his attitude and seriousness. First he must make a firm decision to learn it, and then he must have a strong will to fulfill his intention. He needs perseverance and patience to last to the end. Even if a person has all these virtues, his achievement might still be different from that of another person who has the same qualities and personality. The difference is due to their manner of learning. If a person practices and then ponders every new thing he has learned, and keeps going back to research and master it, he will naturally be better than the person who never explores what he has learned. Both students may learn a method for changing rocks into gold, but only the first one will know why the method works. The former's knowledge will continue to grow and he will soon become a master, the latter will always be only a practitioner.

Tai Chi theory is deep and profound. It takes many years of learning, research, pondering, and practice to gradually grasp the key to the art and "enter into the temple". However, the more you learn, the less you are likely to feel you understand. It is just like a bottomless well or a ceaselessly flowing river. In Appendix A-6 the reader can find an ancient list of five mental keys the student of Tai Chi needs in order to reach the higher levels of the art. It is said: 1. Study wide and deep. 2. Investigate, ask. 3. Ponder carefully. 4. Clearly discriminate. and 5. Work persevering. If you follow this procedure you can learn anything, even how to become a wise and knowledgeable person.

In addition to the above learning attitude, a good master is also an important key to learning the high art of Tai Chi Chuan. In China, there is a saying: "A disciple inquires and searches for a master for three years, and a master will test the disciple for three years". It also says: "A disciple would rather spend three years looking for a good master than learn three years from an unqualified master". A good master who comprehends the art and teaches it to his students is the key to changing a rock into a piece of gold. It is the teacher who can guide you to the doorway by the shortest path possible and help you avoid wasting your time and energy. It is said: "To enter the door and be led along the way, one needs oral instruction; practice without ceasing, the way is through self-practice" (See Appendix A-15). It is also said: "Famous masters create great disciples". On the other hand, a good master will also judge if a disciple is worth his spending the time and energy to teach. A student can be intelligent and practice hard in the beginning, and change his attitude later on. A student who practices, ponders, humbly asks, and researches on his own will naturally be a good successor to the style. Usually a master needs three years to see through a student's personality and know whether he is likely to persevere in his studies and maintain a good moral character.

In the fifty years since Tai Chi Chuan has been popularized, many good Tai Chi books and documents have been published (see Bibliography). A sincere Tai Chi practitioner should collect and read them. Books are the recording of many years of learning, study, and research. If you do not know how to use this literature to your advantage, you will surely waste more time and energy wandering in confusion. However, you should not completely believe what any book says. What is written is only the author's opinions and personal experience. You should read widely, investigate, and then clearly discriminate between the worthwhile and the not-so-worthwhile in what you have read. If you do this well you can minimize confusion and avoid straying too far from the right path.

In addition, you should take advantage of seminars, summer camps, and other ways to come in touch with experienced masters. In this way you will be able to catch many key points and gain a "feeling" for many things which you may have only read about. But remember, you must research on your own in great detail in order to achieve a deeper understanding of the art. Thus it is said "You don't ever want to give up your throat; question every talented person in heaven and earth. If (you are) asked: how can one attain this great achievement, (the answer is) outside and inside, fine and coarse, nothing must not be touched upon" (see Appendix A-5B).

Training Sequence:
Every Tai Chi master has his own sequence of training, emphasizing his methods and content. In this section, the author will list the general training procedures according to his learning experience with three Tai Chi masters and his teaching experience of more than fifteen years. This section is a guide only to the barehand

training procedures of Tai Chi Chuan. The training procedures for Tai Chi weapons will be discussed in a future volume on advanced Tai Chi weapons.

The general sequence of Tai Chi Chuan training is as follows:

1. Understanding the fundamental theory of Tai Chi Chuan.
2. Relaxation, calmness, and concentration practice.
3. Breath training.
4. Experiencing and generating Chi.
5. Chi circulation and breathing.
6. Still meditation.
7. Fundamental stances.
8. Breath coordination drills.
9. Fundamental moving drills.
10. Solo Tai Chi Chuan.
11. Analysis of the martial applications of the sequence.
12. Beginning Tai Chi pushing hands.
13. Fundamental forms of Tai Chi Jing training.
14. Hen and Ha sound training.
15. Fast Tai Chi Chuan.
16. Advanced Tai Chi pushing hands.
17. Advanced Tai Chi Jing training.
18. Chi expansion and transportation training.
19. Martial applications of Tai Chi pushing hands.
20. Free pushing hands.
21. Tai Chi fighting set.
22. Tai Chi free fighting.

Before the Tai Chi beginner starts training, he should ask himself several questions: Why do I want to learn Tai Chi? What benefits do I hope to gain? Am I likely to continue training for a long time? After you have answered these questions you should then ask: Does this Tai Chi style offer what I want? Is this master qualified? Does this master have a training schedule? How long and how deep can this master teach me? Will this master teach me everything he knows or will he keep secrets when I approach a certain level? After I have studied for many years, will I be able to find an advanced master to continue my study? In order to answer these question you have to survey and investigate. You have to know the historical background of the style and the master's experience. Once you have answered the above questions, then you can start your Tai Chi study without any doubt or confusion.

The first step in learning Tai Chi Chuan is to understand the fundamental theory and principles through discussion with your master, reading the available books, studying with classmates, and then pondering on your own. You should ask yourself How does Tai Chi Chuan benefit the body and improve health? How can Tai Chi be used for martial purposes? What are the differences between Tai Chi Chuan and other martial styles? Once you have answers to these questions, you should have a picture of the art, and an idea of where you are going. The next question to arise should be: how do I train the relaxation, calmness, and concentration which are the most basic and important aspects of Tai Chi Chuan? This leads you to the second step of the training.

Usually, if you have the right methods and concepts, you can train your mind to be calm and concentrated and can relax physically in a short time. Keeping this meditative attitude is very important for beginning training. The next step is to train your breathing. The breathing must be deep, natural, and long. If you are interested in health only, you can use Buddhist, or normal breathing. However, if you want to advance to martial applications, you should train and master Taoist, or reverse breathing. You should be able to expand and withdraw the muscles of the abdomen area easily. After you have trained your breath correctly, you should then begin to sense the Chi in your abdomen and Dan Tien. This will lead to the fourth step—generating and experiencing Chi.

Usually, Chi can be generated in two ways: externally and internally. To generate Chi externally is called Wai Dan, and when it is generated internally it is called Nei Dan. Interested readers should refer to the author's book: *Chi Kung-Health and Martial Arts*. Through training Chi generation you will gradually realize what Chi is and why smooth Chi circulation benefits the body. You will also build up your sensitivity to the movement of Chi. The more you train, the more sensitive you will become. After a time, you should then go to the next step-circulating Chi. This is best practiced through still meditation, which will enhance your Chi generation and circulation. Chi circulation is guided by the calm mind and made possible by a relaxed body. You must train your mind to guide the Chi wherever you wish in coordination with correct breathing. First you should develop Small Circulation, which moves the Chi up the spine and down the center of the front of the body. Eventually you should develop Grand Circulation whereby Chi is circulated to every part of your body. When you have completed the above six steps, you should have built a firm foundation for Tai Chi practice. With correct instruction, it should take less than six months to complete the above training (except Grand Circulation).

The above six steps are purely mental training. When you practice these, you can simultaneously practice the fundamental stances, which build the root for the Tai Chi forms. You should be familiar with all the stances and should practice them statically to strengthen your legs. Also, at this stage you can begin fundamental breath coordination drills. These drills are designed for the begining student to train: 1. coordination of breathing and movement, 2. coordination of Chi circulation and the forms, 3. smoothness and continuity, 4. relaxation, and 5. calmness and concentration of the mind. These drills will help you experience Chi circulation and the mood or atmosphere of Tai Chi practice. After you have mastered the fundamental stances and fundamental drills, you should then go on to the fundamental moving drills.

In fundamental moving drills, a few typical forms are selected from the Tai Chi sequence to train proper movement, in addition to the five points mentioned above. These drills are discussed in the author's first Tai Chi book. This step leads the student to the door of the Tai Chi solo sequence.

The Tai Chi solo sequence is constructed with about forty apparent techniques and more than two hundred hidden techniques. It is practiced to enhance Chi circulation and improve health, and is the foundation of all Tai Chi martial techniques. It usually takes from six months to three years to learn this sequence depending on the instructor, the length of the sequence, and the talent of the student. After a student has learned this sequence, it will usually take another three years to attain a degree of calmness and relaxation, and to internalize the proper coordination of the breathing. When practicing, not only the whole of your attention, but also your feelings, emotions, and mood should be on the sequence. It is just like when a musician or a dancer performs his or her art—their emotions and total being must be melted into the art. If they hold anything back, then even if their skill is very great, their art will be dead.

When you finish learning the solo sequence, you should then start discussing and investigating the martial applications of the postures. This is a necessary part of the training of a martial arts practitioner, but it will also help the non-martial artist to better understand the sequence and circulate Chi. With the instruction of a qualified master, it will take at least two or three years to understand and master the techniques. While this stage of analysis is going on, you should begin to pick up fundamental (fixed step) pushing hands.

Pushing hands trains you to listen to (feel) the opponent's Jing, understand it, neutralize it, and then counterattack. There are two aspects of pushing hands training. The first emphasizes feeling the opponent's Jing and then neutralizing it, and the second aspect emphasizes understanding the emitting of Jing and its applications. Therefore, when you start the fundamental pushing hands, you should also start fundamental Jing training. Jing training is usually difficult to practice and understand. A qualified master is extremely important. While training Jing, the coordination of the sounds Hen and Ha become very important. Uttering Hen and Ha can enable you to emit or withdraw your Jing to the maximum and coordinate the Chi with it, and can also help to raise your Spirit of Vitality.

When you finish your analysis of the sequence, you have established the martial foundation of Tai Chi Chuan. You should then start to train speeding up the solo sequence, training Jing in every movement. In fast Tai Chi training, practice emitting Jing in pulses with a firm root, proper waist control, and Chi support. In addition, develop the feeling of having an enemy in front of you while you are doing the form. This will help you learn to apply the techniques naturally and to react automatically. After practicing this for a few years, you should have grasped the basics of Jing, and should start advanced pushing hands and Jing training.

Advanced (moving step) pushing hands will train you to step smoothly and correctly in coordination with your techniques and fighting strategy. This training builds the foundation of free pushing hands and free fighting. Advanced Jing training enables you to understand the higher level of Jing application and covers the entire range of Jing. During these two steps of training, you should continue your Chi enhancement, expansion, and transportation training to strengthen the Chi support of your Jing. The martial applications of pushing hands should be analyzed, and discussed. This is the bridge that connects the techniques learned in the sequence to the real applications. When you understand all the techniques thoroughly, you should then get involved in free pushing hands and learn the two-person fighting set.

The Tai Chi fighting set was designed to train the use of techniques in a way that resembles real fighting. Proper footwork is very important. Once you are moving and interacting fluidly, you can begin to use Jing. The final step in training is free fighting with different partners. The more partners you practice with, the more experience you will gain. The more time and energy you spend, the more skillful you will become.

The most important thing in all this training is your attitude. Remember to study widely, question humbly, investigate, discriminate, and work perseveringly. This is the way to success.

1-7. The Real Meaning of Tai Chi Chuan

People practice Tai Chi Chuan for different reasons. Some practice for health, to cure an illness, for defense, relaxation, or solely for fun. However, when you approach the highest level of Tai Chi Chuan, you will probably feel that the above reasons are not really important any more. At this time, you must seek the real meaning of the practice, otherwise you will soon become satisfied with your achievement and lose enthusiasm for further research. You must ponder what is really behind this highly meditative art. Many religious Taoists practice Tai Chi in their striving to eliminate their grosser elements and become immortal. Many non-religious people practice Tai Chi to gain a peaceful mind and reinvigorate their lives.

However, you should understand that Tai Chi Chuan emphasizes meditation both in movement and in stillness. Through this meditation a Tai Chi practitioner, like a Buddhist priest, trains himself to be calm and concentrated. It is possible to achieve a state of peace and centeredness which allows one to judge things and events in a neutral way, without emotional disturbance. When your mind is truly clear and calm, the spiritual side of things starts to open up. You start to see more deeply into things. A skilled practitioner can sense a person's intentions before they are expressed, and they often develop the ability to look more deeply into people and events in non-martial ways too. Many martial arts masters came to be considered wise men, and were consulted for their insight into the meaning of human life, this world, and the universe. They learned to live in this world without confusion or doubt, and to find peace and happiness. All of this comes through meditation and continuous pondering.

There is a song passed down since ancient times about the real meaning of Tai Chi Chuan (see Appendix A-8). It says: 1. "No shape, no shadow". This means that when you have approached the higher levels of Tai Chi meditation, you find your physical body seems not to exist–you feel that you are a ball of energy, part of the natural world and inseparable from it. Your actions and Self are part of the natural order of things, fitting in smoothly and unobstrusively, seeming to have no independent shape of their own, casting no shadow. 2. "Entire body transparent and empty". When you feel you are only a ball of energy, there is nothing in your mind, no desire or intention. Since your mind and ego are not there to interfere, you can see clearly and respond correctly. 3. "Forget your surroundings and be natural". Once you are transparent you will easily forget your surroundings and your energy flow will be smooth and natural. 4. "Like a stone chime suspended from West Mountain". This implies that your mind is wide open, free, and unrestricted. Like a stone chime suspended from the mountain, all things are clear under you, although your mind is still controlled by you just as the thread suspends the stone chime. 5. "Tigers roaring, monkeys screeching". When you move the energy you have cultivated and built up, it can be as strong as a tiger's roar and reach as far as a monkey's screech. 6. "Clear fountain, peaceful water". Even when your energy is strong, your mind is clear, still, and peaceful. 7. "Turbulent river, stormy ocean". In Tai Chi, if you have to use your energy it can be strong and continuous like a turbulent river or the stormy ocean. 8. "With your whole being, develop your life". During all your practice and meditation, you must concentrate your whole attention in order to develop the highest level of the art. This dedication and concentration carry over to the rest of your life, and the striving for perfection becomes the real inner meaning of Tai Chi.

BIBLIOGRAPHY

1. "太極拳學" (*Study of Tai Chi Chuan*), J. J. Soong, Taipei, Taiwan, 1970.
2. *"Tai Chi Touchstones: Yang Family Secret Transmissions"*, ed. and trans. by Douglas Wile, Sweet Chi Press, 1983.
3. *"Tao of Tai Chi Chuan"*, Jou Tsung Hwa, Tai Chi Foundation, 1981.
4. *"Tao of Meditation"*, Jou Tsung Hwa, Tai Chi Foundation, 1983.
5. *"Tao of I Ching"*, Jou Tsung Hwa, Tai Chi Foundation, 1984.
6. *"Tai Chi Chuan—A Simplified Method of Calisthenics for Health & Self-Defense"*, Cheng Man-Ching, North Atlantic Books, 1981.
7. *"Master Cheng's Thirteen Chapters on Tai Chi Chuan"*, Cheng Man-Ching, trans. by Douglas Wile, Sweet Chi Press, 1982.
8. *"Tai Chi Chuan—For Health and Self-Defense"*, T. T. Liang, Vintage Books, 1974.
9. *"Tai Chi Chuan Principles and Practice"*, C. K. Chu, Sunflower Press, 1981.
10. *"Yang Style Tai Chi Chuan"*, Dr. Yang Jwing-Ming, Unique Publications, 1981.
11. "太極拳刀劍桿散手合編" (*Tai Chi Chuan: Saber, Sword, Staff, and Sparring*), Chen Yen-Lin, Reprinted in Taipei, Taiwan, 1943.

第 二 章
氣與太極拳

CHAPTER 2
CHI AND TAI CHI CHUAN

2-1. Introduction

Once you have learned the postures of the sequence and the basic principles of Tai Chi movement, the next step is to start working on Chi, Yi (Mind), and Jing (power). This chapter discusses Chi, its relationship to health and the martial arts, and how it is controlled by the mind. The role of Chi in Tai Chi Chuan is discussed, as is its relationship with breathing, Spirit, and the Mind. The chapter concludes with general rules of posture, and recommendations for practicing the sequence.

2-2. Chi
General Concepts:

"Chi" in Chinese has two different meanings. The first refers to "Kon Chi", meaning air. The second is "Chi" meaning energy. Many Chinese believe that everything in the universe has its own energy field—every animal and plant, and even inanimate objects like rocks. Living things have a particularly strong energy field circulating through them. When this circulation is disturbed, illness results, and when it stops, there is death. Chi can be transferred from one object to another. In animals this Chi, which is often translated "intrinsic energy", circulates throughout the body to keep every part vital and alive. Chi can be affected by the weather, the season, the food you eat, your mood and thoughts.

Chi is often associated with a feeling of warmth or tingling which many people experience. Some Chi Kung practitioners misunderstand this and believe that Chi is heat, and that this is why they feel warm during meditation or Chi Kung practice. Actually, warmth is an indication of the existence of Chi, but it is not Chi itself. This is just like electricity in a wire. Without a meter, you cannot tell if there is an electric current in a wire unless you sense some phenomenon such as heat or magnetic force. Neither heat nor magnetic force is electric current; rather they are indications of the existence of this current. In the same way, you cannot feel Chi directly, but you can sense the presence of Chi from the symptoms of your body's reaction to it, such as warmth or tingling.

The Chinese have researched human Chi and its relationship with nature for more than four thousand years. This has resulted in acupuncture and in the many exercises and practices which can be used to strengthen the body and improve health and life. Tai Chi Chuan is only one of the many available systems.

Chi and Health:

If you understand the relationship of Chi to health, you will then realize why Tai Chi Chuan is so beneficial. In human or animal bodies, there are two major types of circulation. One is the blood circulation, commonly known in the Western world. Blood vessels and capillaries carry the blood to every part of the body in order to supply oxygen and nutrients, and to carry away waste. The other major circulatory system is that of Chi (internal energy). This Chi circulation supplies energy to the organs and to every cell of the body. There are twelve major pairs of Chi channels (Ching) and eight Chi vessels (Mei). The twelve channels are related to the internal organs, which will function normally when Chi is circulating smoothly, but will degenerate or malfunction when the circulation is disturbed. Of the eight vessels, two are particularly important. These are the Governing Vessel (Du Mei), which goes up the spine and over the head, and the Conception Vessel (Ren Mei), which runs down the center of the front of the body. In addition to the twelve channels and eight vessels, there are numerous small channels called "Lou", which are similar to capillaries. These carry Chi from the major channels to the skin and to every cell of the body. Some of these small channels bring Chi from the main channels to the marrow of the bones, which are also alive and need Chi and blood for growth and repair. Figure 2-1 is an example of a Chi channel (Ching), showing the branches (Lou) through which the Chi can flow laterally to the surface of the skin and deep into the marrow.

In order to maintain and enhance health, the Chi must circulate smoothly and strongly, and it must be balanced. When the Chi circulation loses its balance through stagnation or accumulation in one area, you may become ill. There are many "knots" along the paths of the Chi channels, both the Ching and the Lou, where the flow is constricted. These knots can slow down the Chi circulation and cause serious problems. In addition, stress or injury will cause an accumulation of Chi in the affected area. To heal this, the channels must be opened up and the stagnation removed. The training and practices used to open these knots and strengthen Chi circulation are called Chi Kung. Tai Chi Chuan is a form of Chi Kung, and has been proven to be a safe and effective way to maintain and improve health.

Often imbalances will clear up by themselves, because **CHI ALWAYS SEEKS TO BALANCE ITSELF.** However, it is wise to pay attention to your training and to any activity in your life which influences your Chi circulation. Be careful with anything which may disturb the body's natural circulation pattern, and avoid anything which causes imbalance. For example, if you build up the Chi in your right arm, you should also build up the Chi in your left arm.

Chi Generation:

Generally speaking, there are two ways to generate Chi: externally (called Wai Dan) and internally (Nei Dan). External Chi generation comes from stimulating a part of the body, such as the arms, in order to build up Chi in that area, and then circulating it throughout the body. This circulation is done either through conscious control, or by letting it happen spontaneously.

Methods of external Chi generation include muscular tension, massage or acupressure, and acupuncture:

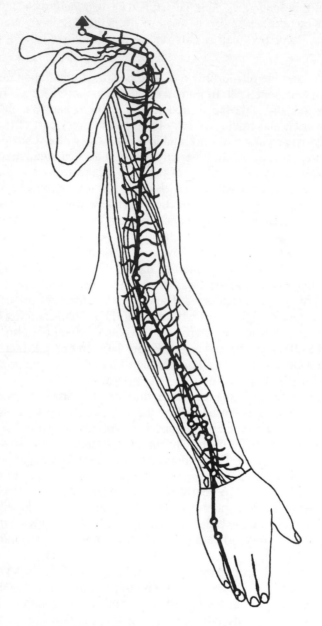

Figure 2-1. A Chi channel and its branches.

1. Muscular tension: The most famous way of generating Chi by muscular tension is Da Mo's system, explained in his book Yi Gin Ching (Muscle Change Classic). In these exercises, the practitioner will repeatedly tense and relax some part of the body, such as the forearms or wrists. When the muscles of a part of the body are tensed, Chi is built up in that area. This accumulation is most commonly felt as warmth. When the muscles are then completely relaxed, the Chi will naturally start to flow to other parts of the body.

2. Massage, Rubbing, and Acupressure: This approach uses external force to stimulate the muscles, skin, or points on the Chi channels in order to normalize or balance the Chi circulation.

3. Acupuncture: This is one of the most common methods in China for adjusting Chi circulation. Needling and other methods are used to balance the system, increasing or decreasing the flow of Chi.

Internal Chi generation comes from exercising the Dan Tien, and uses the mind to guide the Chi:

1. Dan Tien Exercises: The generation of Chi from the Dan Tien has been used by Chi Kung practitioners both for maintaining health and for increasing martial ability. In these exercises, Chi is generated in the Dan Tien by the continual in and out motion of the abdomen. When the Chi has accumulated there to a certain level, the concentrated mind circulates it up the back and down the front of the body, which is called "Small Circulation" (Shao Chou Tien). In the next step, called "Grand Circulation" (Da Chou Tien), the Chi is circulated throughout the whole body.

2. The Mind: The concentrated mind is crucial for generating Chi, and the will and intention lead the Chi throughout the body. A person with extensive Chi Kung experience can concentrate his mind at some area of the body and generate Chi there purely by thinking. The Chi can be affected or disturbed when a person gets nervous, worried, uptight, or in shock. However, this kind of Chi generation is not caused by conscious control and cannot be called Chi Kung.

Chi and the Mind:

Yi has been popularly translated "Mind". However, another Chinese word, Hsin, is also translated "Mind". You must understand and distinguish between them in order to be able to grasp the meaning of the ancient poems and songs translated in Appendix A.

In China, the heart is considered the most vital organ. The direct translation of Hsin is "heart". When Chinese say Juan-Hsin, literally "single heart", they mean "single-minded, with one mind". It is often translated as "concentrated mind". Hsin commonly means "intention, idea, or thought", referring to an idea which is not yet expressed, which lacks the full intention necessary to express it. When this idea is shown or expressed in some way, it is called Yi, and has the meaning of "purpose, intention, or desire". The reader should understand that a person must have Hsin first and then Yi, because Hsin is the source of Yi. If you want to do something, that is called Hsin. When you want it and fully intend to do it, or actually do it, this is called Yi. Sometimes the words are put together: Hsin-Yi. This can be translated "mind" or "intention", and also refers to the intention to do something specific.

The Tai Chi master Chen Yen-Lin wrote: "Somebody said that Yi is Hsin, and Hsin is Yi. As matter of fact, there is some difference between them. Hsin is the master of Yi. Yi is the chancellor of Hsin. When Hsin generates an idea, the Yi is then raised. When Yi is generated, the Chi then follows. In other words, there is linkage and a mutual relationship between Hsin, Yi, and Chi. When Hsin is scattered, the Yi is then dispersed. When Yi is dispersed, then the Chi will float. Conversely, when the Chi is sunken, then Yi is strong; when Yi is strong, then Hsin is steady. Therefore, all three are interrelated and inseparable".

As mentioned, Chi can be affected by your thinking. Consequently, all Chi

Kung styles emphasize calming down the mind and using it to guide the Chi circulation. Therefore, it is said: "Use your mind to lead your Chi" (Yii Yi Yin Chi). Sometimes when you concentrate your mind on the Chi you will find that your body tenses up and adversely affects the Chi circulation. This is because your mind is not calm and relaxed. Remember that your body can only be relaxed if your mind is.

In Chi Kung and Tai Chi Chuan, Yi is probably the most important key to success. If you cannot concentrate your Yi and use it to lead the Chi, all your practice will be in vain.

Chi and the Martial Arts

According to Chinese history, Chi was first noticed four thousand years ago. Later, when its importance to health was realized, methods were researched to enhance its circulation. The Chinese people have used these methods for more than two thousand years to improve their health. Eventually it was realized that this enhanced Chi circulation could be used in the martial arts to support the muscles and strengthen offensive and defensive techniques.

Almost every style trains Chi through Wai Dan, Nei Dan, or both. When Chi is used to support either the muscles (in external styles) or the sinews (in internal styles), the power generated will be greater than if you used only unaided muscular strength. Tai Chi Chuan is an internal martial style and specializes in using Chi to support the Jing which is emitted from the joints, tendons, and sinews, and which is controlled by the waist. The next chapter will focus on the principles of Jing and various training methods.

Chi is also used in Gin Chung Tsao (Golden Bell Cover) and Tiea Bu Shan (Iron Shirt) to train the body to resist strikes without injury. Methods such as Yi Jyy Chan (One Finger Contemplation) and Gin Garn Jyy (Gold-Steel Finger) have been developed to build up high levels of Chi in the fingers. This was used for cavity press (Tien Hsueh) whereby a touch to the appropriate cavity could kill or injure an opponent.

Chi and Hand Forms:

Hand forms play a very important role in Chi Kung and the martial arts. Different hand forms are used for different purposes, and various styles emphasize different forms. It is through your hands that you express your will, whether for martial arts, for health, or for healing. Your hands are the furthest point to which your Chi moves inside your body, and how they are held, and whether any muscles are tensed, influences the flow of energy.

There are six main energy channels which end in the fingers. The thumb and middle fingers each carry a Yin channel (Hand Taiyin Lung and Hand Jueyin Pericardium channels respectively) and the index and ring fingers each carry a Yang channel (Hand Yangming Large Intestine and Hand Shaoyang Triple Burner channels respectively). The little finger has both Yin and Yang channels (Hand Shaoyin Heart and Hand Taiyang Small Intestine channels respectively). Normally, when your Yi leads Chi to your hands, the Chi will be distributed to all the fingers. However, often you would like to concentrate your Chi in specific fingers for some special purpose. For example, you might wish to concentrate the Chi in the index finger for cavity press. In order to do this, a special hand form is used to narrow the other channels while leaving the channel in the index finger open.

Generally speaking, when a finger is extended the Chi will circulate easily to the fingertip and out. This emission of Chi is useful for attacking an enemy's

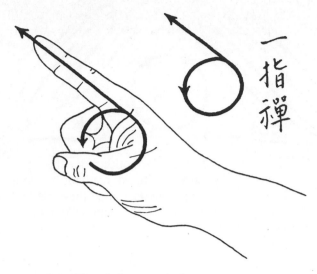

Figure 2-2. One Finger Contemplation

vulnerable points, as well as for healing. An extended finger is usually offensive and is classified as a Yang finger. When the finger is bent and touching the palm, the Chi is less active and will flow back to the palm. This is usually classified as a Yin finger. Sometimes the bent fingers are stiffened to slow down their Chi circulation and make the extended finger(s) stronger. The extended fingers may also be stiffened. This is often seen in external styles where a muscular type of Jing predominates. Conversely, when the extended fingers are relaxed the Chi can move strongly. This is commonly seen in the internal styles where Chi plays a more important role in emitting Jing.

In Chi transportation training, both hands are usually held in the same form in order to keep the Yi and Chi balanced and symmetrical. The exception to this is when one hand is holding a weapon.

We will now discuss the more common hand forms. Most of their names contain the word "Jing" because they use Chi, in coordination with breathing, to generate a flow of energy for either healing or martial purposes. These forms range from ones which only direct Chi, to those which use Chi to support the muscles, and to those in which muscular strength predominates. This will be discussed further in Chapter 3.

A. Yi Jyy Chan (One Finger Contemplation): Yi Jyy Chan is used in both internal and external styles. In this hand form (Figure 2-2), the index finger is straight to allow the free passage of Chi, while the other fingers are bent to slightly restrict the flow. The thumb touching the bent fingers enables the Chi to circle through them, and also helps the Chi to flow strongly to the straight finger. This form is commonly used in cavity press. External styles use special training to stiffen the finger without losing Chi concentration, while internal styles emphasize Chi circulation and minimize the use of the muscles. This form is sometimes also used in healing.

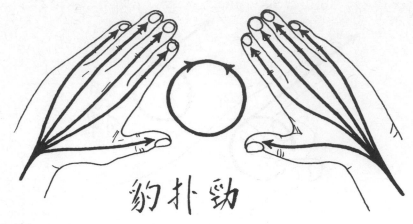

Figure 2-3. Rushing Panther Jing

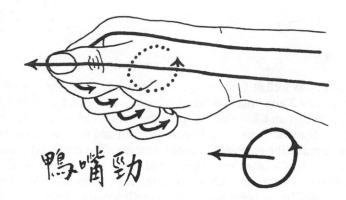

Figure 2-4. Duck's Beak Jing

B. Bao Pu Jing (Rushing Panther Jing): This hand form is said to resemble a panther rushing at something (Figure 2-3). The thumb is separated from the other four extended fingers, dividing the Chi into two major flows—one to the thumb, and the other to the rest of the fingers. This form is commonly used for massage.

C. Ya Tzoei Jing (Duck's Beak Jing): In the Ya Tzoei Jing hand form (Figure 2-4), all the fingers except the thumb are held tightly closed. The channel to the thumb is kept wide open, while the flow to the other fingers is restricted. The thumb in this form is commonly used for cavity press, although it is also often used in massage and Chi Kung healing.

D. Heh Tzoei Jing (Crane's Beak Jing): There are two forms called Heh Tzoei Jing. In the first, commonly used in the Crane martial style, the thumb and index fingers touch while the other three fingers are gently closed (Figure 2-5). Chi is concentrated in the thumb and, index finger, while a lesser flow circles through

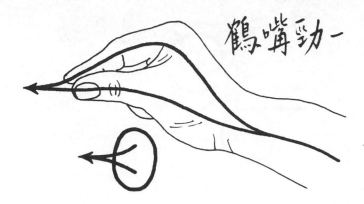

鶴嘴勁一

Figure 2-5. Crane's Beak Jing used in the martial arts

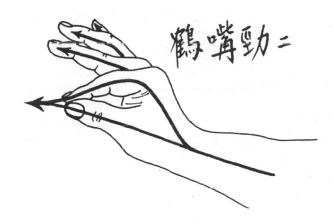

鶴嘴勁二

Figure 2-6. Crane's Beak Jing used in Chi Kung healing

the other three fingers. The second crane's beak form is similar to the first except that the middle, ring, and little fingers are now open (Figure 2-6). Chi is not concentrated as strongly in the thumb and index finger as is the case with the martial crane's beak form. This form is commonly used in Chi Kung healing.

E. Ton Tien Jing (Reach the Heaven Jing): In this form, the middle finger is extend ed, allowing Chi to reach the tip, while all the other fingers are closed, circling and conserving the Chi (Figure, 2-7). The Chi in the middle finger is usually stronger and can reach further than is the case with Yi Jyy Chan. This form is commonly used for healing although it is sometimes seen in the martial arts.

F. Long Shyan Ju Jing (Dragon Holding a Pearl in its Mouth Jing): This form is said to resemble a dragon holding a pearl in its mouth (Figure 2-8). All the fingers except the little one are extended. The Chi is divided into two flows; one to the thumb and the other to the index, middle, and ring fingers. This form is used for attacking the eyes, throat, or armpit, and is also commonly used in massage.

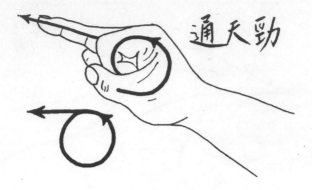

Figure 2-7. Reach the Heaven Jing

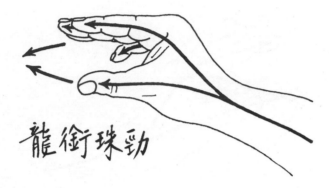

Figure 2-8. Dragon Holding a Pearl in its Mouth Jing

G. Jen Jyue Kai Chi Jing (Secret Sword Opening the Chi Jing): In this hand form, the index and middle fingers are extended, while the other three are closed with the fingertips touching (Figure 2-9). If the palm faces sideward or upward, it is a Yang Jing, and if the palm faces downward, it is a Yin Jing. This form extends Chi to the two straight fingers while allowing a second flow to move through the other three fingers and recirculate.

In sword training it is very important to transport Chi to the end of the sword. In order to do this, while one hand is holding the sword, the other should be in this form to balance the Chi and extend it symmetrically. Without this hand form it is very difficult for the Chi to reach the tip of the sword. Jen Jyue is also commonly used for cavity press and some healing purposes.

H. Sher Tou Jing (Snake Head Jing): In Sher Tou Jing the hand is formed like a snake's head. The index, ring, and little fingers are closed while the thumb and middle finger are extended (Figure 2-10). This form is commonly used in Chi Kung healing.

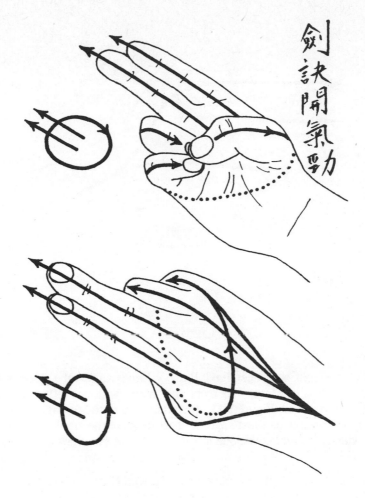

劍訣開氣勁

Figure 2-9. Secret Sword Opening the Chi Jing

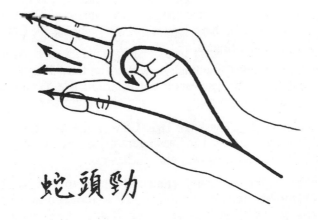

蛇頭勁

Figure 2-10. Snake Head Jing

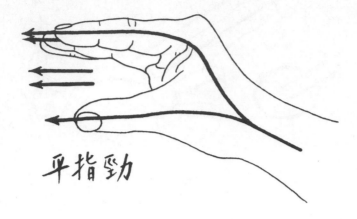

平指勁

Figure 2-11. Flat Finger Jing

I. Pin Jyy Jing (Flat Finger Jing): Pin Jyy Jing is almost the same as Dragon Holding a Pearl in its Mouth Jing mentioned above with one difference: the little finger is also extended (Figure 2-11). It is used to grab the throat, or the muscles located in the armpit or waist area. In order to make the grabbing effective, the Chi is divided into two flows: one to the thumb and the other to the rest of the fingers. This form is also commonly used in massage and Chi Kung healing.

J. Ba Kua Chang (Eight Trigram Palm): Ba Kua Chang is used by the Ba Kua internal martial style, which specializes in using several varieties of this form. In order to make strikes effective, the Chi must be concentrated in the palm. To do this, the fingers are kept extended, and tightened somewhat (Figure 2-12).

K. Ien Jao Jing (Eagle Claw Jing): This is a specialty of the Eagle Claw style, and is used for grabbing. The thumb and fingers are spread and bent like an eagle's claw (Figure 2-13). When this hand form is used for grabbing, the Chi and strength are held in the palm and fingers.

L. Heh Jao Jing (Crane Claw Jing): As with Eagle Claw Jing, this Jing is used by the Crane style for grabbing. The thumb, index and middle fingers are shaped like a crane's claw (Figure 2-14).

M. Fu Jao Jing (Tiger Claw Jing): Tiger Claw Jing is used by the Tiger Claw style for grabbing and clawing. The five fingers are formed like a tiger's claw and tensed to hold the Chi in them (Figure, 2-15).

N. Tan Lang Sou (Praying Mantis Hand): This hand form is used by the Praying Mantis style to hook and grab the enemy. It is also used to attack the opponent's eyes and cavities. The Praying Mantis Hand is formed with the thumb touching the first knuckle of the index finger while the other three fingers are lightly held in (Figure 2-16).

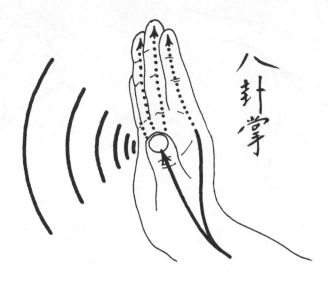

Figure 2-12. Eight Trigram Palm

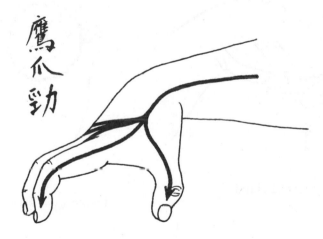

Figure 2-13. Eagle Claw Jing

O. For Sou (Buddha Hand): Buddha hand is popularly used in meditation. It is formed with the thumb and middle fingers touching each other to circulate the Chi back to the body, while the other three fingers are slightly bent (Figure 2-17).

There are many other hand forms used in different martial styles, in meditation, and in healing. Tai Chi Chuan also has its special hand forms. These will be discussed in a later section.

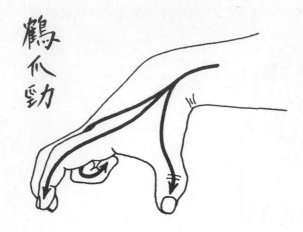

Figure 2-14. Crane Claw Jing

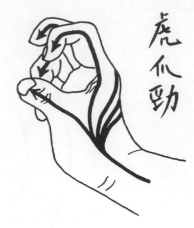

Figure 2-15. Tiger Claw Jing

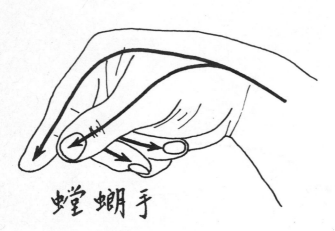

Figure 2-16. Praying Mantis Hand

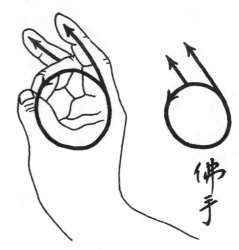

Figure 2-17. Buddha Hand

2-3. Chi and Tai Chi Chuan:

There are several questions which Tai Chi practitioners frequently ask, such as: How do I experience Chi in Tai Chi Chuan? How do I generate Chi? How can Tai Chi Chuan benefit the body and bring me health? How is Chi circulated in Tai Chi Chuan? How do I use my Chi in the martial applications of Tai Chi Chuan? What is the relationship of Chi to Jing? All these questions are very important for the practitioner who wishes to approach the higher levels of Tai Chi Chuan.

Chi Generation and Transportation in Tai Chi Chuan:

Tai Chi Chuan is a style of martial Chi Kung training, so naturally Chi is extremely important. In Chinese martial society there is a saying: "Train muscles,

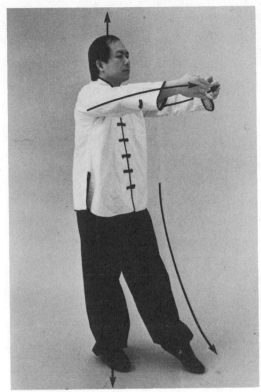

Figure 2-18.

bones, and skin externally, and train Chi internally"(Wai lien gin gu pie, nei lien yi kou chi). However, this raises the questions: How do I generate Chi and how do I experience it?

Chi in Tai Chi Chuan is generated both externally and internally. It is recommended that you do certain exercises, in addition to the sequence, which will help you to understand and develop Chi. An exercise called "Gung Sou" (Arcing the Arms)(Figure 2-18) is commonly used to help beginners generate Chi in the shoulders and back. For this exercise, stand in the False Stance with one leg rooted on the ground and the other in front of it, with only the toes touching the ground. Both arms are held in front of the chest, forming a horizontal circle, with the fingertips almost touching. The tongue should touch the roof of the mouth to connect the Yin and Yang Chi Vessels (Conception and Governing Vessels respectively). The mind should be calm and relaxed and concentrated on the shoulders; breathing should be deep and regular.

When you stand in this posture for about three minutes, your arms and one side of your back should feel sore and warm. Because the arms are held extended, the muscles and nerves are stressed and tense. Chi will build up in this area and heat will be generated. Also, because one leg carries all the weight, the muscles and nerves in that leg and in one side of the back will be tense and will thereby generate Chi. Because this Chi is generated in the shoulders and legs rather than in the Dan Tien, it is considered "local Chi". In order to keep the Chi generation and the flow in the back balanced, after three minutes change your legs without moving the arms and stand this way for another three minutes. After the six minutes, put both feet flat on the floor, shoulder-width apart, and lower your arms

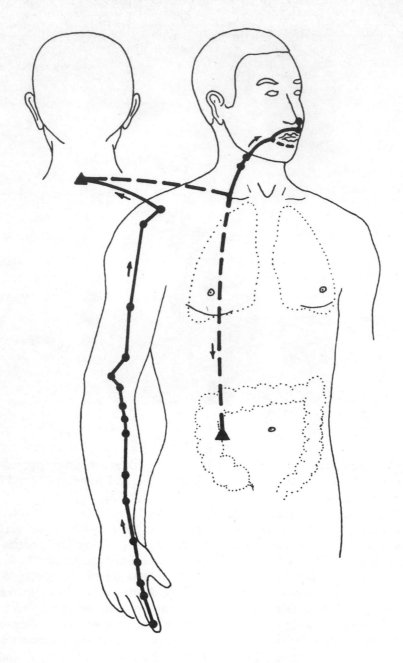

Figure 2-19. Hand Yangming Large Intestine Channel

slowly. The withheld Chi will then flow out naturally and strongly. It is just like a dam which, after accumulating a large amount of water, releases it and lets it flow out. At this time, concentrate and calm the mind and look for the feeling of Chi flowing from the shoulders to the palms and fingertips. Beginners can usually sense this Chi flow, which is typically felt as warmth or a slight numbness.

Sometimes Chi is felt on the upper lip. This is because there is a channel (Hand Yangming Large Intestine) which runs over the top of the shoulder to the upper lip (Figure 2-19). However, the feeling is usually stronger in the palms and fingers

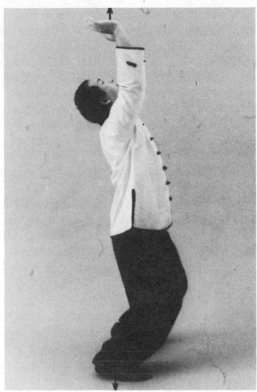

Figure 2-20.

than in the lip, because there are six Chi channels which pass through the shoulder to end in the hand, but there is only one channel connecting the lip and shoulder. Once you experience Chi flowing in your arms and shoulders during this exercise, you should also find that you can sense it in your back.

After you have developed your Chi circulation you should practice directing it into both arms as you exhale. The energy goes out each arm, exchanges at the fingertips, and comes in through the opposite arm as you inhale, circling in both directions simultaneously. Because the arms and hands form a circle, the Chi is always flowing from each hand into the other and back to the body. Since the energy is withheld or conserved within the body, the Gung Sou posture is considered Yin. In addition to increasing the circulation of Chi in the arms and shoulders, the Gung Sou exercise will also improve the flow in the spine, which is particularly important in Tai Chi Chuan.

This exercise is one of the most common practices for leading the beginner to experience the flow of Chi, and some Tai Chi styles place great emphasis on it. If a Tai Chi practitioner does not know and experience the feeling of Chi flow, how can he really understand Chi?

Another common form is called Tou Tien (Supporting the Heavens)(Figure 2-20). This exercise has been discussed in the author's first Tai Chi book *Yang Style Tai Chi Chuan*, and will not be repeated here. There are many other forms which are used to teach beginners about Chi. The reader should consult different Tai Chi and Chi Kung books for further ideas.

After you understand what you are looking for, there are two basic sets of exercises you should practice. These exercises increase the generation of Chi, balance it, and train the coordination of breath with movement and the transporting of Chi. The mind is all-important, and the beginner will find visualizations extremely helpful. For the beginner, **THE GENERATION AND TRANSPORTING OF CHI COMES FROM THE CONCENTRATED IMAGINING THAT YOU ARE PUSHING A HEAVY OBJECT WITH RELAXED MUSCLES**. At first, most beginners will not feel the energy flow, but with time and practice most will start feeling warmth in the palms. It is important also to **KEEP THE YI FURTHER THAN THE CHI**. You know that when you walk you must keep your Yi (mind, attention, intention) ahead of you, rather than on your feet, or else you won't be able to take the first step. Similarly, when you want to transport Chi you must keep your Yi ahead of where the Chi is in order to move it.

The first set of these exercises trains the coordination of Chi and breath, balances energy, and opens up the Chi channels in the arms and legs. The exercise consists of standing stationary and moving the arms in simple movements—up and down, in and out—in coordination with the breathing. This set has been mentioned in the author's first Tai Chi book and will not repeated here.

After you have practiced this set for a while and can move Chi to your limbs, you can start the second set, which coils the Chi throughout your body and out to the skin. In these exercises, your muscles are tensed by the twisting of your limbs and body, and then relaxed. The Chi which is generated in these tensed areas is led by the mind to coil out to the extremities and spiral out to the skin. This coiling motion helps to increase the penetration of your Jing and brings the Chi out to the skin, opening all the little Chi channels (Lou). This slows degeneration and increases the efficiency of your muscles. This is what is meant by the saying: "Transport Chi as though through a pearl with a 'nine-curved hole', not even the tiniest place won't be reached" (Appendix A-3).

In pushing hands and in fighting, victory is frequently decided by who has the greatest skill in what is called "listening". When Chi is circulating smoothly to your skin, you will be able to sense or "listen" to your enemy's power and intention. Also, after many years of Chi development, you may be able to pass your Chi into another person's body through the cavities on his Chi channels in order to injure or heal.

Once you have accomplished Grand Circulation, you can use these exercises to circulate energy from the Dan Tien out to the extremities, instead of just using local energy.

Before starting this exercise, calm down and meditate for a minute. The tongue should be touching the roof of the mouth, and the entire body should remain relaxed throughout the exercises. The thumbs and little fingers should be pulled back slightly to direct the Chi to the palms. In order to build the Chi to a high level, repeat each form ten to twenty times, then go on to the next form without stopping.

In these exercises, inhale as you bring your hands toward your shoulders, and exhale as you move your hands away from your shoulders. As in all of Tai Chi, the arms are never extended fully—you should always maintain a slight bend in the elbow. As you inhale, imagine that you are drawing energy in through your hands and feet, and condensing it in your Dan Tien and spine. As you exhale, move the Chi from your Dan Tien and spine out through your hands and feet. When you exhale you should notice five flows of Chi—two out the arms, two out the legs, and one from the Dan Tien down to the tailbone. As always, imagine that you are moving against resistance, and that your feet are pushing against the floor.

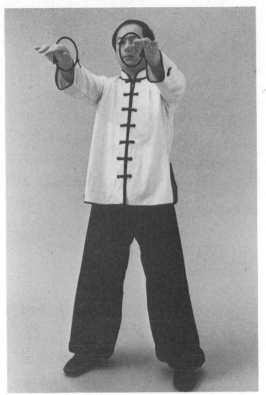

Figure 2-21.

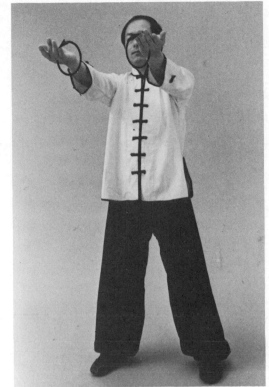

Figure 2-22.

Chi Coiling Exercises:

Form 1 (Figures 2-21 and 2-22): This is the beginning warm-up form. Hold both arms extended in front of the chest. Rotate your palms downward as you inhale, and imagine drawing energy into your bones. Rotate the palms upward, exhaling and using the mind to lead the Chi from the inside of the arms to the surface in a coiling, expanding motion. When a hand faces down-ward it is considered a Yin Palm, and when it faces upward it is a Yang Palm. After doing this form ten to twenty times, you should feel your forearms and shoulders getting warm. This form helps you to generate a feeling of coiling Chi from inside your arms to the surface of the skin.

Form 2 (Figures 2-23 and 2-24): This is the second warm-up form. Continuing from the last exhale form, inhale and bring the hands in to the chest in a twisting motion. Then exhale, stretching the hands out in a screwing mo-tion. The right hand moves in a regular screwing motion, clockwise forward and counterclockwise backward, while the left hand reverses this, twisting counterclockwise forward and clockwise backward. Finish this form with the arms in and both palms facing down. This form practices a forward drilling motion in addition to the coiling motion of the first exercise.

Form 3 (Figures 2-25 and 2-26): Continuing from the last inhale form, keep the palms down and exhale as you lower your hands to the waist. Imagine that you are pushing something downward, but do not tense your muscles. Turn your palms

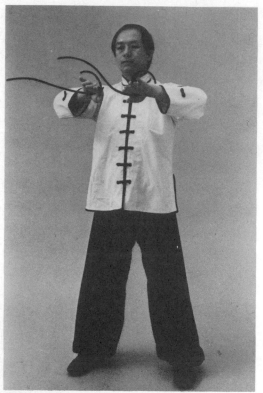

Figure 2-23.

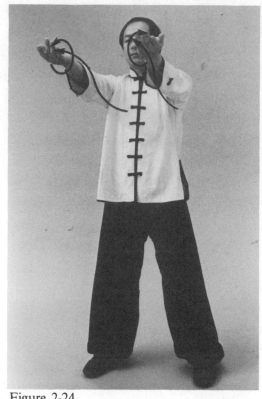

Figure 2-24.

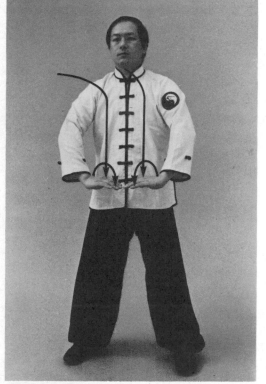

Figure 2-25.

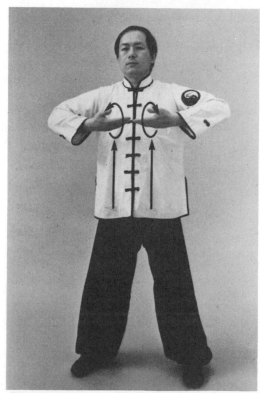

Figure 2-26.

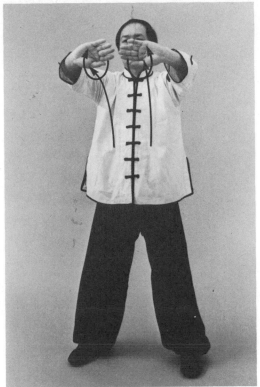

Figure 2-27.

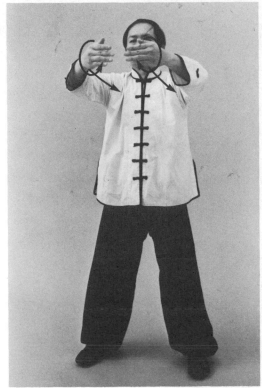

Figure 2-28.

up and raise them to the chest as you inhale. Turn the palms down and repeat. In this form keep the fingers and palms of both hands in a line with each other, rather than pointing out to the front. This increases the twisting motion. This form builds up Chi in the forearms through the alternate twisting and relaxing of the muscles. The Chi thus generated is coiled outward to the surface of the skin.

Form 4 (Figures 2-27 to 2-29): After the last inhale of the previous form, exhale and push the arms out in front of the chest while rotating the palms forward. Inhale and bring the hands in, palms facing the chest, then exhale and let the hands sink down, palms down. Raise them again, palms up, as you inhale. This form has two complete breaths and four motions: forward, back, downward, and upward. Keep the fingers of both hands in line while moving the hands upward, forward, and back, but let them relax to a natural angle while sinking. When you are moving your hands forward, imagine that you are pushing a heavy object, and also visualize the counterforce into your feet.

Form 5 (Figures 2-30 to 2-33): Continuing from the last exhale form, inhale and raise the hands to the chest, palms up, fingers pointing forward. Exhale and extend your arms forward until they are almost straight, with the palms facing sideward. Inhale and move your arms in a big circle out, back, and forward again to your chest. Exhale while extending the arms forward, continuing the exercise in a swimming motion. When you exhale, you should have a flow of Chi reaching out through the fingertips of both hands in a drilling or screwing motion.

Form 6 (Figures 2-34 to 2-37): After the last inhale form, exhale and push your

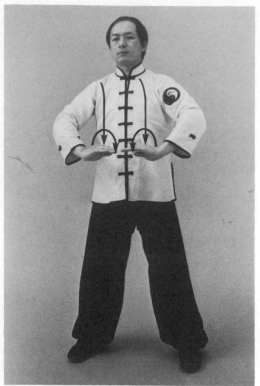

Figure 2-29.

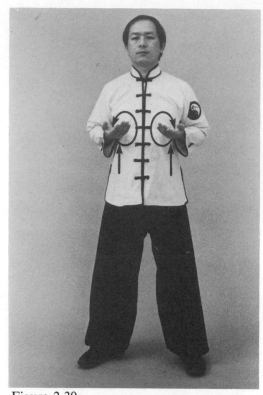

Figure 2-30.

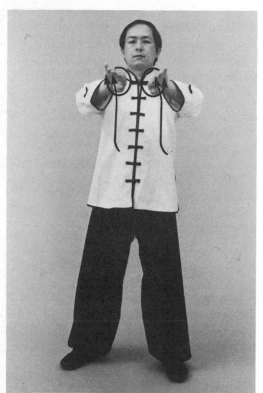

Figure 2-31.

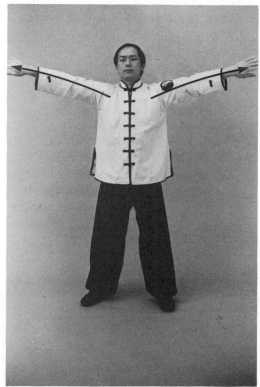

Figure 2-32.

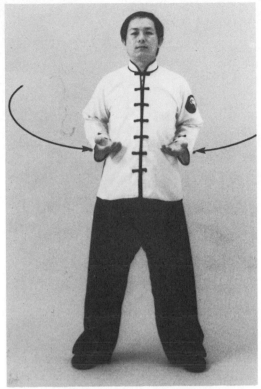

Figure 2-33.

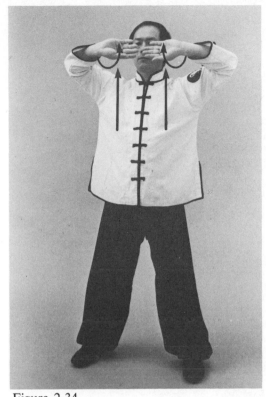

Figure 2-34.

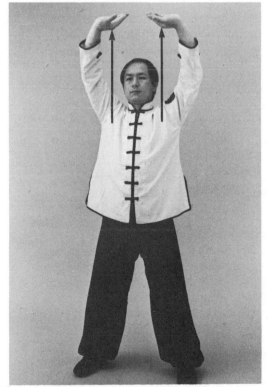

Figure 2-35.

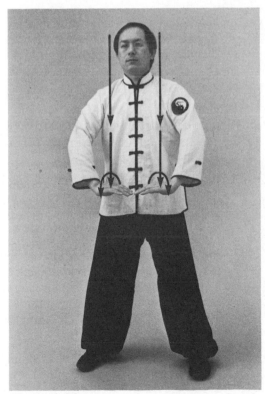

Figure 2-36.

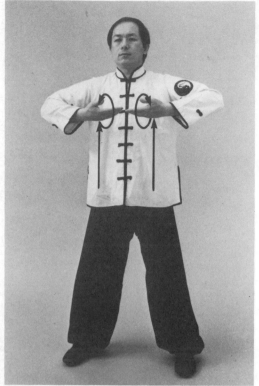

Figure 2-37.

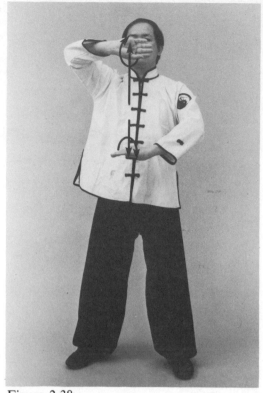

Figure 2-38.

hands over your head, palms up. As you inhale, turn the palms down and bring them to your chest. Exhale and lower your hands to your waist, inhale and raise them again to your chest. This form has two complete breaths and four motions.

Form 7 (Figures 2-38 to 2-41): When the last inhale form is finished, exhale and separate your palms. One palm continues to push upward while the other pushes downward in front of the abdomen. Inhale and draw both hands toward each other, exhale and repeat the motion with the opposite hands raising and lowering. Inhale and draw both hands toward each other. This form trains the Chi to balance in both arms.

Form 8 (Figures 2-42 to 2-44): Continue the same motion as the last form except this time the lower hand goes behind the body in the hip area, palm down. This twists the shoulder of the back hand and coils the Chi through it.

Form 9 (Figures 2-45 to 2-48): Continue the previous exercise with one addition— rotate the body in the direction the upper hand is moving. While the right hand is rising, rotate the body to the left as far as possible. Similarly, while the left hand is rising, rotate the body to the right. As you twist your body to the rear, exhale and extend your Chi out through your fingertips, rather than your palms. This is similar to the last form, except that twisting the body coils the Chi around the body.

Form 10 (Figures 2-49 to 2-52): Continuing from the last inhale form, extend the legs somewhat wider than shoulder width. This exercise is essentially the same as the last form, except that when you turn to the side, let the feet turn into a

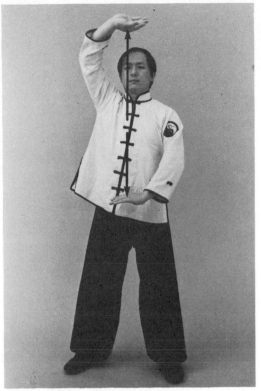

Figure 2-39.

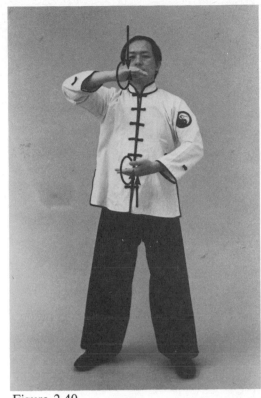

Figure 2-40.

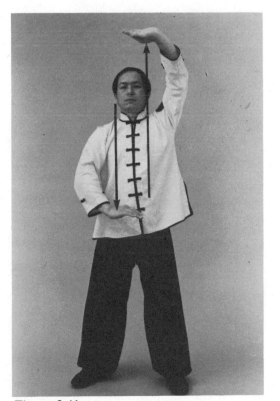

Figure 2-41.

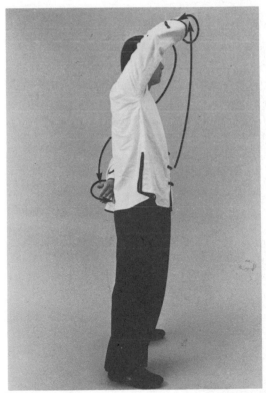

Figure 2-42.

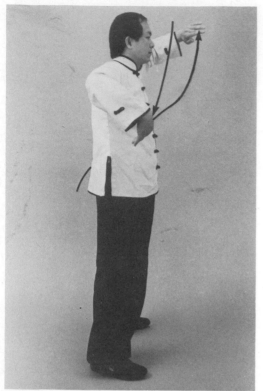

Figure 2-43.

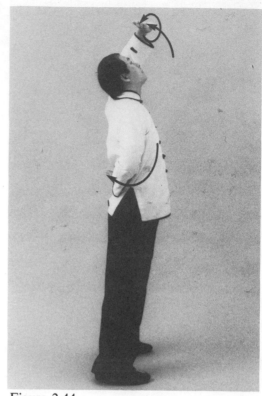

Figure 2-44.

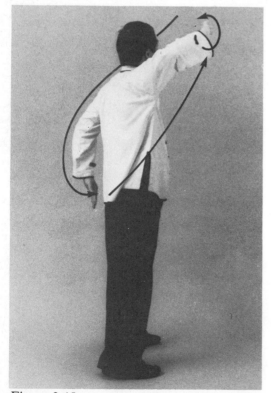

Figure 2-45.

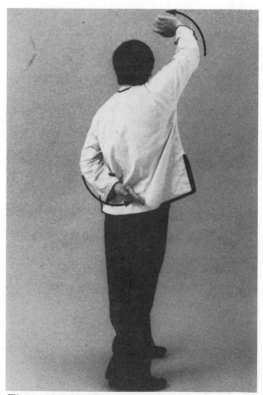

Figure 2-46.

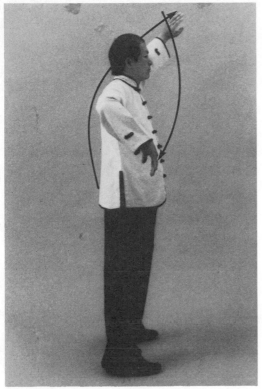

Figure 2-47.

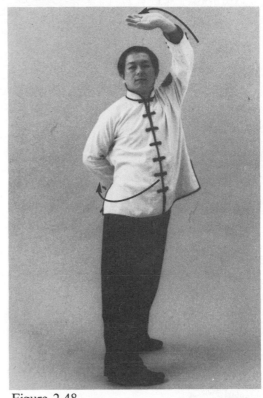

Figure 2-48.

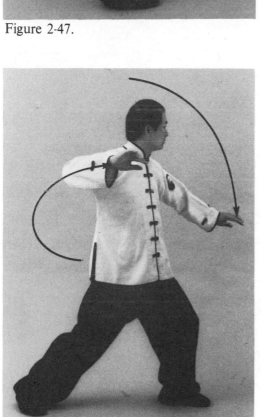

Figure 2-49.

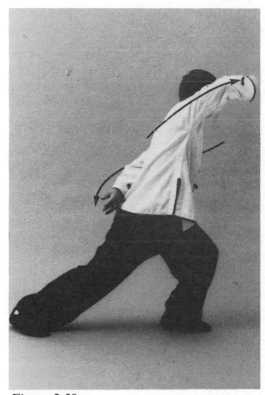

Figure 2-50.

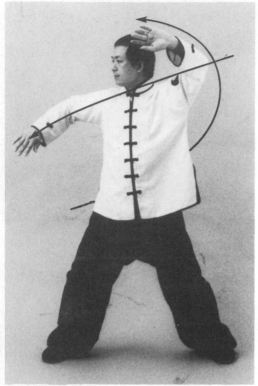 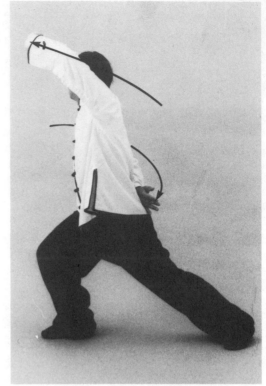

Figure 2-51.   Figure 2-52.

Bow and Arrow stance, and tilt the body. This form coils the energy around the whole body even more than theprevious form.

Form 11 (Figures 2-53 to 2-62): After the last exhale form, inhale and rotate your body to the front while bringing the legs back to shoulder width, and return both hands to the waist, palms up. Exhale while raising the hands and turning the palms forward. Inhale, and rotate the body all the way to the rear into the Sitting on Crossed Legs stance, while bringing the hands to the chest, palms facing in. Exhale while turning and lifting the body to the front and raising the hands above the head, palms forward. Inhale and repeat the same motion, turning to the other side, and on the exhale return again to the front. This form trains coiling Chi through the whole body as well as screwing the body up and down.

Form 12 (Figures 2-63 and 2-64) After completing the above exercises, you should have built up and transported quite an amount of Chi to your skin. Let your hands drop down naturally and rotate them in both directions in coordination with your breathing for a minute or so to continue feeling the Chi flow. This form will help you to balance your energy after the exercises.

With continued practice, these Chi transportation exercises will teach you to build up and circulate Chi in the local areas which are being stressed. After a while you should be able to apply the principles of these Wai Dan Chi Kung exercises to the Tai Chi solo sequence. However, this is only a part of the Chi Kung training which Tai Chi Chuan uses. A skilled Tai Chi artist generates Chi in the Dan Tien and circulates it throughout his body. This is called Nei Dan (a Taoist

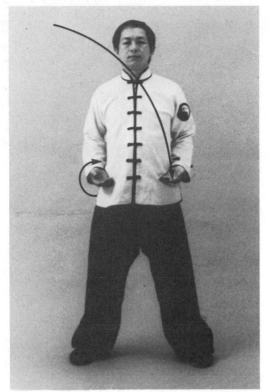

Figure 2-53.

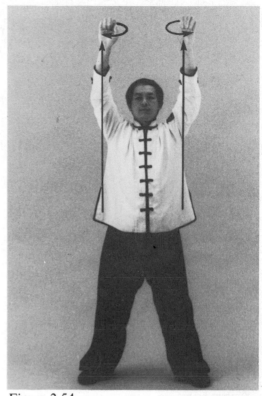

Figure 2-54.

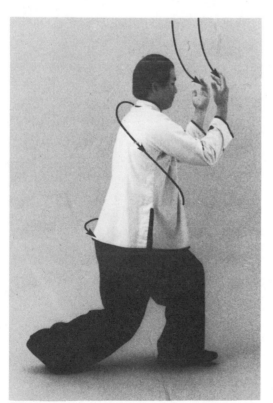

Figure 2-55.

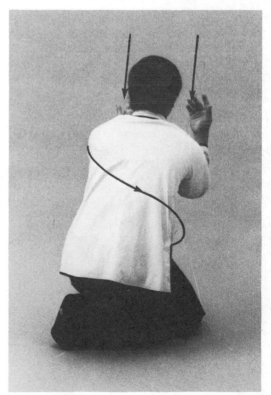

Figure 2-56.

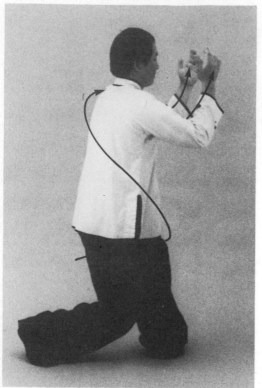

Figure 2-57.

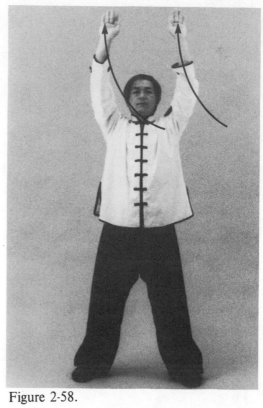

Figure 2-58.

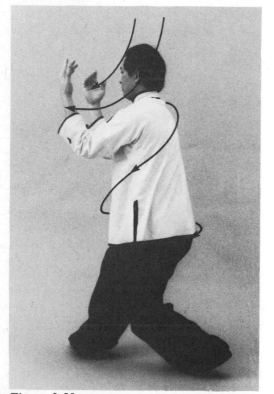

Figure 2-59.

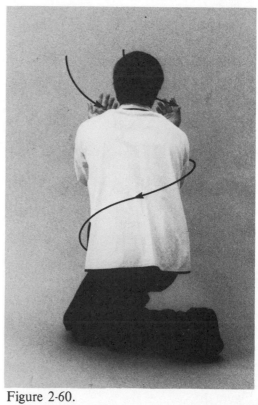

Figure 2-60.

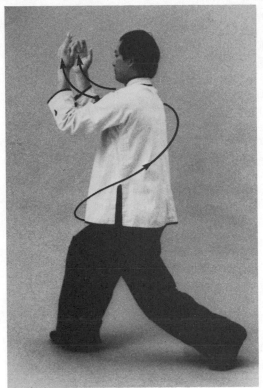

Figure 2-61.

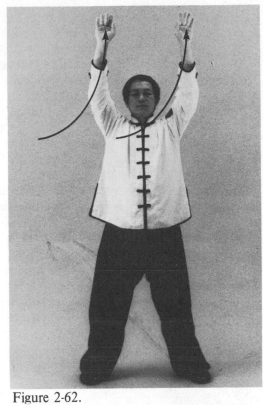

Figure 2-62.

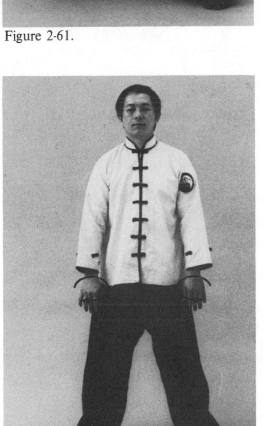

Figure 2-63.

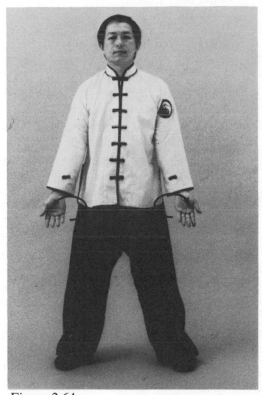

Figure 2-64.

term meaning Internal Elixir), and is the foundation of Tai Chi Chuan. The classics refer to this frequently: "The Chi is sunk to the Dan Tien" (Appendix A-2), "Grasp and hold the Dan Tien to train internal Kung Fu" (Appendix A-13), and "The Dan Tien is the first chancellor" (Appendix A-5A). If you keep part of your attention on your Dan Tien while doing the sequence, you will gradually build up your internal circulation from this area. If you wish to develop your Dan Tien circulation more rapidly, see the author's book *Chi Kung–Health and Martial Arts*.

Once you can generate Chi in the Dan Tien, you begin circulating it through the Small Circulation (the Conception and Governing Vessels). After you have accomplished this, you can work on Grand Circulation, which circulates Chi through the arms and legs and clears obstructions in the twelve main channels. One of the best ways to do this is through doing the Tai Chi sequence. The final step is to move the Chi from the channels to the skin through the small channels (Lou). The Chi flow should be smooth, continuous, strong, and animated, but yet condensed. There are many references to this in the classics: "Chi should be full and stimulated" (Appendix A-1); "(You) want the entire body's Chi to circulate smoothly, (it) must be continuous and non-stop" (Appendix A-5B); "Don't be broken and then continuous, refine your one Chi" (Appendix A-13); "Chi (circulates) in the entire body without the slightest stagnation" (Appendix A-15); "Third saying: Chi condenses. When the appearance of Chi is dispersed and diffused, then it is not conserved, and the body can easily be scattered and disordered. In order to make Chi condense into the bones your exhalation and inhalation must flow agilely (smoothly). The entire body is without gap" (Appendix A-12).

Once you have built up your Chi circulation you should begin to train using it to support your fighting techniques. For this the Chi must be able to flow readily to the arms and legs in coordination with the breath. This will be discussed in the next section.

After you have worked for a while on circulating your Chi with the exercises mentioned above, you should start practicing individual forms from the sequence. Wardoff, Rollback, Press, and Push can be practiced together as a unit. You can also use Brush Knee and Step Forward, Diagonal Flying, Wave Hands in Clouds, Step Back and Repulse Monkey, and Step Forward, Deflect Downward, Parry and Punch. Individual forms should be practiced repeatedly, emphasizing root, stability, and balancing the Chi.

It is important to balance the Chi accurately so that the Jing will be able to reach its maximum. In order to do this, the Yi must be balanced first. You know that when you push a heavy object, you must push the rear leg back in order to push the object forward. In the same way, when you wish to lead Chi forward, you must think of the rear foot in order to lead the Chi forward efficiently. It is very important to remember: **THE CHI MUST BE BALANCED TO THE OPPOSITE SIDE, OR IT WILL BE WEAK AND INEFFICIENT**. Thus it is said: "If there is a top, there is a bottom; if there is a front, there is a back; if there is a left, there is a right" (Appendix A-1). Therefore, in the beginning, the mind should concentrate on balancing the Chi flows. If you persevere in this practice, the balancing will begin to occur naturally, and you will no longer have to think about it. When you use this balanced Chi to support Jing, the Jing will be able to reach its maximum.

In conclusion, Tai Chi Chuan uses both Wai Dan (external) and Nei Dan (internal) Chi circulation. A wise Tai Chi practitioner will use Wai Dan to open the channels and branches locally in the limbs, and at the same time build up his internal Nei Dan Chi in the Dan Tien. One day, when he has completed the Small

Circulation, he will be able to accomplish Grand Circulation quickly and easily because he has already opened the channels in the limbs. Remember, even if you don't have internal (Nei Dan) Chi circulation, you can still circulate Chi locally in the limbs with the Wai Dan exercises. This will benefit your internal organs, though not as much as the internal Nei Dan circulation will.

Chi and Breathing:

Breathing plays a very important role in Chi Kung and Tai Chi practice. Breathing with the right method calms down the mind and relaxes the body. This makes it possible for the Chi to circulate smoothly, and helps the Yi to generate and lead Chi wherever desired. Breathing should be deep, relaxed, and regular. In Chi Kung, there are two common ways of breathing. The Buddhist method uses the normal breathing in which the abdomen expands as you inhale, whereas the Taoist method uses "reverse" breathing in which the abdomen expands as you exhale. Tai Chi Chuan was developed according to the Taoist method and therefore uses reverse breathing. Because detailed theory and training methods have been discussed in the author's books *Yang Style Tai Chi Chuan* and *Chi Kung—Health and Martial Arts*, we will not repeat them here. We will only discuss the essential points of breathing in Tai Chi practice.

In Tai Chi, the breathing coordinates with Chi and the fighting techniques. There are several stages of coordinating breath and Chi. The first stage uses meditation, usually sitting, to develop Small Circulation. This trains you to bring the Chi up the Governing Vessel from the tailbone to the roof of the mouth and down the Conception Vessel from the tongue to the tailbone. This can be done with either two cycles of inhalation and exhalation (Figure 2-65) or only one cycle (Figure 2-66).

In the second stage, after you have developed Grand Circulation, you can coordinate Chi with your technique. On the inhale, bring Chi up the spine from the tailbone to the point between the shoulder blades, and also from the roof of the mouth down to the Dan Tien (Figure 2-67). In this way you are accumulating energy in the back and Dan Tien. When you exhale, bring Chi from your back out your arms, and from your Dan Tien out your legs. On the exhale the Chi also moves over your head and from the Dan Tien to the tailbone to complete the circuit of the Small Circulation. This method is considerably more complicated than the Small Circulation because there is more than one single focus point of attention and Chi.

In the third stage, once the Chi moves quickly and easily wherever you want it, you can use a much simpler visualization. When you do a defensive move, inhale and accumulate energy in your Dan Tien and spine. When you do an offensive technique, exhale and send Chi out your arms and legs. Your abdomen becomes firm as you move Chi in both directions. It is said: "Inhalation is storage, and exhalation is emitting. That is because inhalation lifts up naturally (the Spirit of Vitality). It can also lift (control) the opponent. (When you) exhale, then (your Chi) can sink naturally. (You) also can release (Jing) out to the opponent. That means use Yi (your mind) to move your Chi, don't use Li (strength)" (Appendix A-12).

It is said: "Every form of every posture follows smoothly; no forcing, no opposition, the entire body is comfortable. Each form smooth" (Appendix A-10). In the sequence, breathing coordinates with the forms. Since some of the forms are long and some are short, you must vary the length of your breaths to keep the speed of the sequence uniform. If a form in the sequence is too long for one

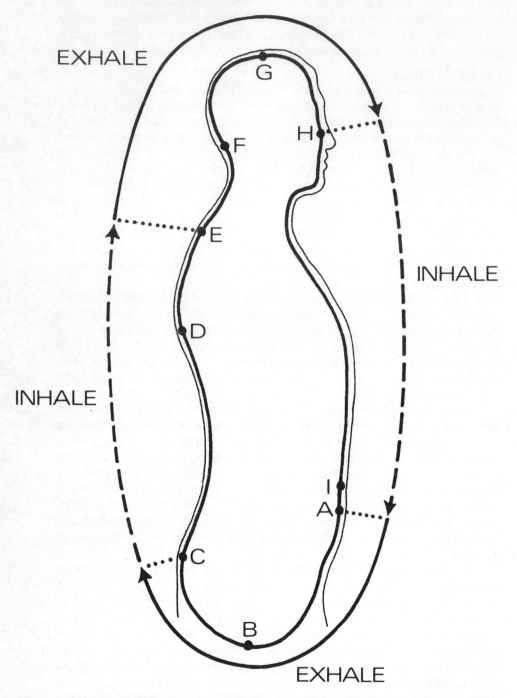

Figure 2-65. Small Circulation with two cycles of inhalation and exhalation

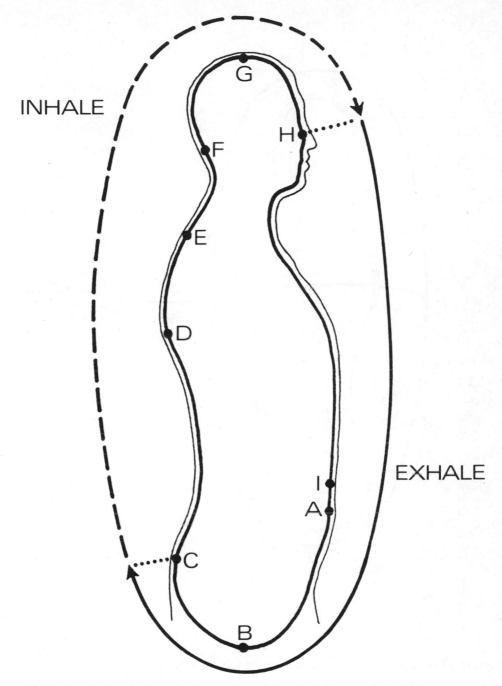

INHALE

EXHALE

Figure 2-66. Small Circulation with one cycle of inhalation and exhalation

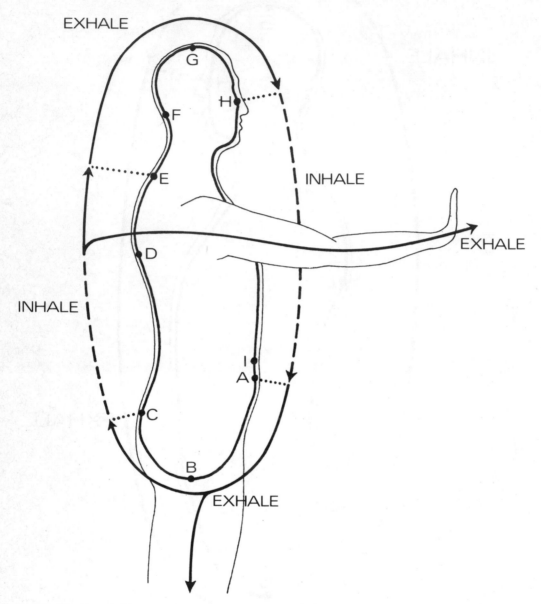

Figure 2-67. Grand Circulation—coordinating Chi with your techniques

breath, add another. **YOUR BREATHING SHOULD BE RELAXED—DO NOT HOLD IT, DO NOT FORCE IT**. Don't hold your breath, because your lungs will tighten and your body will tense. This not only slows the Chi circulation, but also damages lung cells.

ONCE YOUR BREATHING NATURALLY COORDINATES WITH THE MOVEMENTS, YOU SHOULD NO LONGER PAY ATTENTION TO YOUR BREATHING. It says in the classics: "(Throughout your) entire body, your mind is on the Spirit of Vitality (Jieng-Shen), not on the breath. (If concentrated) on the breath, then stagnation. A person who concentrates on breath has no Li (strength); a person who cultivates Chi (develops) pure hardness (power)" (Appendix A-3). The reason for this is that the mind must be ahead of the Chi in order to lead it, and you cannot do this if your mind is on your breathing. If you develope a sense of having an enemy in front of you, the Spirit of Vitality is raised and the mind is kept ahead of the Chi, leading it naturally in support of your movements.

Chi and Shen:

Before we discuss the relationship of Chi and Shen, the reader should understand three concepts: Shen, Jieng, and Jieng-Shen.

In China, Shen means Spirit, one's higher nature, or the soul. Shen is the divine part of man, his inner nature which is in contact with the divine nature. When you act in harmony with your Shen, you are in harmony with yourself and all around you. Shen is the vital part of your being, the alert aliveness, the consciousness within which the mind and thought function. It is the force behind your attitudes, thoughts and actions. The Chinese believe that when a person with a strong will and Spirit dies, his Shen lives on. Many Chinese still worship these spirits of the dead. A person's Spirit may be good or evil, and this will carry over into death.

Jieng in Chinese means essence. It is what is left after something has been refined and purified. In Chinese medicine, Jieng can mean semen, but generally refers to the basic substance of the body which the Chi and Spirit enliven. Jieng is inherited from your parents, and the amount of Jieng that you have inherited determines the strength of your constitution. Generally speaking, the amount of Jieng is fixed, although it can be weakened by illness or dissipation, and it can be augmented through diet and certain meditational practices, including Tai Chi.

When the term Jieng-Shen is used in Tai Chi it means "the essence of the Spirit", and is sometimes translated "Spirit of Vitality". The Chinese also commonly use just Shen to express Jieng-Shen. When a person has a strong Jieng-Shen it is usually visible in how he holds himself and moves. He is concentrated, active, alive, vigorous, and often highly spiritual. Strong Spirit often shows in the brightness and alertness of a person's eyes. When a person lacks Jieng-Shen he is dull and listless, without will or enthusiasm.

In China, Jieng, Chi, and Shen are called the "San Bao", or Three Treasures, because they are so important. In Tai Chi practice, the highest of these is Shen, because it can control the others. It is the Spirit which stimulates the Chi, causing it to condense, and which guides it throughout the body. This is especially important when Tai Chi is used for fighting. A person who has a strong Jieng-Shen will be able to use his condensed and stimulated Chi to support his Jing in a fight.

It is said: "The Spirit of Vitality is threaded and concentrated" (Appendix A-12). Just as you must thread your Chi throughout your body, so too must you thread your Spirit. You should be able to expand your consciousness to fill your body without any gaps or dark spots. At the same time, you must be able to concentrate your awareness wherever you wish.

It is said: "Chi should be full and stimulated, Shen (Spirit) should be retained internally" (Appendix A-1). Retaining the Spirit internally means to be centered and to avoid unnecessary actions of the body, mind, and eyes. Thus concentrated, you will be able to use your mind to act quickly and efficiently, and you will avoid betraying your intentions to the opponent.

It is also said: "(If) the Jieng-Shen (Spirit of Vitality) can be raised, then (there is) no delay or heaviness (clumsiness)" (Appendix A-3). When Chi is sunken and concentrated, it is possible for the Spirit of Vitality to rise to the top of the head. This clears the mind and allows the body to move lightly and without inhibition. The Song of Five Key Words talks of the importance of a calm heart, an agile body, condensed Chi, and integrated Jing, and then goes on to say: "All in all, (if) the above four items (are) totally acquired, it comes down to condensing Shen (Spirit). When Shen condenses, then one Chi (can be) formed, like a drum. Training Chi belongs to Shen" (Appendix A-12).

Chi and the Mind in Tai Chi Chuan:

The mind, both Yi (Mind) and Hsin (Heart), controls the actions of the Chi, and it is the Chi which controls the actions of the body. It is said: "Use the heart (mind) to transport the Chi, (the mind) must be sunk (steady) and calm, then (the Chi) can condense (deep) into the bones. Circulate the Chi throughout the body, it (Chi) must be smooth and fluid, then it can easily follow the mind.....Yi (Mind) and Chi must exchange skillfully, then you have gained the marvelous trick of roundness and aliveness.....The Hsin (heart, mind) is the order, the Chi is the message flag" (Appendix A-3). It is also said: "If asked, what is the standard (criteria) of its (thirteen postures) application, (the answer is) Yi (mind) and Chi are the master, and the bones and muscles are the chancellor" (Appendix A-15).

From the above sayings, it is clear that the ancient masters placed great emphasis on the mind and Chi. A Chi Kung proverb says "Use your mind to lead your Chi" (Yii Yi Yin Chi). This is the key to using Chi, because it tells you that if you want to move your Chi somewhere, your mind must go there first. Remember: **FIRST THERE IS YI, THEN THERE IS CHI**.

The Highest Level of Chi Transportation:

Once you have achieved Grand Circulation you have opened up the twelve channels and the two major vessels, but this doesn't mean that you have opened up all the channels in your body. There are the thousands of small Chi branches (Lou) which spread from the main channels out to the skin and in to every part of the body. The benefits of opening these branches can be explained from both the health and martial arts points of view.

From the point of view of health, the stagnation of Chi in the Lou will not significantly affect the functioning of the organs, but it will affect your overall health in some ways. If there is stagnation in some of the Lou, the Chi may not be able to reach the skin, and this will be reflected in the condition of the skin. For example, when people get old, Chi is not easily transported to the skin, and this shows as age spots. In Chinese medical diagnosis, the appearance of the skin is commonly used to judge a person's health and the balance of his Chi. When a person is sick his Chi flow loses its balance. Since the Lou are connected to the Chi channels, the appearance of the skin will then show symptoms of the illness. Conversely, because the main channels are connected by these branches to the skin, stimulation of the skin is commonly used to generate Chi to compensate for imbalances in the channels and organs. A common method is rubbing the skin, as in massage.

In order to be healthy your Chi should reach every cell of your body, from deep inside the bones out to the skin. It is believed that if you can circulate Chi smoothly throughout the body, there will be no danger of getting cancer. One of the leading causes of death in this country, cancer is the uncontrolled growth of certain cells in the body. It is believed that this is caused by unbalanced Chi flow. For further discussion, interested readers should refer to the author's Chi Kung book. Once you can transport Chi to your skin, you may then start developing the ability to transport it beyond your body. When this goal is reached, you can then use your Chi for healing by removing excess Chi from a person or by reinforcing his deficient Chi.

For the martial artist, there are two reasons for circulating Chi to the skin: defense and offense. In defense, a Tai Chi martial artist must build the sensitivity of his skin to "listen" to his enemy's Jing. Listening Jing is one of the most decisive factors in Tai Chi fighting. The better a Tai Chi fighter's ability to sense the enemy, the better his fighting art will be. When two Tai Chi artists fight, skill in "Listening Jing" is usually the main factor in deciding the winner. It is said that when your Chi can be transported strongly to your skin, it will cover the body like a cloud of energy. The better you are, the thicker this cloud will be.

For offensive purposes, a martial artist wants to build up his Chi as much as possible, both to support his Jing and also for use in cavity strikes. The highest level of Tai Chi martial application is to have your Chi overflow into the opponent's body when you touch one of his cavities. For example, if you can transport Chi beyond your skin, you can strike or touch the cavity in the opponent's armpit and shock his heart through the heart channel. It takes many years of correct practice to reach this level.

When you can extend Chi beyond your body, you can also move it to the tip of weapons such as the sword or spear. It is said that the sword is king of the short weapons and the spear is leader of the long weapons. This is because these two weapons require Chi rather than muscle for the higher levels of the art.

Now let us discuss how to transport Chi to your skin. First, you must open as many of the Lou as possible. Most of these branches are already open, but if you use only these branches to transport your Chi to the skin you will be no different than any run of the mill martial artist. But how do you open these branches? You must build up your Chi so that the branches which are already open cannot handle the flow, and the Chi overflows into the other branches and opens them. The stronger your Chi is, the more branches you will open. In order to strengthen your Chi, you must train your Dan Tien continuously so that it is full of Chi like a drum or a balloon. You must also train your Chi to extend out to the furthest parts of your body, to fill every nook and cranny, to extend from the marrow of the bones to beyond the skin. Thus, it is said: "Transport Chi as though through a pearl with a 'nine-curved hole', not even the tiniest place won't be reached" (Appendix A-3).

There are several ways to work at expanding your Chi out to the skin, but in every method the most important point is to use your Yi. Do the Chi coiling exercises and visualize the Chi spiralling out to the skin. Another good method that you can use while doing the form, meditating, sitting at work, or just walking down the street, is to feel when you exhale that Chi is expanding from the Dan Tien into a sphere which is larger than your body. You can also visualize that you are inflated with Chi, and your limbs and body are rounded and full like a balloon. An especially good way to train extending your Chi further is to increase the length of your breath. When you coordinate your Yi, Chi and breath, the longer your breath is, the further your Chi will extend. This is why the solo Tai Chi sequence is normally done so as to take 18 to 20 minutes. The breath is coordinated with each movement, and the mind leads the Chi inward with each inhale and extends it outward to the maximum with each exhale. To train and extend the Chi further, the sequence should be done slower, without adding any breaths.

2-4. Posture and Tai Chi Chuan

Since Tai Chi Chuan is an internal Chi Kung martial style, correct posture is one of the most important essentials. Incorrect postures can cause many problems: a tight posture can stagnate the internal Chi circulation, wrong postures may expose your vital points to attack, floating shoulders and elbows will break the Jing and reduce Jing storage.

Tai Chi students are generally taught to make the postures large at first. This helps the beginner to relax, makes it easier to see and feel the movements, and also helps him to sense the Chi flow. Furthermore, because large postures are more expanded and relaxed, the Chi flow can be smoother. Large posture Tai Chi was emphasized by Yang Chen-Fu and has been popularly accepted as the best Tai Chi practice for health.

Large postures also make it easier to train Jing. It is more difficult to learn Jing with small postures because the moves are smaller and quicker, and they require more subtle sensing Jings. Large postures build the defensive circle larger and longer than small postures, which allows you more time to sense the enemy's Jing and react. It is best to first master the large circles, and only then to make the circles smaller and increase your speed. Thus, the poem of Thirteen Postures: Comprehending External and Internal Training states: "First look to expanding, then look to compacting, then you approach perfection" (Appendix A-3).

In addition, when you begin Tai Chi, you should first train with low postures and then gradually get higher. When you first start Tai Chi you cannot build your root by leading your Chi to the Bubbling Well point (Yongquan) on the soles of your feet. Without this firm foundation you will tend to float and your Jing will be weak. To remedy this problem, you should first train with low postures (though not so low as to make you tense), which will give you a root even without Chi, and simultaneously develop your Chi circulation. Only when you have accomplished Grand Circulation and the Chi can reach the Bubbling Well can you use it to build the internal root. This is done by visualizing the Chi flowing through your feet and extending into the ground like the roots of a tree. At this time you may start using higher postures and relaxing your leg muscles. This will facilitate the Chi flow, which in turn will help you to relax even more. In the higher levels of Tai Chi Chuan, muscle usage is reduced to the minimum, and all the muscles are soft and relaxed. When this stage is reached, Chi is being used efficiently and is the predominant factor in the Jing. Usually it takes more than thirty years of correct training to reach this level. Train according to your level of skill—start with the larger and lower postures, and only move to the smaller and higher postures as your skill increases.

To summarize: build your Chi both externally and internally, and circulate it through the entire body. After the internal Chi can reach the limbs, use this Chi to support your Jing. Gradually deemphasize the use of the muscles, and rely more and more on using the mind to guide the Chi to lead the body. Train the postures from large to small, low to high, slow to fast, and easy to hard. First build the defensive circle large, then make it smaller. For maximum Jing, strengthen the root, develop power in the legs, balance your Yi and Chi, exercise control through the waist, and express your will through your hands.

Now, let us discuss the general rules of posture:

Hands and Wrists: The most common hand forms used in Yang style barehand practice are the Tai Chi palm and the Tai Chi fist. The open palm hand form is done in two ways, depending on the style one is practicing. In one style, the little finger is pulled slightly back while the thumb is pressed forward (Figure 2-68). The hand should be cupped. The other open palm hand form is similar to the first except that the thumb is pulled back slightly instead of pushed forward (Figure 2-69). Here, the hands should be shaped as if you were holding a basketball with the palms, without the thumbs and little fingers touching the ball. In Yang style Tai Chi Chuan this hand form is called Wa Sou (Tile Hand) because it is curved like a Chinese roof tile. In both hand forms, the thumbs and little fingers are slightly tensed to restrict the Chi flow to these fingers and increase the flow to the middle fingers and palms.

The open palm hand form is classified as a Yang hand in Tai Chi. When palms are used to attack, the fingers are loosely extended and the wrists settled (dropped slightly) in order to allow the Jing to reach the palms and exit easily. It is said: "Settle the wrists, extend the fingers" (Appendix A-10).

The Tai Chi fist should be formed as if you were holding a Ping-Pong ball lightly in the center of the hand (Figure 2-70). When striking, the fist closes momentarily, but the fingers and palms are kept relaxed to allow the Chi to circulate. The fist hand form guides the energy back to the palm and is classified as a Yin hand in Tai Chi.

Elbows and Shoulders: The Tai Chi classics say: "Sink the shoulders, drop the elbows" (Appendix A-10). There are several reasons for this—first, it allows the elbows and shoulders to be loose and the muscles relaxed. Second, dropping the elbows seals several vital cavities, such as the armpits. Third, when the elbows and shoulders are sunk, Jing can be effectively stored in the postures, as well as emitted naturally from the waist without being broken (see next chapter for a more detailed discussion). Fourth, dropped elbows and shoulders help to keep the postures stable and the mind more centered.

Head: The head should be upright. It is said: "An insubstantial energy leads the head (upward)" (Appendix A-10). When your head is upright and feels suspended from above, your center will be firm and the Spirit of Vitality will be raised up. In addition, the eyes and mind should concentrate. It is said: "The eye gazes with concentrated Spirit" (Appendix A-10).

Chest: It is said: "Hold the chest in, arc the back" (Appendix A-10). Remember that Yi leads the Chi, so whenever you inhale, pull your chest in and arc your back to store Jing in the posture, and visualize as vividly as possible that you are storing Yi and Chi.

Waist, Hips, and Thighs: The waist and hips are particularly important in Tai Chi martial applications. The waist is the steering wheel which is used to direct the neutralization of the enemy's attack and the emission of Jing. The waist must be relaxed and the hips should be as if sitting, so that the pelvis is level and the lower back straight. This will let your movements be agile and alive. As you move, your waist should generally stay the same distance from the floor—unnecessary

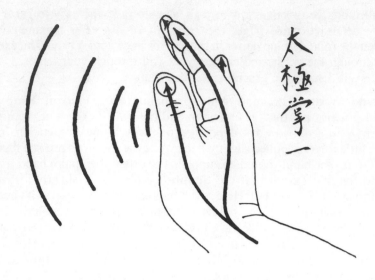

Figure 2-68. Tai Chi Palm with little finger back and thumb forward

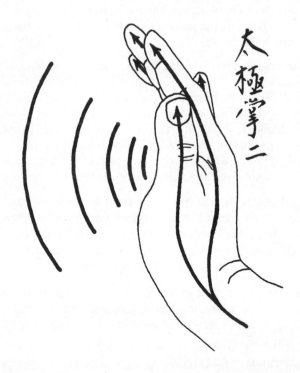

Figure 2-69. Tai Chi Palm with both thumb and little finger back

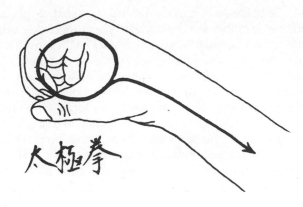

Figure 2-70. The Tai Chi fist

up and down movement will disturb your root. The Dan Tien in the abdomen is the source of Chi. It must be stimulated in order to fill it up with Chi so that the abdomen is tight like a drum. However, the muscles in this area must be relaxed in order to pass the Chi which you have generated in the Dan Tien down to the Sea Bottom cavity, and then up the spine and out to the hands. The hips and thighs connect the waist to the legs where the Jing is generated. In order to pass this Jing to the waist, the hips and thighs must be relaxed and stable, otherwise the Jing will be broken and the Chi stagnant. In addition, if the hips and thighs are tight, the Chi generated in the Dan Tien will have difficulty reaching the legs. Thus, it is said: "Relax your waist and relax your thighs" (Appendix A-10).

Legs, Knees, and Feet: The legs and knees must be loose and alive, then you can generate Jing from the tendons and sinews. The muscles should not be tensed, for this will obstruct the generation of Jing. However, the legs and knees cannot be completely loose and relaxed. They must be slightly tensed in order to keep your foundation stable. You should look loose but not be loose, look relaxed but not be relaxed.

When your weight is on the front foot, the rear leg should not be straightened, but should have a slight bend, and the front knee should generally not go past the front toe. The exception to this is when you are emitting Jing. In this case the knee may momentarily go past the toe, but should immediately pull back, and the rear leg may momentarily straighten, but should immediately bend again.

In Tai Chi, the weight is almost never distributed evenly on both legs. Rather, it is always more on one foot than the other, and it is always shifting from one foot to the other. Once you learn to use the muscles and tendons in your legs correctly, and learn the exchange of substantial and insubstantial, you will not lose your root, and will be able to generate Jing efficiently. Thus, it is said: "The knees look relaxed, but are not relaxed" (Appendix A-10).

The feet are the root of all the postures and the source of mobility. The feet must firmly stick to the ground. It is said: "Soles touch the ground" (or "Feet flat on the ground") (Appendix A-10). In order to do this, your Yi must be directed into the ground and the Chi must be able to reach the Bubbling Well cavity. It takes a great deal of practice to develop a good root, but gradually you will grasp the trick and your root will grow deeper and deeper.

In conclusion, the entire body must be relaxed, centered, stable, and comfortable, and should not lean forward or backward nor tilt to either side. It is said: "Postures should not be too little or too much (i.e. neither insufficient nor excessive). They (the postures) should seek to be centered and upright" (Appendix A-10). Every form must be continuous, smooth, and uniform, then the Spirit will be calm, the Yi concentrated, and the Chi will flow smoothly and naturally. Also: "Every form of every posture follows smoothly; no forcing, no opposition, the entire body is comfortable. Each form smooth" (Appendix A-10). Chang San-Feng's Tai Chi Chuan treatise says: "No part should be defective, no part should be deficient or excessive, no part should be disconnected" (Appendix A-1). Yi, Chi, Jing, the postures, top and bottom, inside and outside, front and back: all must act as one unit. When you reach this level, you will no doubt be a real Tai Chi expert.

2-5. How to Practice the Tai Chi Chuan Sequence

This chapter has discussed the two most basic aspects of Tai Chi Chuan practice: Chi and postures. Normally, it takes at least three years to learn to circulate Chi smoothly in coordination with the breathing and postures. You should then learn to transport Chi, and develop Chi balance. Even after you have accomplished this, there is still more to learn before you can be considered a proficient Tai Chi martial artist. You must learn how to strengthen your Chi through practice, you must develop a sense of having an enemy in front of you during the sequence, and lastly, you must learn how to train Jing during the sequence.

In Tai Chi Chuan, Chi plays a major role in Jing. When Chi is strong and full, then the Jing will also be strong. An important way to strengthen and extend your Chi is to **PRACTICE THE SEQUENCE SLOWER AND SLOWER**. If it usually takes 20 minutes to finish the entire sequence, increase the time to 25 minutes, then 30 minutes, and so on. Do not add any more breaths. Everything is the same except that every breath, which is used to lead the Chi, gets longer and longer. In order to do this you must be very calm and relaxed, and your Chi must be full like a drum or balloon, first in your abdomen, and later in your whole body. If you can extend a sequence which normally takes 20 minutes to one hour, your Chi will be very full and fluid, your mind calm, and the postures very relaxed. When you do the sequence at this speed, your pulse and heartbeat will slow down, and you will be in a self-hypnotic state. You will hardly notice your physical body, but instead will feel like a ball of energy.

Even when you can do the form very well, it may still be dead. To make it come alive you must **DEVELOP A SENSE OF ENEMY**. When practicing the solo sequence, you must imagine that there is an enemy in front of you, and you must clearly "feel" his movements and his interaction with you. Your ability to visualize realistically will be greatly aided if you practice the techniques with a partner. There are times when you will not actually use visualizations, but every time you do the sequence your movement must be flavored with this knowledge of how you interact with an opponent. The more you practice with this imaginary enemy before you, the more realistic and useful your practice will be. If you practice with a very vivid sense of enemy, you will learn to apply your Chi and Jing naturally, and your whole Spirit will melt into the sequence. This is not unlike performing music. If one musician just plays the music, and the other plays it with his whole heart and mind, the two performances are as different as night and day. In one case the music is dead, while in the other it is alive and touches us.

If you don't know how to incorporate Jing into the forms, then even if you do the sequence for many years it will still be dead. In order for the sequence to be meaningful, Jing and technique must be combined. An important way to do this is to **PRACTICE FAST TAI CHI CHUAN**. Once you can do the sequence of movements automatically, and can coordinate your breathing and Chi circulation with the movements, you should practice doing the form faster. Remember, if you ever get into a fight, things are likely to move pretty fast, so you have to be able to respond fast in order to defend yourself effectively. If you only practice slowly, then when you need to move fast your Chi will be broken, your postures unstable, and your Yi scattered. If any of this happens, you will not be able to use your Jing to fight. Therefore, once you have developed your Chi circulation you should practice the sequence faster until you can do it at fighting speed. Make sure you don't go too fast too soon, or you will sacrifice the essentials such as Yi concentration, Chi balance, breath coordination, and the storage of Jing in the postures. When doing fast Tai Chi, do not move at a uniform speed. Incorporate the pulsing movement of Jing so that you are responding appropriately to the actions of your imaginary enemy. It is difficult to develop the pulsing movement of Jing solely by doing the sequence, so you should also do Jing training either before or concurrently with the fast Tai Chi. This will be discussed further in Chapter 3.

第三章
勁

CHAPTER 3
JING

3-1. Introduction

Jing training is a very important part of the Chinese martial arts, but there is almost nothing written on the subject in English, and very little even in Chinese. Many instructors have viewed the higher levels of Jing as a secret which should only be passed down to a few trusted students. Also, it is unfortunately the case that many instructors don't understand Jing very well themselves. It is a difficult subject to explain and, like the poetry and songs in the appendix, it is even harder to express in English. While the author's understanding of Jing is still incomplete, he feels it is better to publicize the available information to help the serious martial artist get on the right track, and to encourage further study and research. Information in this chapter is drawn from the available Chinese literature on the subject, oral instruction from the author's two Shaolin masters and three Tai Chi teachers, and from the author's research and discussion with his students. This chapter is not meant to be the final authority on the subject, but rather a catalyst to research. Rather than a monument, this chapter should serve as a stone generating ripples in the minds of the readers.

Many martial artists nowadays do not understand what Jing is, or think that it is trained in only a few particular styles. Some even brag that the style they have learned is the only style which has Jing training. In fact, almost all Oriental martial styles train Jing. The differences lie in the depth to which Jing is understood, in the different kinds of Jing trained, and in the range and characteristics of the emphasized Jings. For example, Tiger Claw style emphasizes hard and strong Jing, imitating the tiger's muscular strength; muscles predominate in most of the techniques. White Crane, Hsing Yi, and Ba Kua are softer styles, and the muscles are used relatively less.

In Tai Chi Chuan and Liu Ho Ba Fa, the softest styles, soft Jing is especially emphasized and muscle usage is cut down to a minimum. This often confuses people, and they ask: If the muscles are not used for fighting, where does the power to win the fight come from? Hopefully, once you have read this chapter you will know the answer, and will have grasped the key to the traditional Chinese martial arts.

The application of Jing brings us to a major difference between the Oriental martial arts and those of the West. Oriental martial arts traditionally emphasize the training of Jing, whereas this concept and training approach are relatively unknown in other parts of the world. In China, martial styles and martial artists are judged by their Jing. How deeply is Jing understood and how well is it applied? How strong and effective is it, and how is it coordinated with martial technique? When a martial artist performs his art without Jing it is called "Far chuan shiou twe", which means "Flower fist and brocade leg". This is to scoff at the martial artist without Jing who is weak like a flower and soft like brocade. Like dancing, his art is beautiful but not useful. It is also said "Lien chuan bu lien kung, tao lao yi tsang kong", which means "Train chuan and not kung, when you get old, all emptiness". This means that if a martial artist emphasizes only the beauty and smoothness of his forms and doesn't train his Kung, then when he gets old, he will have nothing. The "Kung" here means "Chi Kung", and refers to the cultivation of Chi and its coordination with Jing to develop the latter to its maximum, and to make the techniques effective and alive. Therefore, if a martial artist learns his art without training his "Chi Kung" and "Jing Kung", once he gets old the techniques he has learned will be useless, because he will have lost his muscular strength. The author is saddened to see that for the last thirty years Jing Kung has been widely ignored while the beauty of the art has been emphasized. Many of the martial artists today tend to train dance-like forms and acrobatic skills and ignore the major part of Kung Fu training.

This unfortunate tendency is also common in Tai Chi society today. Since the great majority of people do Tai Chi for health, the martial aspect is being more and more ignored. An example of this is that most people only practice Tai Chi slowly. How can Jing be developed this way? How can martial applications be learned? When a person attacks you he will move fast and hard, so unless you have trained with speed and Jing, you will be unable to defend yourself.

Jing has been considered a secret transmission in Tai Chi society. This is so not only because it was not revealed to most students, but also because it cannot be passed down with words alone. Jing must be experienced. It is said that the master "passes down Jing". Once you feel Jing done by your master, you know what is meant and are able to work on it by yourself. Without an experienced master it is more difficult, but not impossible, to learn about Jing. There are general principles and training methods which an experienced martial artist can use to grasp the keys of this practice. If you read this chapter carefully and practice patiently and perseveringly, and remember to remain humble, to question and ponder, you will no doubt be able to learn Jing and become a real master.

Section 2 of this chapter will define Jing according to the author's best understanding. Jing, Chi and Li will be compared and contrasted, and the range of Jing will be explained. Section 3 will discuss the general theory of Tai Chi Jing and the keys to its generation. Section 4 will discuss the accumulation of Jing in your postures. Section 5 is a summary of the key points to Tai Chi Jing. Section 6 will explain the different kinds of Jing and offer exercises to help you discover and train your Jing. Finally, section 7 will summarize the training methods which have been explained in the preceding sections.

3-2. General Definition of Jing

Before you can understand Jing, you must first understand Li. Li, which is defined as muscular strength, is usually visible as big muscles. It is considered "post-birth" energy because it goes through the cycle of increasing as you mature and then weakening as you grow old. Muscular Li can be long and slow, and can be used to push a car or hold a heavy object. When Li is used, the muscles are tensed and stiff.

Now let us define Jing. The Chinese dictionary gives two main meanings of Jing. The first is "strong, unyielding, muscular", and is usually applied to powerful, inanimate objects. For examples, "Jing Gung" means a strong bow, and "Jing Fong" means a strong wind. It can also be applied to more abstract feelings of strength, as in "Jing Tee" which means a strong enemy. These examples illustrate the first difference between Jing and Li. Li is explicit and is shown externally, while Jing is more implicit and internal—you must feel it to sense its strength. You can't tell the strength of a bow by looking at it, rather you must pull it to see if it has the potential to generate a lot of power. Once it emits an arrow, the strength of its Jing is shown by the power (Li) of the arrow. (For inanimate objects, Li refers to manifest strength or power.) Another quality often associated with Jing is the feeling of a strong, pulsed, flow. An example is "Jing Fong" (a strong wind)—never steady, it moves this way and that, over and around obstacles, and when it surges, trees bend and houses are knocked down.

The second dictionary definition of Jing is "Chi-Li" (or "Li-Chi"), which refers to muscles which are supported by Chi. Using only your muscles is considered Li. However, when you use your Yi (mind) and concentration to lead the muscles to do something, Chi will flow to where you are concentrating and enliven the muscles. This is considered Jing. The Chinese martial arts emphasize using Yi and concentration, so whenever Jing is mentioned in this book, it means "Chi-Li".

There are many types of Jing, but the one thing they all have in common is that they all deal with the flow of energy, one aspect of which is Chi. The most obvious type of Jing is "manifest Jing", where you can see something happening, as when you push someone. Sensing another person's motion or energy is also considered a type of Jing. In fact, in the highest levels of the "sensing Jing" you actually sense the Chi flow of your opponent and thereby know his intentions. These sensing Jings are enhanced by increasing the Chi flow to your skin. Many of the hand forms described in Chapter 2 are called Jings—they direct the Chi flow in particular ways, or rely on Chi support for use in martial techniques. In general, the higher the level of Jing, the more Chi and the less Li is used.

In the martial arts, it is said that Jing is not Li. This means that although you must use your muscles (Li) every time you move, Jing is more than just muscular strength. There are several different kinds of manifested Jing. When you rely primarily on muscular strength, but also use Chi and your concentrated mind, it is considered "hard" Jing. This kind of Jing is usually easily visible as tensed muscles. When muscle usage is reduced, and both Chi and muscles play equal roles in the Jing, it is called "soft-hard" Jing. When muscle usage is reduced to a minimum, and Chi plays the major role, it is called "soft Jing". Soft-hard Jing, and especially soft Jing, are usually expressed in a pulse. Soft Jing is often compared to a whip, which can express a great deal of force in a very short time, concentrated in a very small area. When you snap a whip, it stays loose as it transmits a wave or pulse of energy along its length to the tip. In the same way, when you use soft Jing your muscles stay relatively relaxed as you transmit a pulse of energy through your body. This is done with the tendons and the ends of the muscles, supported by Chi. A more detailed discussion of this will be given later in this section.

Most of the Tai Chi Jings are of the soft variety. The emission of Jing is a relatively short, smooth, and relaxed pulse of energy, without any angular changes in direction. The pulse can be long or short, near the body or at a distance. It can be a sudden contraction and expansion as you bounce the opponent away, or an even sharper "spasm" as you strike or break something. In all of this, Jing uses Li, because Li is necessary any time you move, but the muscles must be supported by Chi.

Figure 3-1 may help you understand the difference between Jing and Li. In this figure, the vertical coordinate represents the depth to which power can penetrate, and the horizontal coordinate represents the elapsed time. The areas under the curves represent the power generated for each curve. We assume that the areas under the curves are the same, i.e., the power generated for each curve is equal. In curve 1, the power is generated, reaches its maximum, stays at the maximum for the time t1, and then drops to zero. Without Chi, this is a typical example of Li—muscular strength predominates and penetration is limited. With Chi, it is considered "hard" Jing. In curve 2, both muscles and Chi are involved, and the power is at its maximum for the shorter time t2. Since the power generated is the same as with curve 1, the peak has to reach higher, which means there is greater penetration. In order to do this, the muscles must be relaxed to allow the Chi from either the local area or the Dan Tien to flow smoothly to support them. This is the general idea of "soft-hard" Jing. In curve 3, the time t3 in which the power is generated is even shorter. The muscles must be extremely relaxed to generate and express this sharply penetrating power. Naturally, Chi plays the predominant role in this "soft" Jing. Curve 3 is typical of Tai Chi Jing. From the point of view of muscle usage, curve 1 is like a wooden staff, curve 2 is like a rattan staff, and curve 3 is like a whip. The wooden staff is stiff like tensed muscles, the rattan is more flexible, and the whip is soft, its power sharp and focused.

Even curve 3, which is a very high level of power, is still not the highest power in the martial arts. As mentioned in the last chapter, this is when pure Chi is used, which can be represented by line 4. When a martial artist has reached this level, he can transport his Chi into his enemy's body through the acupuncture cavities to shock the organs and cause damage or death instantly. The time used is extremely short and the penetration is deeper than is possible with Jing or Li.

The Difference between Jing and Li:

Li is said to derive from the bones and muscles. Jing comes from the tendons, and is supported by Chi which is generated either in the Dan Tien or the local area. Since the tendons are emphasized, the muscle fibers are able to be relaxed, allowing the Chi to flow through them and support them. If your force is derived from the bones, there is a strong tendency for you to resist and meet your opponent's force directly. When your force is derived from the tendons it is easier to be flexible and elusive, to disappear in front of the opponent's attack and to appear at his weak spot.

Li has shape, while Jing has no shape or form. This means that Li can be seen, but Jing must be felt. The storing of energy and the preparation for moves, as well as the actual emission of energy, can be more subtle with Jing because it is done with the body and Dan Tien rather than the arms. With Li the muscles of the arms and shoulders tend to be the source of energy, and this is more easily seen.

Li is square, whereas Jing is round. In Chinese, square means clumsy, stiff, stubborn, and straightforward; whereas round implies smooth, flexible, alive, and tricky. This means when Li is used, it is sluggish and stiff, whereas when Jing is used, it is smooth, agile and alive.

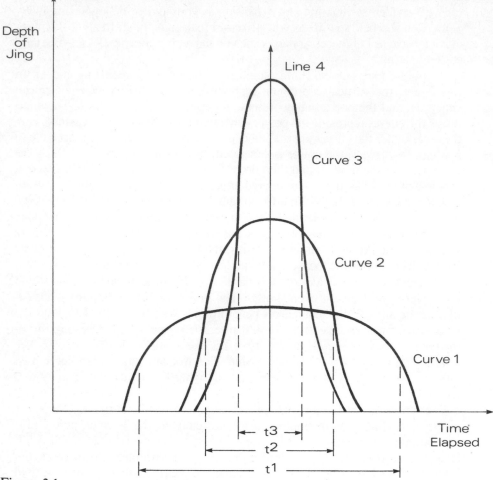

Figure 3-1.

It is said that **Li is stagnant and Jing is fluid.** It is also said that Li is slow, but Jing is swift. Because Li emphasizes muscular contraction, the muscles are stiffer and respond more slowly. Since Jing is more relaxed it is easier to change direction. The actual emission of energy is more restrained and controlled, so you can be more subtle and can deal more easily with changes in the situation.

With Li, power is diffuse, but the power of Jing is concentrated. When using just the muscles, it is hard to concentrate the energy. When you train Jing you emphasize relaxation and moving from the center of your being. This allows you to concentrate all of your energy into a very small space and time.

It is said that **Li floats, but Jing is sunken.** This has two interpretations. First, when you use muscular strength you emphasize the arms and shoulders, and your movements tend to be angular and jerky. This makes it easier to lose your connection with the ground. With Jing, especially in Tai Chi Chuan, the arms and body are relaxed, and energy is derived from the waist, legs, and Dan Tien. When your attention is on your legs, it is easier to keep firmly in contact with the ground. Since your center and source of motion are more removed from the opponent than is the case with Li, it is easier to avoid throwing yourself at the opponent, which would break your root. A second interpretation of this saying is that with Li the power is more from the surface, while with Jing the power is more internal. That is, the tendons, from which Jing is derived, are relatively more internal than the muscles. After long training, the Chi which supports Jing comes from deep within the body.

Finally, it is said that **Li is dull, but Jing is sharp.** This implies that Li's power stays on the surface while Jing penetrates deeply. Since the approach and the methods of training Jing are more refined and internal than is the case with Li, it is possible to be more precise in the application of force, and to have the force penetrate more deeply into the opponent.

The Range of Jing:

The concept of Jing covers quite a wide range. As mentioned before, when muscles are used without any particular Chi support, the power generated is called Li. This is the most basic power, the post-birth strength which grows as you grow and reaches its maximum when the muscles have developed to their maximum. When you get older, the strength of the muscles lessens, and Li is lost. However, if you learn to concentrate your Yi (mind) on the muscles used, the Chi will be generated naturally in the local area, i.e., the muscles being used. Chi is the pre-birth energy which flows in the human body. When you concentrate your Yi, the Chi will naturally follow, invigorating the muscles being used and raising them to maximum energy. When this pre-birth energy is involved, the force produced is called Jing. If the muscles predominate, it is considered a low level of Jing. This energy, which still shows most of the characteristics of Li, is called "Ying Jing" (hard Jing). Tiger Claw is a typical example of a martial style which specializes in hard Jing.

External stylists frequently train their local Chi to support the muscles. This training can not only enable the muscles to express power more efficiently, but can also enable the Chi-filled muscles to resist blows without injury. The latter training is called "Iron Shirt" or "Golden Bell Cover".

If you know how to train your Yi to become stronger and stronger, your Chi will become correspondingly stronger as well. In order to have this stronger Chi flow smoothly in support of the muscles, the muscles must be relaxed. The more the muscles are relaxed, the more easily the Chi can flow, allowing the muscles to do the job more efficiently. After many years of training, you will rely primarily on the ends of the muscles near the tendons, which allows the bulk of the muscle to stay relaxed and soft. In China it is not uncommon to see old men do feats of strength with apparently soft muscles. This is only possible after long years of Jing training which develops Yi, Li, and Chi. Such skills can grow with age, which makes it possible for an old man to successfully defend himself against a strong, young man. The main factor in such a victory remains, however, the ability to concentrate Yi and Chi sufficiently so that the muscles can reach maximum efficiency. You have probably experienced trying to push a heavy object that seemed immovable . If you stop for a moment, relax your muscles, and visualize the object moving, you will often find that you can now move it. This is because Chi is now playing a greater role.

When Chi and the muscles are involved in equal amounts, the Jing is considered mid-level and is called "Roan Ying Jing" (soft-hard Jing). This is considered a higher level of Jing expression than hard Jing, both in theory and technique. When using this Jing, the muscles are entirely relaxed to allow the Chi to flow. Right before the target is reached, the muscles are suddenly tensed to get the stored Jing out.

Some martial styles specializing in this kind of Jing are White Crane, Snake, and Praying Mantis.

The next stage is to relax the muscles as much as possible. The more the muscles relax, the more the Chi can be used, allowing the tendons to take over control of the motion and keep it flowing smoothly. In order to emit power without relying on the muscles, the force is used in a pulse-like fashion. When this fluid, tendon-oriented Jing is the main source of power instead of the muscles, it is called "Roan Jing" (soft Jing). It is considered the highest type of Jing, in regards to both theory and technique. Tai Chi Chuan and Liu Ho Ba Fa are styles which use this kind of Jing.

However, the Jing just described is still of a low level if the supporting Chi is generated from the local area. For higher levels of Jing the Chi must be generated from the Dan Tien. When the Chi comes from the local area, the Jing is called "Wai Jing" (external Jing), and when the Chi is generated from the Dan Tien, it is called "Nei Jing" (internal Jing).

Some martial artists use a kind of "jerking power" and believe that it is Jing. This jerking power is only a part of Jing. It is considered "Wai Jing" because it relies upon locally generated Chi to reinforce its power. Even with external Jing, in order to develop maximum power you must still build the root in the feet, generate Jing from the legs, use the waist to control the Jing, and store power in the postures.

When a person trained in Chi development has achieved Small Circulation and Grand Circulation, he can use the Chi generated at the Dan Tien. The energy passes through the Sea Bottom cavity and is led to the feet, and it is also led up the spine and out to the hands. When Chi from the Dan Tien is used to support the tendons, the Jing can reach a high level. Naturally, the root, legs, waist, and postures must also be considered. This kind of Jing is called "Nei Jing" (internal Jing) and is the goal most Tai Chi martial artists aim for.

The final level of Tai Chi power is not Jing, but is using pure Chi to affect the enemy. This is the highest level of Tai Chi Chuan and is rarely seen today. When you train Tai Chi correctly for thirty years or more, your Chi will grow stronger and stronger. One day you may reach the point where you are able to pass your Chi out of your body or take in Chi from the enemy by touch. This is the highest level of Tien Hsueh (cavity press). At this level, with a touch to an enemy's vital cavity you will be able to upset his body's energy balance or shock the organ which corresponds to the cavity.

We have seen that Jing can range from external to internal. In the spectrum of energy, one end is Li and the other is Chi. Jing is in the middle, using both Li and Chi. The Jing used by beginning Shaolin is generally the external variety which relies mostly on Li and local Chi. However, when a Shaolin martial artist reaches a high level of achievement, his Jing will tend to be softer and Dan Tien Chi will take the place of local Chi.

Tai Chi Chuan stresses the internal Jing first. The muscles are relaxed so that Chi from the Dan Tien can circulate and support the muscles. However, when a Tai Chi martial artist has reached a high level of internal Jing, he should also master external Jing to cover the entire range of Jing training. In Chinese martial society there is a saying: "Shaolin from hard to soft, Tai Chi from soft to hard—the approaches are different, but the goal is the same". For this reason section 6 of this chapter will include both hard and soft Jings.

3-3. General Theory of Tai Chi Jing

The last few sections have given you a general idea of Jing. In this section we will discuss the theory and important points of the soft Tai Chi Jings. The theory and emphasis of hard Jings and soft-hard Jings are somewhat different, and will be discussed in a later volume.

Categories of Jing:

There are many ways to categorize Jing. To help you understand the Jings discussed in this volume, the author has organized them in the way shown in Table 3-1. The types of energy can be divided into two groups: sensing Jing (Jywe Jing) and manifested Jing (Hsing Jing).

Sensing Jing can be divided into active sensing Jing and passive sensing Jing. Active sensing Jing is the ability to generate a strong Chi flow which, in coordination with your Yi and breath, can be led in a wave into the opponent's body. This pulsing Chi flow is usually used to support hand forms (see section 2-3) for either attacking or healing. In external styles, this Chi flow is coordinated with techniques such as grabbing or poking, in which case they are more properly classified as manifested Jings. In internal styles the Chi flow is harder to see since it is not combined with Li, and can usually only be felt. An example of this internal Jing is Graze Skin False Critical Jing (see next section).

Passive sensing Jing is the capability of perceiving the opponent's energy. For example, one of the passive sensing Jings is called "Listening Jing", in which you use your skin and Spirit to sense the opponent's energy. The advanced stage of this is called "Understanding Jing" where, upon listening to the opponent's energy, you understand his intention. It is confusing to Westerners to call the ability to listen to the opponent's Jing a form of Jing. It becomes clearer when you understand that listening to Jing is not entirely passive. You have to stick with the opponent and move with him, almost matching his moves. When he emits Jing you must be able to deal with it easily and comfortably, which demands a degree of skill, sensitivity, Chi flow, and the ability to use Jing in your own movements.

Manifested Jing can be broken down into active Jing which is called Gong Jing (Offensive Jing) or Fa Jing (Emitting Jing), and passive Jing which is called Shoou Jing (Defensive Jing) or Huah Jing (Neutralizing Jing).

Active Jing is considered Yang, and is the emitting of power from the body, usually for attack. Yang Jing can also be discriminated into pure Yang Jing (Chwen Yang Jing) or pure offense Jing (Chwen Gong Jing), and Yang with some Yin Jing (Yang Jong Dai Yin Jing) or offense with some defense (Gong Jong Dai Shoou Jing).

Passive Jing is considered Yin and deals with the ability to yield to, lead, and neutralize the opponent's Jing. Yin Jing is usually used for defense and is in turn divided into pure Yin Jing (Chwen Yin Jing) or pure defense Jing (Chwen Shoou Jing), and Yin with some Yang Jing (Yin Jong Dai Yang Jing) or defense with some offense Jing (Shoou Jong Dai Gong Jing). In addition, there is a type of Jing which is neither Yin nor Yang (Fei Gong Fei Shoou Jing), and is normally used for Jing training and raising the Spirit of Vitality.

Almost every Jing classified above can again be divided into near (Gin) or far (Yeuan) Jing, and long (Chang) or short (Doan) Jing. Near or far refers to the distance from your body that the technique is done. Long and short refers to the distance that your hands travel while actually emitting energy. Long Jing normally requires more time to emit and is used to bounce the opponent away without hurting him. Short Jing is normally sharp and fast and is usually used to injure

Table 3-1.

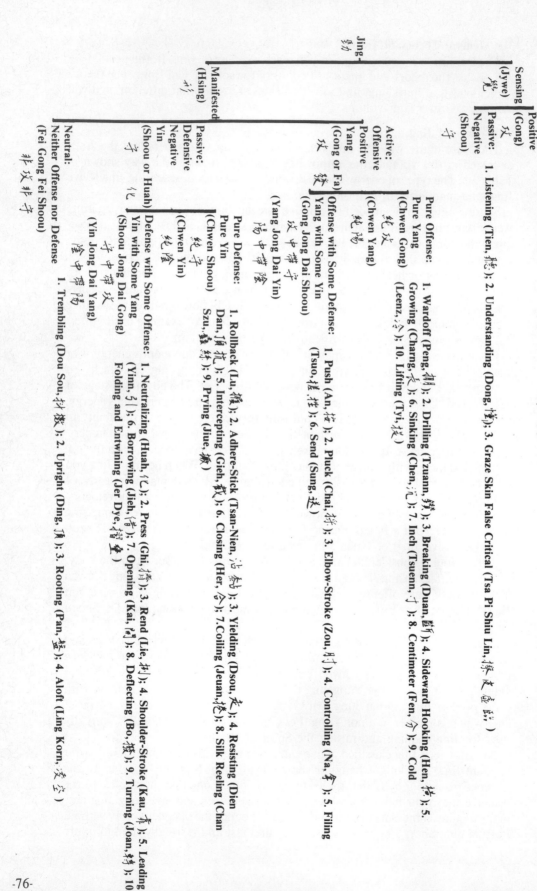

Jing- 勁

Sensing (Jywe) 覺

- **Active:** Positive (Gong) 攻
  1. Listening (Tien, 聽); 2. Understanding (Dong, 懂); 3. Graze Skin False Critical (Tsa Pi Shiu Lin, 擦皮虛臨)

- **Passive:** Negative (Shoou) 守
  1. Graze Skin False Critical (Tsa Pi Shiu Lin, 擦皮虛臨)

Manifested (Hsing) 形

- **Active:** Offensive Positive Yang (Gong or Fa) 發 (Chwen Yang) 純陽

  - Pure Offense: Pure Yang (Chwen Gong) 純攻
    1. Wardoff (Peng, 掤); 2. Drilling (Tzuann, 鑽); 3. Breaking (Duan, 斷); 4. Sideward Hooking (Hen, 橫); 5. Growing (Charng, 長); 6. Sinking (Chen, 沉); 7. Inch (Tsuenn, 寸); 8. Centimeter (Fen, 分); 9. Cold (Leenz, 冷); 10. Lifting (Tyi, 提)

  - Offense with Some Defense: Yang with Some Yin (Gong Jong Dai Shoou) 攻中帶守 (Yang Jong Dai Yin) 陽中帶陰
    1. Push (An, 按); 2. Pluck (Chai, 採); 3. Elbow-Stroke (Zou, 肘); 4. Controlling (Na, 拿); 5. Filing (Tsuo, 挫); 6. Send (Sung, 送)

- **Passive:** Defensive Negative Yin (Shoou or Huah) 化 (Chwen Yin) 純陰

  - Pure Defense: Pure Yin (Chwen Shoou) 純守
    1. Rollback (Lu, 捋); 2. Adhere-Stick (Tsan-Nien, 沾黏); 3. Yielding (Dsou, 走); 4. Resisting (Dien Dan, 頂抗); 5. Intercepting (Gieh, 截); 6. Closing (Her, 合); 7. Coiling (Jeuan, 卷); 8. Silk Reeling (Chan Szu, 纏絲); 9. Prying (Jiue, 撅)

  - Defense with Some Offense: Yin with Some Yang (Shoou Jong Dai Gong) 守中帶攻 (Yin Jong Dai Yang) 陰中帶陽
    1. Neutralizing (Huah, 化); 2. Press (Ghi, 擠); 3. Rend (Lie, 挒); 4. Shoulder-Stroke (Kau, 靠); 5. Leading (Yinn, 引); 6. Borrowing (Jieh, 借); 7. Opening (Kai, 開); 8. Deflecting (Bo, 撥); 9. Turning (Joan, 轉); 10. Folding and Entwining (Jer Dye, 折叠)

- **Neutral:** Neither Offense nor Defense (Fei Gong Fei Shoou) 非攻非守
  1. Trembling (Dou Sou, 抖擞); 2. Upright (Ding, 頂); 3. Rooting (Pan, 蟠); 4. Aloft (Ling Korn, 凌空)

or kill the enemy. Both long and short Jing can be done either near to the body or at a distance.

Jing and Yi:

Jing and Yi (mind, will) are probably the most important keys to success in Tai Chi. You should understand that if there is no Yi, the Chi will be stagnant, and if the Chi is stagnant, then it cannot be applied to Jing. Therefore, **WHEREVER THE JING IS TO GO, THE YI MUST GO FIRST, AND THE CHI WILL NATURALLY FOLLOW**. When you use your Yi to lead Chi in support of Jing, the Yi should always be further than the Jing, otherwise the Jing will be restrained and not completely expressed. This is best done by maintaining a sense of having an enemy in front of you. Imagination is the key here. If you only put your attention on your hands, the energy will have difficulty reaching them. When you put your mind on an imaginary opponent in front of you, the Chi will more easily reach your hands and pass through them. Therefore, it is said: "Jing (can be) broken, mind not broken" (Appendix A-3).

Jing, Muscles, and Chi:

As mentioned in the previous sections, almost all Jings require using the muscles. Muscles play the major role in hard Jings, a lesser role in soft-hard Jings, and a relatively small role in the soft, pulsing Jings used in Tai Chi. As the role of the muscles decreases, the role of the tendons gradually increases, and the expression of Jing changes from the slower muscular version to a fast pulse strike.

In Chinese martial arts, all of these Jings require Chi support. How does this Chi support work? Let us digress for a moment and consider several factors affecting muscular strength. Most people know that we use only a portion of the capacity of our brains. The same situation prevails with our muscles, for we use only about forty percent of their capacity. There are several ways to increase this percentage. The will (Yi) is important, sometimes to an astounding degree. When people are confronted with emergencies, they can sometimes do things far beyond their normal, everyday ability. When you decide you MUST do something, your body follows your will. Another factor which increases muscular strength is concentration. You have probably already observed that concentration increases the effectiveness of your exertion. When all of your mind is on what you are doing, and none of your attention is distracted by extraneous matters, all of your efforts and energy can be focused on one target.

Wherever your mind is, your Chi is. Once you have developed Grand Circulation, you should be able to move your Chi from your Dan Tien to any part of your body. When you put your mind (Yi) on a particular technique, for example a push, your Chi will go to the muscles being used. The stronger your imagination is, and the greater your concentration, the more the Chi will flow and fill the active muscles. This energizes them the way a surge of electricity brings an electric motor to life. It will also increase the flexibility and elasticity of the muscles and make them feel inflated and capable of resisting a punch or generating a lot of power. The more disciplined your will and concentration are, the more effectively you can move your Chi. Western science reports that concentration generates a chemical reaction in your muscles that increases the power much more than usual. I do not doubt that this is caused by the Chi that this concentration of the mind brings.

When you have trained your Chi and muscles, you will find that you can generate the same power with less muscle tissue. You will be able to relax your muscles, which will let the Chi flow even more easily. The main bulk of the muscle fiber, which is in the middle of the muscle, will relax, and you will rely more on the ends of the muscles near the tendons. It is said that Tai Chi Jing comes from the tendons. This demands great skill and control on your part. To move in the loose, fluid, almost boneless fashion of Tai Chi, you have to be able to place every part of your body in the correct relationship to each other part, the ground, and the target. The force generated by your legs is bounced off the floor and coiled through your body. The force cannot pass through any kinks or around any corners. Tension in any muscle will hinder the flow of force and Chi. The tendons, which are the connectors of the parts of the body, transmit the force from each part to the next. The ends of the muscles use the minimum amount of effort to keep the flow going and direct it.

Most people have parts or patches of their bodies that they are not really aware of. This may show up as, for example, a place on your thigh where you are not as sensitive as elsewhere. This means that your Spirit (Shen) doesn't normally reach everywhere in your body, and consequently, your Mind and Chi don't go there either. You must train your Spirit, Mind, and Chi to fill your body like a thread passing through every part of the pearl with the nine-curved passage. Only when your consciousness and Chi suffuse your muscles can you really control them and your movement.

There are several ways you can fill your body with Spirit and Chi after you have completed Grand Circulation. You can visualize that you are a balloon being inflated with energy and awareness. However, the main way that Tai Chi uses is doing the sequence slowly. When the form is done at a slow, steady pace you have a chance to pay attention to the movement of Chi without sacrificing anything else. Accumulate Chi in your Dan Tien and coordinate it with your movements through your breathing.

You will always use some muscular energy (Li) when you move. It is impossible to move without it. Similarly, there is always Chi moving in your body. It only stops when you die, or a part of your body dies. An external stylist can develop Chi to strengthen his movements, but it is local Chi, developed in the arms and shoulders. Since this kind of movement uses tensed muscles, the Chi from the Dan Tien cannot reach the arms. An external style of Kung Fu like Tiger style uses this kind of local Chi to greatly strengthen the hands and arms. A soft-hard style like White Crane uses this local Chi to strengthen the arms, and balances it with attention to the waist and Dan Tien. Most of the time, however, the Chi in the Dan Tien is not circulated up the back and into the arms. External styles exhale to get the air out, and coordinate it with the energy, but it is stiff energy, not the soft energy of Tai Chi.

Jing and the Feet:

One of the most important factors in expressing Jing through the palms and fingers is the root. Your root is like the root of a tree: without it, the tree will fall. If you do not have a good root when you apply techniques, they will float and have no power. It is like trying to push a heavy object while wearing roller skates. The root of Jing and all techniques comes from the feet. The feet must be stable. To develop this stability **YOU MUST VISUALIZE YOUR ROOT A FEW INCHES BENEATH YOUR FEET**. If your thought is only on your feet, the connection between your feet and the ground is broken and the root will not grow deep into the ground. Almost all Chinese martial styles train root at the very beginning of the martial training. Without a good root, all the techniques are weak and ineffective. Thus, it is said: "The root is in the feet" (Appendix A-1); and also: "The foot and sole are the third chancellor" (Appendix A-5A).

The classics also mention: "(If) the Bubbling Well (Yongquan cavity) has no root, the waist has no master, (then) you can try hard to learn until you almost die, you will still not succeed" (Appendix A-14).

Jing and the Legs:

Once a martial artist has his root, the next step is to look to the legs. The legs are the main source of Jing, so investigate carefully how they bend and straighten to generate energy. When emitting Jing, you must balance force and counterforce with your legs. The rear leg usually generates the force and transmits the counterforce back into the ground. Without balancing the force through your legs in this way, it is difficult to generate power. This should be apparent to anyone who has ever tried to push a car or other heavy object. Therefore, it is said: "(power is) generated from the legs" (Appendix A-1).

Jing, the Waist, and the Spine:

Once you have a firm root and can generate Jing, the next step is to control and direct it. The most important factor in the application of Jing is probably the waist and spine. It is said: "The waist and the spine are the first master" (Appendix A-5A). Also: "(Jing) controlled by the waist" (Appendix A-1). It is also said: "The mind is the order, the Chi is the message flag, and the waist is the banner.... The Chi is like a cartwheel, the waist is like an axle"(Appendix A-3). All of these sayings emphasize that it is the movement of the waist which directs the force being emitted by the whole body.

The Song of the Thirteen Postures says: "The tailbone is central and upright" (Appendix 15). To have the tailbone central means that the body is balanced above it, not leaning to either side or to the front or rear. To have the tailbone upright means that most people must pull their buttocks in. When this is done, the lower spine loses its usual curve and straightens out. Most people do this when they sit down. When this is done properly, the bowl that is the pelvis is even, instead of tilting forward (Figure 3-2). This lets the organs in the abdomen rest comfortably within and on top of the pelvis instead of hang out the front. Proper posture eases strain on the organs, and allows the motion of your breathing to gently massage them. Also, when the lower spine is straight it is easier to transmit force through it, and you have a better chance of avoiding strain.

For a number of Jings, a jerking movement of the waist is needed to lead the Jing from the legs to the hands. In order for the Jing to be integrated and strong, there should not be any stagnation in the waist area. When Jing is stagnant, its strength will be broken or reduced. Therefore, the timing must be right and, above all, the waist must be relaxed. It is said: "Relax your waist and relax your thighs" (Appendix A-10).

Another important reason for the emphasis on the waist is that it is the location of the Dan Tien, which is the original source of the Chi used in Tai Chi Chuan. The Chi generated there is led to the legs, as well as up the spine, out the arms, and to the palms and fingers to support Jing. Without this Chi, the Jing will remain at a low level, perhaps supported only by local Chi. The spine acts not only as a conduit for the Chi, but also as a storage area. After long and correct training, Chi will accumulate in the marrow of the spine. Thus, it is said: "Power is emitted from the spine" and "(The mind) leads the Chi flowing back and forth, adhering to the back, then condensing into the spine" (Appendix A-3); "In every movement the heart (mind) remains on the waist, the abdomen is relaxed and clear, and Chi rises up" (Appendix A-15).

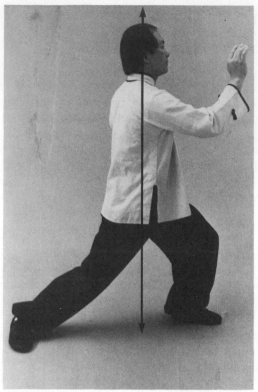

Figure 3-2.

Jing and the Hands:

In Tai Chi fighting, the palms and fingers are extremely important. These are the parts which most often touch the enemy. From this touch, a Tai Chi martial artist will sense or feel the enemy's power, understand his intention, neutralize his power, and finally counterattack with Jing. Therefore it is said: "The root is in the feet, (power is) generated from the legs, controlled by the waist and expressed by the fingers" (Appendix A-1). It is also said: "The fingers and palms are the second chancellor" (Appendix A-5A).

Jing and Sound:

Almost all martial styles use different sounds in practice and fighting. There are two sounds, Hen and Ha, which are especially important in Tai Chi Chuan. These sounds serve several purposes. During a fight, a loud sound can scare the enemy and disturb his concentration. Yelling can raise your fighting spirit and help increase your concentration. **A YELL CAN RAISE THE SPIRIT OF VITALITY TO THE MAXIMUM, AND HELP THE CHI MOVE QUICKLY AND SMOOTHLY.** The Hen sound, when made on the inhale, is Yin and can help to store Chi and condense it in the bone marrow. When the Hen sound is made on the exhale it is a mixture of Yin and Yang, and will help you emit energy while still conserving some to support the defense. The exhaled Ha sound is extremely Yang, and can be used to raise the Jing to its maximum. It is said: "Grasp and hold the Dan Tien to train internal Kung Fu. Hen, Ha, two Chi's are marvelous and infinite" (Appendix A-13). It is also said: "The throat is the second master" (Appendix A-5A). Sound training will be discussed in Chapter 3 of Volume Two.

Balancing Jing:

Balancing your Jing includes balancing your Yi, Chi, and posture. When Yi is balanced, the mind is centered and able to handle all directions. Upward and downward must also be balanced or you will lose your root. It is said: "Up and down, forward and backward, left and right, it's all the same. All of this is done with the mind, not externally. If there is a top, there is a bottom; if there is a front, there is a back; if there is a left, there is a right..."(Appendix A-1). Furthermore, Yi is the leader of Chi, and if the Chi is not balanced, then the force and counterforce relationships in the body are not balanced. Finally, you should use the balanced Chi to support the tendons and muscles when expressing Jing externally. With this balance and support the Jing can reach its maximum. It is like when you push a heavy object—you need to mobilize your Yi, and to direct power backward in order to push the object forward. It is said:"(When you) wish the foot to go forward, you must push off from the rear (foot)"(Appendix A-14). Thus, it is understood that **FIRST YOU MUST HAVE BACKWARD, THEN YOU CAN HAVE FORWARD. YOU MUST HAVE DOWNWARD FIRST, THEN YOU CAN HAVE UPWARD.**

Lastly, balancing your posture is extremely important. In regards to Jing, this means balancing the forces inside your body: If you want to push forward with a certain amount of force, you must push backwards with exactly the same amount of force in order to counterbalance it. You also need to balance the upward and downward forces, otherwise you will lose your root and push yourself up and away from your opponent. It is also necessary to balance forces in your two hands. When your posture is balanced the body is centered and stable, and the root is firm. This allows the power from the legs to be fully transmitted to the hands. Thus it is said: "When standing, the body must be centered, calm and comfortable, so you can handle the eight directions" (Appendix A-3). It is also said: "Postures should not be too little or too much (i.e., insufficient or excessive). They (the postures) should seek to be centered and upright" (Appendix A-10). **IF YOU CAN GRASP THE KEY OF BALANCING YOUR YI, CHI, AND POSTURE, YOU WILL HAVE GAINED THE SECRET OF PUSHING HANDS AND TAI CHI FIGHTING.**

Jing's Substantial and Insubstantial:

A very important part of Tai Chi fighting strategy is the principle of substantial and insubstantial. It applies to Jing, postures, and techniques. In this section we will discuss Jing; the latter two will be discussed in the second volume.

In the Tai Chi diagram, where one side is heavy the other side is light, and where one side is light the other side is heavy. In Tai Chi Chuan, this means that where your opponent attacks (is substantial), you yield and neutralize (are insubstantial). The other side of this is that you attack (are substantial) where the opponent is weak (insubstantial). To attack where the opponent is strong is called "mutual resistance". This is inefficient, and contrary to Tai Chi principles. You must train so that you automatically meet the opponent's substantial (attacking) Jing with an insubstantial (defensive) Jing. As you defend, you may simultaneously counterattack, or set yourself and your opponent up for your counterattack.

Offensively, attack where the opponent is weak. This does not mean where he is insubstantial, because you would be falling into a trap. Instead, attack when he is switching from a substantial Jing to an insubstantial, or vice versa. If you catch him just before he emits an offensive Jing, or just after he has emitted Jing and before he can switch to a defensive Jing, you will be certain to succeed.

Substantial and insubstantial Jings are determined by your Yi (mind). When you sense the opponent's intention, your Yi can change your actions from substantial to insubstantial, and vice versa. To facilitate this, **DO NOT EMIT ALL YOUR ENERGY. RATHER, CONSERVE SOME SO THAT YOU CAN EASILY SWITCH FROM ONE TECHNIQUE TO ANOTHER.**

If you can switch easily and quickly between attack and defense, you will be able to conceal your techniques so that the opponent cannot understand what you are doing. When you look like you are attacking, you should not necessarily be attacking, and when you look like you are withdrawing, you should not necessarily be withdrawing. Your opponent should not be able to sense your intention from how you express your Jing. This is called skillfully exchanging substantial and insubstantial. After a great deal of practice with many partners, your opponent will not be able to understand what you are doing, whether you are attacking or feinting, resisting or neutralizing, and he will not perceive how you are going to attack. This is reflected in the saying: "false-false, real-real, real-false, and false-real".

When you fight against an opponent who has mastered Listening, Understanding, and Neutralizing Jings, it is very hard to apply your Jing to his body. This is because when you store your Jing for an attack, your opponent has already sensed your intention. Therefore, you must **SHORTEN THE TIME OF JING STORAGE.** If you can store Jing in a very short time, and can skillfully exchange substantial and insubstantial, you will be hard to beat. Therefore, the classics say: "Suddenly disappear, suddenly appear. When there is pressure on the left, the left becomes insubstantial; when there is pressure on the right, the right becomes insubstantial. Looking upward it seems to get higher and higher; looking downward it seems to get deeper and deeper. When (the opponent) advances, it seems longer and longer; when (the opponent) retreats, it becomes more and more urgent. A feather cannot be added and a fly cannot land. The opponent does not know me, but I know the opponent. A hero has no equal because of all of this" (Appendix A-2).

3-4. Accumulating Jing in the Postures

Before you can emit Jing you must first generate or accumulate it. This is done through your Yi, Chi, and posture. Yi must lead the way. Jing is generated through understanding the enemy's intention and neutralizing his power. When you neutralize the opponent's attack you may see an opportunity or the possibility of an opportunity to counterattack. As you sense the opponent's intention, your Yi is stored and raised. As shown in Figure 3-3, your Yi will then lead you to store Chi in your Dan Tien. This perception of the opponent's attack will help you to coil your body as you evade in such a way as to accumulate power in the posture. Therefore, as you neutralize the opponent's attack your mind draws in to accumulate energy, and your Chi and body follow. Remember: **THE MIND LEADS, THE CHI FOLLOWS THE MIND, AND THE BODY FOLLOWS THE CHI.** Jing accumulation is facilitated by inhaling. If you inhale with the Hen sound it will help the Chi condense deep into the bones. **WHEN YOU KNOW HOW TO STORE YI, CHI, AND POSTURAL ENERGY, YOU HAVE BUILT THE FOUNDATION OF JING.**

Many people know how to store Yi and Chi, but don't know how to use their posture correctly. Everything must be done correctly and coordinated properly at the right time; a lapse in any area will cut down the effect of the whole effort. Jing can be stored in the bend of a joint, a twist of the body, the arcing of the chest, and even in the sinking of the body. In this section we will discuss the ways in which Jing is stored in the body. Once you understand this, you should be able

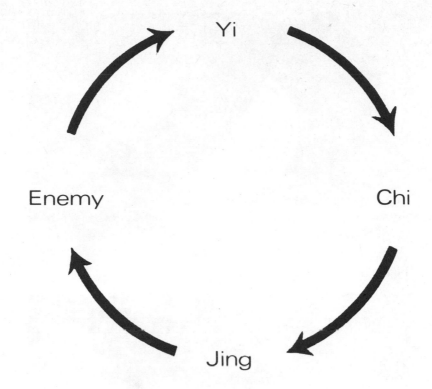

Yi

Chi

Enemy

Jing

Figure 3-3.

to discover the best ways to store energy for the different Jings discussed in the next section.

Legs

The legs are the major source of manifested Jing, and control how much Jing is emitted. In order to function effectively, the feet must be firmly rooted; the posture of the legs, especially the knees, must be correct; and the thighs must be relaxed. Jing can be stored in either the front or the rear leg. When the front leg is used to store Jing, it is bent (Figure 3-4), and when the Jing is expressed, the leg pushes forward to generate the backward Jing (Figure 3-5). When Jing is stored for this backward Jing, the front knee should not pass over the toes. Backward Jing is usually used to pull the opponent or to neutralize his attacking Jing.

When Jing is stored in the rear leg, the knee is also bent (Figure 3-6). When Jing is emitted, the knee straightens out, though not completely (Figure 3-7), as the leg pushes downward. When the Jing is emitted to its maximum, the front knee may pass the toes for an instant. In order to prevent your opponent from using this overextension, your knee must immediately bounce back to restore the body's stability and equilibrium. It is just like a spring which stretches out to emit force, but immediately moves back to its equilibrium position. Similarly, the rear leg may straighten out at the final moment of expressing your Jing, but it must move back to its bent and relaxed state right after the Jing reaches its maximum. Naturally, most of the time you won't be making an all-out attack, and so the front knee will not pass over the front toes and the rear leg will remain slightly bent.

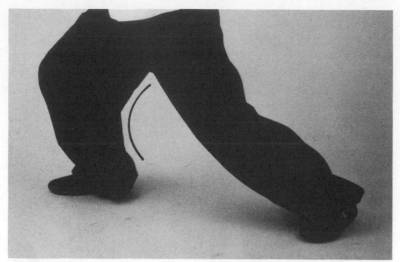

Figure 3-4.

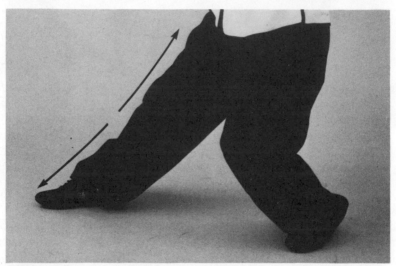

Figure 3-5.

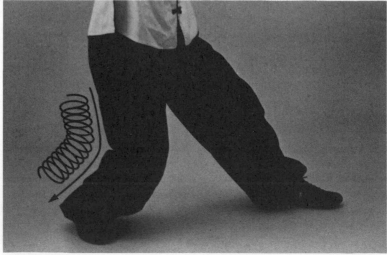

Figure 3-6.

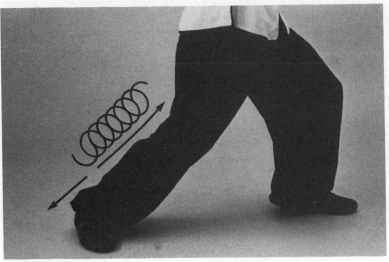

Figure 3-7.

The push by the front leg or rear leg builds the root from which the Jing is bounced backward or forward. The Jing passes through the thigh and hip, joins the Jing from the waist, and reaches the final target.

The legs can also generate sideward Jing. In this case the legs generate a twisting force (Figure 3-8) which is enhanced by the twisting force of the waist before it is expressed through the hands.

Hips

The hips do not usually play an important role in generating Jing in Tai Chi. However, in some styles such as wrestling and Judo, where the body or hips are generally in contact with the opponent, they take most of the credit for the techniques. A twist or bounce of the hips, in coordination with Jing from the legs, can pull up the opponent's root or bounce him away (Figures 3-9 and 3-10). In Tai Chi Chuan, the hips are sometimes used to absorb the opponent's force and then rebound it. In all of these, the hips move in one direction to accumulate Jing, and in the opposite direction to emit it.

A sitting down motion of the hips can be very useful in coordinating your upper body and legs when emitting Jing. When you shift your weight from the rear foot to the front foot, sit down slightly as you sink into the front foot (Figures 3-11 and 3-12). This sitting and sinking motion is precisely coordinated with the emitting of Jing through the hands. It may feel as if you are shifting weight or force from the rear leg, and bouncing it off your front foot into your hands. The hips are also used in a sinking motion to prevent the opponent from pulling you up. Remember, the Jing generated in the legs passes through the hips, so they must be relaxed and flexible.

Waist

The waist is the most important part of the body in the expression of Jing. The success of almost every Jing depends upon the right movement and timing of the waist. It directs Jing to the right place at the right time, and controls the degree of force used and the way that Jing is expressed. The waist can also generate Jing and add it to the force which has been generated by the legs. Your posture must be correct so that the waist can move freely to transmit both the Jing of the legs as well as its own. Usually this is done with a jerking motion—a sudden pulse

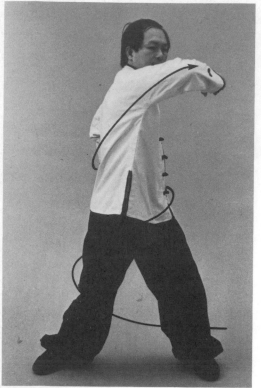

Figure 3-8.

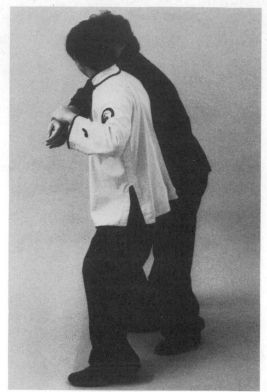

Figure 3-9.

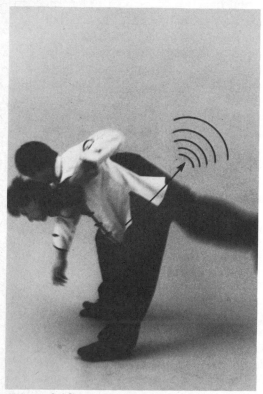

Figure 3-10.

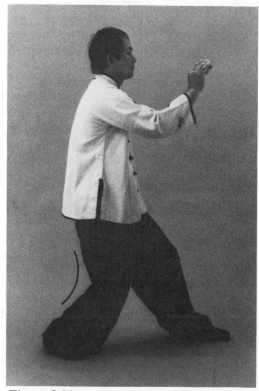

Figure 3-11.

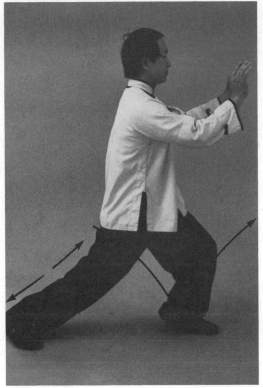

Figure 3-12.

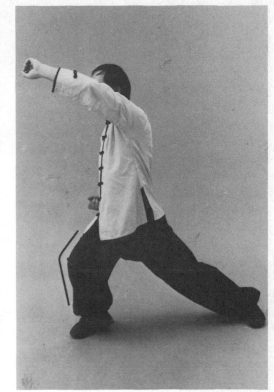

Figure 3-13.

which transmits force from the legs to the shoulders and on to the hands. Every part of the body moves together, with the waist in the center coordinating it all. The waist usually moves first in one direction to accumulate the Jing (Figure 3-13), and then in the other to emit it (Figure 3-14). The accumulation phase can be done very subtly, so that it is part of the motion of neutralization or of stepping toward the opponent. The waist can also fold in to store Jing (Figure 3-15) and straighten out to emit Jing in coordination with the Jing of the legs (Figure 3-16). Usually this is done when both hands are used simultaneously for attack. The emitting motion is done suddenly, in exact coordination with your shoulders, as you match the force of action toward the opponent with the reaction into your root. You can experiment with generating Jing from the waist by jerking your waist while standing on roller skates. This will give you a feel for generating force only with the waist, and also demonstrates how necessary a firm root is.

Torso

The torso is also an important place to store Jing, and once you catch the knack of it your Jing will gain in strength. You store Jing by hollowing the chest as if embracing someone, and by arcing the back slightly (Figure 3-17). The body acts like a bent bow, ready to shoot an arrow. When emitting Jing, the body straightens and the chest opens up (Figure 3-18). The classics refer to this, saying "Hold the chest in, arc the back" (Appendix A-10). This arcing of the back and hollowing of the chest, along with condensing Chi in the spine is referred to as closing. Straightening the body and emitting energy is known as opening (See Appendix A-12, Fifth saying). There may also be some rotation of the body, which

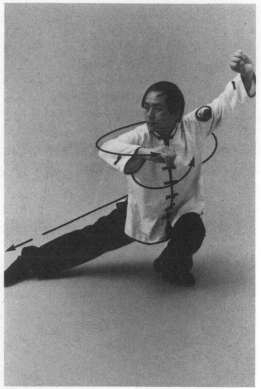

Figure 3-14.

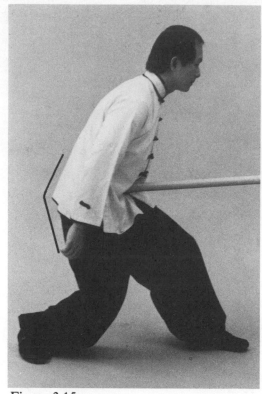

Figure 3-15.

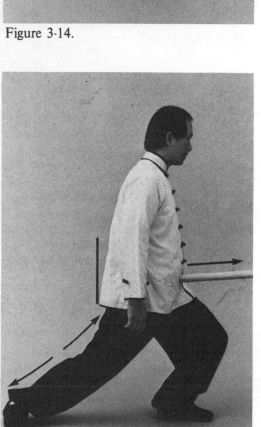

Figure 3-16.

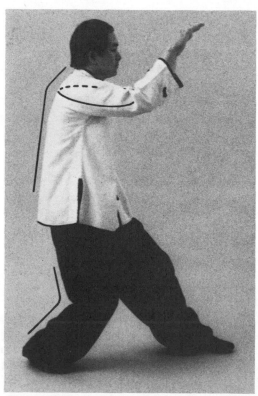

Figure 3-17.

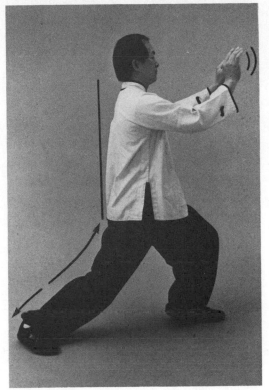

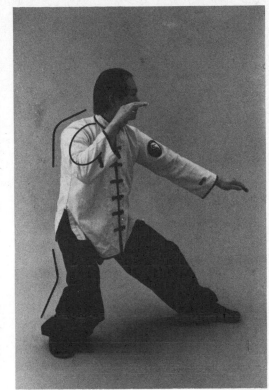

Figure 3-18.   Figure 3-19.

acts like an axle in that it rotates to neutralize the opponent's Jing or to emit Jing sidewards or forward. When this is done, the chest is held in as the waist rotates the body to accumulate Jing (Figure 3-19), and then the chest opens up as the Jing is expressed (Figure 3-20).

Shoulders

The shoulders can move in a number of ways to accumulate and emit Jing. Sometimes a shoulder moves back first to store Jing (Figure 3-21), and then jerks forward with the waist as the root to emit the Jing (Figure 3-22). Sometimes the shoulder curves inward toward the chest to store Jing (Figure 3-23), and then opens outward to emit Jing (Figure 3-24). To get a feel for the role of the shoulders, sit on a table so your feet are off the ground, and then move your shoulder back and jerk it forward. Experiment with different techniques. Then try curving your shoulders in and arcing your chest to accumulate Jing, and then suddenly opening as you emit the force. Also try rolling your shoulder outward to accumulate force, then closing your shoulders in to compress this force, and then expanding your shoulders as you emit the force directly forward. This last movement is used in Press and in Brush Knee and Step Forward. If you experiment this way, you should be able to easily understand the principle of using the shoulder to store and emit Jing.

When you do not have a good root or cannot use the waist, you can still generate some Jing and express it with the arms and shoulders alone. Naturally, this Jing generation is local and will not be as strong as the Jing generated from the legs and controlled by the waist. When the Jing is generated locally, the shoulder acts

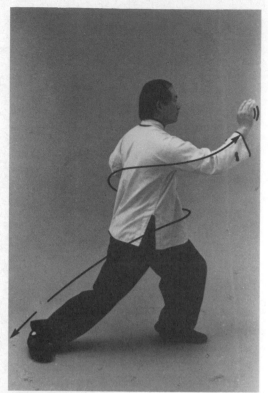

Figure 3-20.

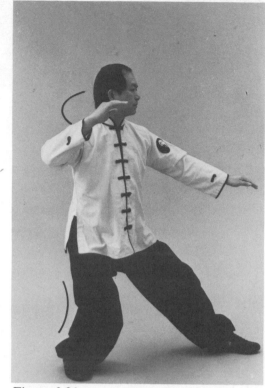

Figure 3-21.

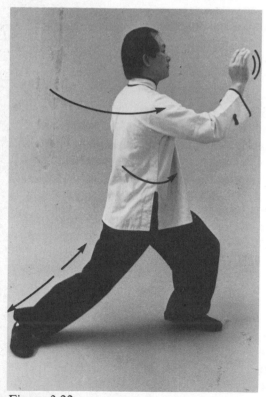

Figure 3-22.

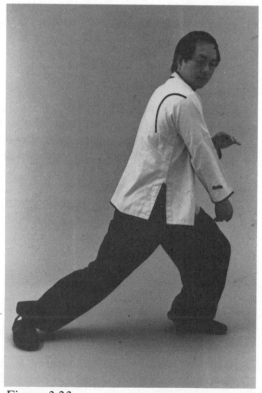

Figure 3-23.

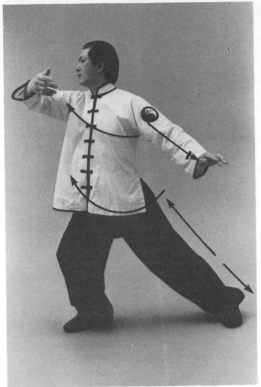

Figure 3-24.

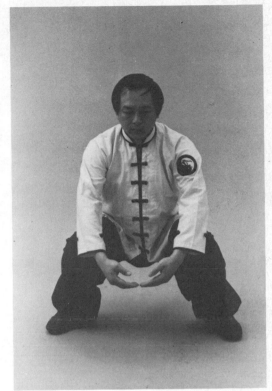

Figure 3-25.

like the legs and generates the Jing, and the elbow acts like the waist and directs and controls the expression of the Jing. In this case the root is in the waist.

Some Jings are used to lift the opponent and destroy his root, such as in Embrace Tiger, Return to the Mountain. In this case the shoulders are lowered to store Jing (Figure 3-25) and raised slightly as you lift the opponent (Figure 3-26).

Elbows

The elbow usually bends to store Jing in the arm (Figure 3-27), and straightens to direct its Jing and the Jing of the whole body out to the hand (Figure 3-28). Thus it is said: "Find the straight in the curved; accumulate, then emit" (Appendix A-3). When you emit Jing, the elbow must remain sunken. This not only seals several vital areas but also increases your stability and your control of the Jing. This is analogous to sinking the waist when it is being used to direct the Jing. Since your elbow directs the Jing, its movement and position will strongly influence a number of Jings, especially Adhere-Stick, Coiling, Silk Reeling, and Rotation. When you know how to store Jing in your elbow and how to use your elbow to lead the Jing effectively, you have learned the important knack of expressing local Jing.

In some cases, the elbow will accumulate Jing when straight, and bend to emit. This occurs when pulling the opponent, or when pulling your hand out of his grasp.

Wrists

The wrist has three ways of storing Jing. The first posture is used to store Jing when it is going to be expressed forward, the second when you are going to pull your hand back, and the third is for when the Jing is going to be expressed in

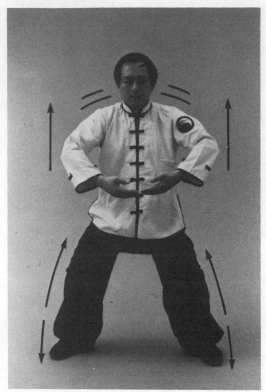

Figure 3-26.

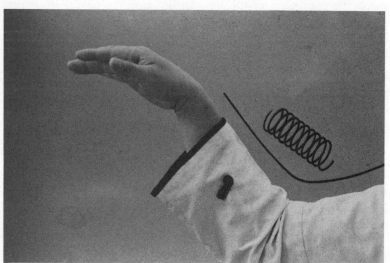

Figure 3-27.

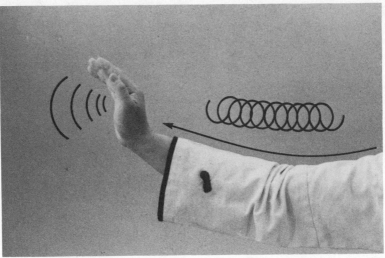

Figure 3-28.

coiling, drilling, rotating, and silk reeling. In the first case the hand is curved slightly while the wrist may be either straight or bent slightly (Figure 3-29). When Jing is expressed forward, the bottom of the palm will snap forward as the fingers straighten and rise (Figure 3-30). This is what is meant by "Settle the wrists, extend the fingers" (Appendix A-10). The second Jing is commonly used to withdraw from the opponent's hooking or grabbing. The hand form in this case is just the reverse of the last one. When storing, the wrist is settled (Figure 3-31), and when Jing is expressed the hand and fingers are curved in and the wrist is straightened. In order to escape from the opponent's grasp, the wrist must be jerked back quickly. The rotation of the wrist is important (Figures 3-32 and 33). Experience will show the best direction and timing for various situations.

In coiling, drilling, rotating, and silk reeling, the whole arm is generally turning, including the wrist. It may move in a short, sharp motion as you pull out of the opponent's grasp or drill forward in a strike, or it may be a longer motion with no particular focus point as you coil around your opponent. In either case the storing and emitting of Jing is expressed not by the bending, but rather by the rotating of the wrist. This turning of the wrist is also involved when the focus of energy is moved to various parts of the arm, or when energy is stored in the body and brought out as needed.

Hands

The fingers are the furthest point to which your Jing travels inside your body. From them the Chi can flow to a weapon or to the opponent's body. With your hands you can sense the opponent's Jing and even his intention, or you can grasp and control him. If your finger position is wrong, you may not be able to store Jing and Chi effectively.

Tai Chi Chuan's most common hand form is called Wa Sou (Tile hand)(see section 2-4), in which the fingers and palm are curved in the shape of a Chinese roof tile. The hand flattens and the fingers straighten out when Jing is expressed, and the hand curves in to store Jing or to grasp something. When the fingers are extended while emitting Jing, the muscles of the hand are tensed somewhat to hold the Chi in the hand so that it may be coordinated with the Jing. When grabbing, the muscles are also tensed slightly to keep the Chi in. When accumulating energy, the hand is curved in slightly and relaxed so that the Chi can move back to the body.

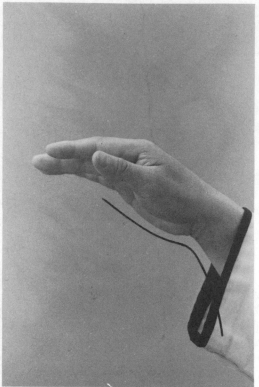

Figure 3-29.

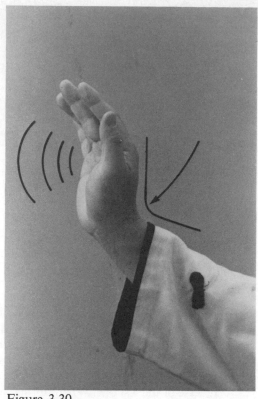

Figure 3-30.

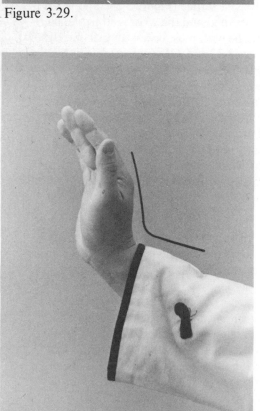

Figure 3-31.

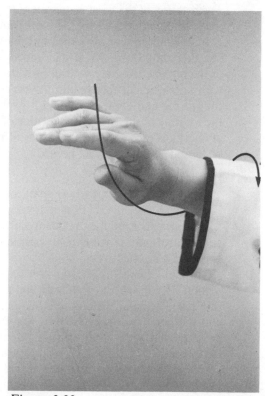

Figure 3-32.

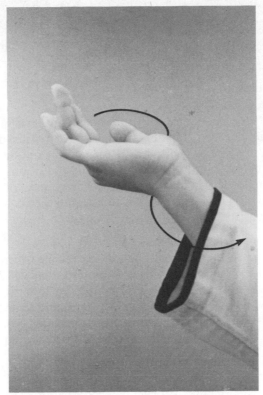

Figure 3-33.

From the above discussion you can see that there are three major places where you can generate Jing—the legs, waist, and shoulders. A number of other places, such as the torso, elbows, hands, wrists, and hips can store Jing, however it is difficult to generate Jing by using these places alone. Although the legs, waist, and shoulders can generate Jing independently, their Jings will still be weak unless they are coordinated with each other. To express Jing strongly and effectively, you must first generate Jing in your rooted legs, combine it with the Jing of the waist, where the combined flow is controlled, and route this flow through the shoulder. The shoulder adds its own Jing, and makes any adjustments necessary to express the total Jing out the arm.

The most common difficulty beginners have in coordinating these three places is the timing. When emitting Jing, the legs, waist, and shoulder move right after each other, without a break. When there is a lag between two parts, the Jing is broken, and the technique will be weak. In order to connect these three Jings, you need to use other places such as the chest and elbows, where Jing can be stored in the postures. For example, when you pass your Jing from your leg to your waist, your hips must be loose and relaxed, and they must be in the best position to store and emit their own Jing, as well as lead the leg Jing to the waist. In the same way, to connect the waist Jing to the shoulders, your chest and back must be in the correct posture, otherwise, the Jing will be weak or even broken. It is said: "The root is in the feet, (power is) generated from the legs, controlled by the waist and expressed by the fingers. From the feet to the legs to the waist must be integrated, and one unified Chi" (Appendix A-1). It also discussed in the Five Key Words: "Fourth saying: Jing is integrated. The entire body's Jing, (when) trained, becomes one family (one unit). Distinguish clearly insubstantial and substantial. Emitting Jing must have root and origin. Jing begins at the foot's root, is controlled by the waist, expressed by the fingers, emitted by the spine and back..." (Appendix A-12).

3-5. The Key Points of Tai Chi Jing
First, Jing is integrated:

It is said:"Jing is integrated; The entire body's Jing, (when) trained, becomes one family (one unit)...Emitting Jing must have root and origin. Jing begins at the foot's root, is controlled by the waist, expressed by the fingers, emitted by the spine and back" (Appendix A-12). It is also said: "From the feet to the legs to the waist must be integrated, and one unified Chi. When moving forward or backward, you can then catch the opportunity and gain the superior position" (Appendix A-1).

Second, Chi supports Jing.

In order to use Jing, you must be able to circulate Chi at will throughout your body. With Chi suffusing your muscles, they will be more efficient and responsive to your will. You must learn to move so as not to interfere with the flow of your Chi. As your mind leads the Chi, so your Chi leads the body. After a great deal of training, your Chi will come from the Dan Tien naturally, and flow deeply within your bones.

Third, the Spirit of Vitality enlivens the Jing.

When the Spirit of Vitality is raised, the Chi will be highly stimulated and able to move faster, stronger, and more naturally to support the Jing. The Hen and Ha sounds can condense the Chi deep into the bones and help to raise the Spirit of Vitality."(If) the Spirit of Vitality (Jieng-Shen) can be raised, then (there is) no delay or heaviness (clumsiness). That means the head is suspended" (Appendix A-3).

Fourth, Jing is balanced.

Every action has a reaction. When you emit force in one direction, there is a counterforce in the opposite direction. These must be carefully balanced not only in your posture, but also in your mind (Yi) and Chi flow. This will keep your body centered and stable, and your root firm.

Fifth, Jing must be accumulated before it can be emitted.

Emitting Jing is like shooting an arrow from a bow—you must draw the bow first. This is done in your posture by coiling your body, hollowing your chest, and slightly arcing your back. You must vividly visualize yourself drawing your body's total energy inward, compressing and coiling it like a spring.

Sixth, when Jing is used, the body is relaxed.

To enable Chi to circulate smoothly and support Jing, the muscles must be relaxed. This allows Chi from the Dan Tien to reach and support them. The tendons should be used to transmit force so that it springs through the limbs. It is said: "When emitting Jing, be calm and relaxed, concentrated in one direction" (Appendix A-3).

Seventh, soft Tai Chi Jing is emitted in a pulse.

The ends of the muscles connected to the tendons play the major role in generating soft Jing, and the tendons transmit it through the body.

This power is best expressed in a pulsed, whip-like motion, rather than in a long, sustained motion.

Eighth, your Jing should be mysterious to the opponent.
Insubstantial and substantial strategy should be used skillfully in order to confuse the opponent. The time used to accumulate Jing should be as short as possible, so that you don't telegraph your intention.

Ninth, Jing is not a form or technique, it is a way of expressing power.
Each Jing is a different manner of expressing power, and can be used in many different techniques. Also, most techniques use several different Jings.

3-6. The Different Jings and Their Applications

Jing can be expressed by the hands, elbows, shoulders, hips, knees, legs, or even the body itself. Tai Chi Chuan emphasizes the upper limbs and the body, and uses the legs and feet as secondary weapons. In this section we will discuss the major areas first, and then the secondary areas.

As mentioned before, excluding leg and foot Jings, there are more than forty different kinds of Jing. They can be distinguished into sensing Jings and manifested Jings. Sensing Jings include passive sensing Jings, which are the ability to sense the opponent's power, and active sensing Jings, which are the ability to move Chi into or out of another person's body. Manifested Jings visibly exhibit the use of force and can also be divided into Yang Jings or offensive Jings (Gong Jing), Yin Jings or defensive Jings (Shoou Jing), and Neutral Jings or neither Yin nor Yang Jings (Fei Gong Fei Shoou Jing)(Table 3-1). Because offensive Jings usually emit force onto the opponent's body, they are also called Emitting Jings (Fa Jing). Defensive Jings usually neutralize the opponent's power, and thus are generally called Neutralizing Jings (Huah Jing).

Offensive Jings can be subdivided into pure offensive Jings and attack with some defense Jings (Gong Jong Dai Shoou Jing). The first is strongly Yang and can be represented by three solid lines (☰). The second is also Yang, but with some Yin, and can be represented by two solid lines and one broken line (☱ , ☲ , or ☳).

Defensive Jings can also be subdivided. First there are purely defensive Jings which are extremely Yin and are characterized by three broken lines (☷). Then there is defense with some attack Jings (Shoou Jong Dai Gong Jing). These are Yin but have some Yang and can be represented by two broken lines and one solid line (☴ , ☵ , or ☶). Almost every Jing, both offensive and defensive, can be used as a hard or soft Jing, long or short Jing.

In this next section we will list some important precautions which the beginner to Jing training should observe, and then list and explain all the different Jings. Sensing Jings will be discussed first, and then manifested Jings. Manifested Jings will be divided into active Jings, passive Jings, and neutral Jings. Active Jings will be subdivided into pure offensive Jings, and offense with some defense Jings. Similarly, passive Jings will be divided into purely defensive Jings and defense with some offense Jings.

In the discussions, the basic theory of each Jing will be explained and training methods will be given, along with examples drawn from the Tai Chi Chuan sequence and pushing hands. Many of the concepts are advanced, so if you are a beginner and are having difficulty understanding them, don't give up hope. Select a few basic techniques and keep working on them, slowly adding new ones when you are ready. Remember: the most important key to learning is perseverance.

Before you start to study, you should know that many Jings are mixtures of two or more other Jings. For example, Growing Jing is a mixture of Controlling, Neutralizing, Resisting, Drilling, and Coiling Jings. Before you can understand a complex Jing like this you must first learn the simpler ones. Second, you should understand that when most Jings are used they are usually coordinated with other Jings, either to set up the opponent or to enhance the Jing being applied. For example, in pushing hands, you must use Yielding, Neutralizing, and Leading Jings first before you can apply Controlling Jing. Third, some of the Jings are very similar to others, and you may find it difficult to differentiate between them. However, if you persevere in your practice and pondering, and continue to humbly seek the answer, you will eventually come to understand them.

Precautions for Beginners to Jing Training:
1. When you generate Jing, do not hold it in the body.

If you hold your energy in, and restrict its passage through your body, you can injure yourself. Knowing how to generate Jing is like knowing how to start a car. If you do not know how to control the car or the generated power, it can be very dangerous for you. With a car you must know how to use the steering wheel, and with Jing you must know how to use your waist. It is very common for beginners to get strains and injuries, especially in the waist, or in joints, particularly the shoulders, elbows, and wrists. This is most likely to happen when you haven't learned how to use your waist to control and transmit the Jing to your hands or legs, or when some part of your body is tight and is restricting the smooth passage of the Jing. Jing is usually emitted in a sudden, but smooth, jerking motion. If your stomach muscles are tight, this jerking motion will stress them, and sometimes cause strains or pulls. More seriously, if the generated Jing is strong it can damage the internal organs. It is for this reason that most Chinese martial arts masters will not teach Jing to beginning students until they know that their martial knowledge, in addition to their morality and personality, have reached a certain level.

It is sometimes desirable when emitting Jing to hold some of the energy in the body, and not emit all of it. This should not be encouraged in beginners. If energy stagnates in the body, the internal organs can be damaged. If Jing is held in a joint, the joint muscles, ligaments, and tissue can be damaged. Only when you understand Jing well, and can control it skillfully, should you start to hold part of it in. At that time you will find that it is often desirable to retain part of your Jing for tactical reasons, e.g., to counterattack, or to defend against a counterattack.

It is not uncommon for people to injure their joints when they can generate a great deal of Jing but do not know how to tense the muscles when the Jing reaches the hand or foot. When Jing reaches the end of the limb, it keeps on going and continues to exert a pull on the joints. At this time the muscles must be tensed slightly for a second to prevent injury to the joints.

In external styles, it is very common to use a belt to hold the stomach in and prevent injury. This is seldom seen in Tai Chi, because the abdomen must be completely relaxed in order to generate Chi in the Dan Tien and circulate it around the body. If this area is held tightly, the Chi will not be generated naturally and may stagnate. Therefore, in the first few years of Tai Chi training, soft Jings are practiced in which none of the energy is restrained. Soft and long range training is emphasized, and the Jing is transmitted completely out. Only after you have mastered this should you learn to hold in Jing for fast and short range Jings.

In external styles, the approach is different. Usually hard Jings are trained first, and short Jing is emphasized at the same time as long Jing. Local Chi is used to support the Jing, and Dan Tien Chi is not absolutely necessary. A belt is usually necessary to prevent waist injury. Once you have approached a high level of Jing, you will then turn to the soft Jing training and a belt will not be necessary. Naturally, Dan Tien Chi also becomes important at this stage. Thus it is said: **INTERNAL STYLES FROM SOFT TO HARD, AND EXTERNAL STYLES HARD TO SOFT. THE APPROACHES ARE DIFFERENT BUT THE PRINCIPLES AND GOAL ARE THE SAME.**

2. From Soft to Hard, Easy to Difficult, and Slow to Fast.

It is very common for a beginner to look high and walk low. That is, he has high expectations and looks to the highest goal, but he is lazy in his training. This frequently causes injury and deviation from the right path. Before you put too much time and effort into the more difficult techniques, you should understand the easier ones. Therefore, you should start with the soft, easy, and slow. Only after you have mastered these should you go on to the harder techniques. If you follow this general rule, you will avoid most injuries.

3. If you have stopped training for a while, go slow.

If you stop training for a while, and then start again, you should take it slow and easy. Experienced martial artists sometimes injure themselves when they forget this. When you take a long break from practice, the muscles which you built up in coordination with the Jing weaken. However, your knowledge of how to generate Jing does not decrease. When you do a hard technique, the muscles will still be able to generate a lot of force, but they may have lost just enough of their edge so that they cannot fully control the force. This puts a lot of strain on the joints and ligaments, particularly the elbows, shoulders, and knees. Therefore, after a break you should take it easy and let your muscles rebuild their strength.

4. Do not practice just before or after a meal.

You should not practice Jing when you are hungry or right after a meal. Hunger will make your mind scattered and a full stomach will cause pain in the waist when you jerk.

5. Do not practice when you are in a bad temper.

When you are in a bad mood, your Yi is stimulated, and the Chi will not be condensed and controlled. When this Chi is used in Jing, it can go astray and harm you. As a matter of fact, whenever you are in a bad temper you should not build up or circulate your Chi.

6. Do not practice right after drinking alcohol.

As with meditation, you should not practice after drinking. When you drink, your Chi is floating and your mind is not clear. Under these circumstances, Chi circulation may be harmful.

Table 3-2

Jings

I. Sensing Jings:

1. TIEN JING (Listening Jing)

Listening Jing is not done with the ears, but rather with the skin. You use your sense of touch to pay very close attention to the opponent's motion and energy. This skin listening capability is generally obtained from training Adhere-Stick (Tsan Nien) Jing, and from paying careful attention during Pushing Hands. After much practice you develop a sense for precisely what it feels like to have the opponent try each particular technique, and what it feels like when you do a technique on him.

Listening is done with the skin of the entire body. Any part of your body may be touched or attacked during a fight, and almost any part may be used for an attack. For example, if your chest is pressed by your opponent, you must be able to listen to this press, understand it, and react with yielding, neutralizing, or other defensive strategy. Offensively, many parts of the body can be used for attack when the right opportunity occurs. For example, your hip can be a very powerful weapon for hitting or bouncing the enemy away. However, regardless which technique you use, success is largely determined by how well you can sense the opponent's energy and chose the right timing for offense or defense.

There are three places where listening is particularly important. The first place is the forearm, the second is the palm, and the third is the soles of the feet. The forearm is usually the first part of the body to come in contact with the enemy when you are attacked. It is very important to build up the capability of listening on the forearm. If you can accurately sense the opponent's Jing from the first touch, you can neutralize it, and then continue your control of the situation by using Adhere-Stick and other Jings.

When Adhere-Stick Jing is applied, the palm and the forearm are equally important. They are not used only for defensive sensing (listening), but also for offensive sensing. When you attack your enemy, he will generally react with a block, neutralization, or yielding in any one of a number of ways. When this happens, you must keep listening alertly to understand his further intention. Without this listening, your attack is blind, and it is likely to be nullified or countered. Good Listening Jing can help you to direct your offensive Jing in the right direction and apply it at the right time. The better your listening Jing is, the better you can understand your opponent's Jing. If you can sense the enemy's intention before his Jing is emitted, you will be able to defend with certainty. The highest Listening Jing is demonstrated when Borrowing Jing (Jieh Jing) is used by a master. In Borrowing Jing, Listening Jing is the key to success. The reader can refer to the Borrowing Jing section for details.

The third place which is considered important in Listening Jing is the soles of the feet. The feet are your root, without which all your techniques would float and be useless. You should always listen to the exchange of energy between your feet and the ground. To build up Listening Jing in your feet is to build up your root and develop your balance. The more you can feel your root, the more stable you will be.

The best way to train Listening Jing is through pushing hands practice. In pushing hands, you first learn Adhere-Stick Jing. Practice following the opponent, not letting go and not separating from him. The more automatically you can do this, the more easily you can pay attention to the opponent instead of yourself. The Tai Chi ball is sometimes used for building up Listening Jing. The reader should refer to Chapter 3 of the second volume for pushing hands and Tai Chi ball training.

2. DONG JING (Understanding Jing)

Dong Jing comes from practicing Adhere-Stick (Tsan Nien) Jing and Listening (Tien) Jing. As a matter of fact, Listening Jing and Understanding Jing cannot be separated in practice, because you must listen before you can understand. If you cannot listen to and understand the opponent, you are blind to him. When you listen, your Yi must be wholly concentrated on listening and understanding. If your mind is scattered, you will not be able to understand your opponent's intention and you will miss the purpose of listening. As is the case with Listening Jing, Dong Jing has two aspects, one for defense and the other for offense. Defensive Understanding Jing is the capability of understanding the opponent's offensive intention. Offensive Understanding Jing is just the reverse. It is the capability of understanding the opponent's defensive ability and intention when you are attacking him. If you lack this double-sided understanding, you will not be able to skillfully change your strategy and Jing from substantial to insubstantial and vice versa.

When you practice adhering, sticking, and listening for a long time, you will gradually be able to understand with just a light touch what the opponent is going to do. The greater your understanding, the less of a hint you will need in order to know where, when, and how the attack is coming, and the more easily you will be able to defend yourself. But it takes a long time. Wang Dsung-Yueh said:"After you have mastered techniques, then you can gradually grasp what 'Understanding Jing (Dong Jing)' means. From 'Understanding Jing' you gradually approach enlightenment (spiritual understanding) of your opponent's intention. However, without a great deal of study over a long time, you cannot suddenly grasp this spiritual understanding of your opponent". He also said:"To adhere means to yield. To yield means to adhere. Yin not separate from Yang. Yang not separate from Yin. Yin and Yang mutually cooperate, (understanding this) is 'Understanding Jing'. After Understanding Jing, the more practice, the more refinement. Silently learn, then ponder; gradually you will approach your heart's desire"(Appendix A-2).

Before you achieve Dong Jing, it is easy to resist, to lose balance, to lose contact with the enemy, or to use force against force. When you almost have Dong Jing you will still have trouble with broken Chi, tightness, and with leaning forward or backward. Practice until you can listen accurately, then you will know when to use power and when not to, when to be Yin (insubstantial) or Yang (substantial). The highest level of Dong Jing is when you understand the opponent's intentions before he moves. Thus, it is said:"Light, agile, and alive, seek Dong Jing (to understand Jing); Yin and Yang cooperate mutually without the fault of stagnation" (Appendix A-11).

Understanding Jing is best trained through pushing hands. Pay very close attention to what your skin feels. The more you practice, the more you will be able to tell by feel what the opponent is doing or even what he is planning.

3. TSA PI SHIU LIN JING (Graze Skin False Critical Jing)

This Jing is probably the hardest Jing to understand and practice. Tsa Pi in Chinese means to lightly rub the skin or to graze the skin. Shiu means false and not real. Lin means critical. Shiu Lin refers to the feeling of standing precariously on the edge of a cliff. In Tai Chi Chuan and some other internal Chinese martial arts, this Jing is the highest art and skill. Tsa Pi Shiu Lin Jing is the capability of sensing and understanding the opponent's energy (Chi) pattern with only a touch or even with just being near him. When two skillful internal martial artists are fighting, Chi in the bodies of both fighters is stimulated to the highest level. Chi is vital in the application of Jing. Usually, Yi leads Chi to support Jing. If you can sense the opponent's Chi flow before it is shown in Jing, you should be able to recognize the opponent's Yi and intention. Therefore, by sensing the opponent's Chi, you know his intentions even before his Jing is emitted. The two master fighters will seem to the average observer to be doing very little. However, they may in fact be maneuvering through repeated attacks and counterattacks on a very subtle level which seldom reaches visibility.

The highest level of Graze Skin False Critical Jing can be both active and passive. Usually, if you are able to sense the opponent's Chi, you should be able to pass Chi into him or drain it out in order to shock his internal organs. To do this you must be able to understand his Chi pattern with a touch, or even without touching. The passive aspect of this Jing is the ability to sense the opponent's intention, and resist his Chi attacks. When this kind of battle is occuring, the participants are probably not even aware of their bodies, but instead are putting their whole attention into the flow and exchange of energy. It is unlikely that anyone in today's martial society has reached this level, and so unfortunately the training methods are probably lost.

II. Manifested Jings:
A. Offensive (Yang) Jings:
a. Purely Offensive (Yang) Jings:
1. PENG JING (Wardoff Jing)

Wardoff Jing is a strong Yang Jing that is used offensively even in defense. In principle, it behaves like a large rubber ball--when pressure is applied it compresses (Figure 3-34), and when a certain point is reached it bounces the outside force away (Figure 3-35). The opponent's force is often directed upward, as you lift his attack the way water lifts a boat. This Jing is often emitted at maximum strength in coordination with the sound Ha. It may be done at all ranges, and is often used to bounce the opponent away. This application is forceful, but not directly destructive.

Defensively, this Jing absorbs the opponent's attack and then

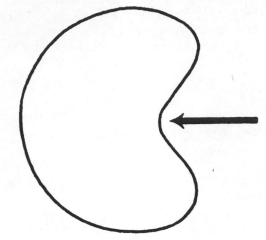

Figure 3-34.

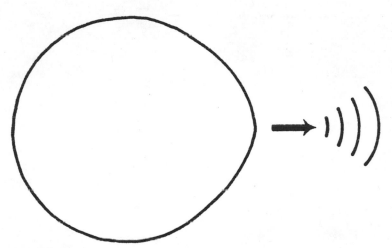

Figure 3-35.

bounces him away. In this application, your forearm does not generally come into contact with the opponent's body, but instead functions through his attacking arm. Specifically, you absorb some of the opponent's force either at the very beginning or at the end of his attack, and give the force back to him through his stiff arms (also read Borrowing Jing). Wardoff is commonly used against a punch, in which case it directs the attack upward and seals the arm (Figure 3-36).

Offensively, Wardoff is used as a strike, most often to the opponent's chest or arm. When this Jing is used to attack the chest, some other neutralization is usually used first in order to set up the attack. For example, if the opponent attacks with a right punch, you may deflect with your left hand (Figure 3-37) and strike his chest with your right forearm (Figure 3-38). When this Jing is used to attack the opponent's arm, his attack must be neutralized downward and sealed first. For example, when the opponent attacks with a right punch, deflect his attack to the right and down with your right arm (Figure

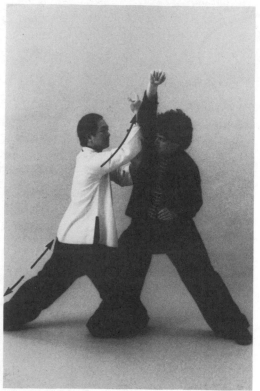

Figure 3-36.

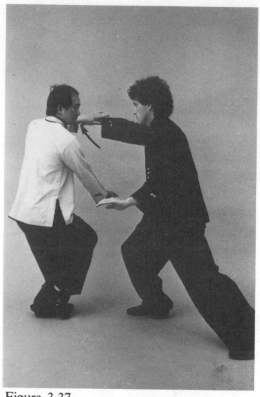

Figure 3-37.

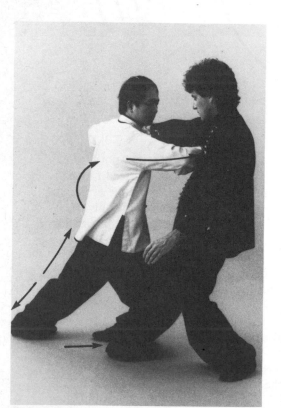

Figure 3-38.

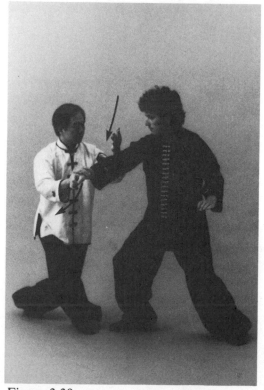

Figure 3-39.

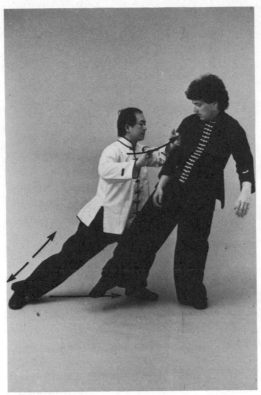

Figure 3-40.

3-39). Then step behind his right leg with your left, while your left arm covers his right arm and then attacks forward (Figure 3-40).

In order to bounce the opponent away, you must first destroy his root to upset his stability and balance. This is done by directing the force of your Wardoff slightly upward (Figure 3-41) or sideward (Figure 3-42). Your body must be sunken in order to build up your own root, stability, and upward power. Wardoff is sometimes done as a sort of double technique. First, apply a small push to the opponent, or deflect his attack and lead him to an unbalanced position. If he rises up a little and his root becomes unstable you should immediately apply a second, stronger push to knock him away. If, on the other hand, he resists and pushes forward, withdraw slightly and lead his momentum upward. As soon as you succeed in leading him, immediately emit your force to knock him away.

As with most of these techniques, muscular force will predominate in the beginning, but as you gain skill the reliance on muscles will lessen and you will do these techniques with arms that are more and more relaxed. Indeed, you will find that you cannot really do these techniques well with tensed muscles because this interferes with accurate sensing and precise control.

There are several ways to train Wardoff Jing. A good way is to use a bag, first a light one, and later heavier ones. You can practice striking with the Wardoff, and you can practice pushing. To do the latter, you can place your forearm against the bag and push it slight-

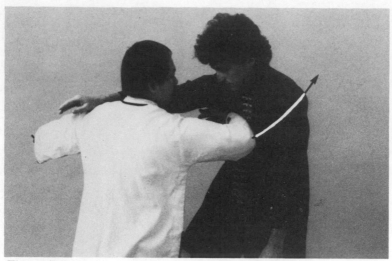

Figure 3-41.

ly to get it moving."Catch"the bag on your forearm as soon as it starts to move toward you, and immediately bounce it away. You can swing the bag and"catch"it near the end of its swing and bounce it, or move the bag around in circles and use Wardoff to redirect it sharply away from you.

You can also practice Wardoff on a partner. When you do this, it is best for the person being pushed to protect his chest with his forearms to prevent injury (Figure 3-43). Another exercise is for one person to stand in the Wardoff position, and the other to push the extended forearm with both hands in a somewhat stiff-armed fashion (Figure 3-44). The first person either absorbs some of the force, directs it into his root, and then bounces it back, or else emits force just as the other person is about to push.

When doing Wardoff, the body must be centered and stable, and your Yi of attacking must be further than the target. Yi, Chi, and Jing must be balanced between the attacking arm, the other arm, and the rear foot.

2. TZUANN JING (Drilling Jing)

Drilling Jing is an offensive Jing which twists as it penetrates. When your hand touches the opponent's body, your arm and hand rotate clockwise (Figures 3-45 and 3-46) or counterclockwise (Figures 3-47 and 3-48) in a screwing motion, which makes the power penetrate more deeply than with a regular attack. The power, which is generated by turning the waist and shoulder, is usually directed forward, although it can also be used sideward. The fist, finger, or knuckle are usually used for attack, frequently against vital cavities. The muscles must be tensed somewhat to direct the Jing and to insure that it penetrates, and also to protect the hand against injury. Also, your Yi must be concentrated inside his body in the organ or cavity being attacked. Drilling Jing is also occasionally used to pull your arm out of the opponent's grasp. Here too the shoulder and waist are the source of the Jing.

Because Drilling Jing is used in both external and internal styles,

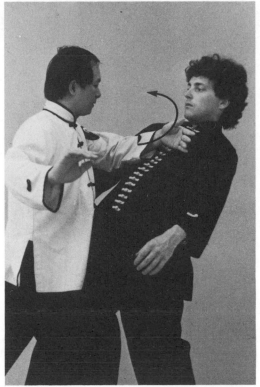

Figure 3-42.

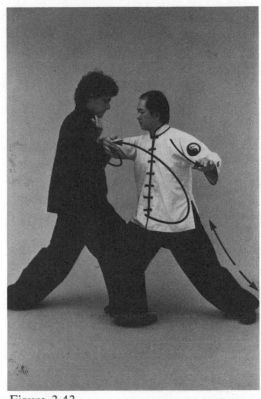

Figure 3-43.

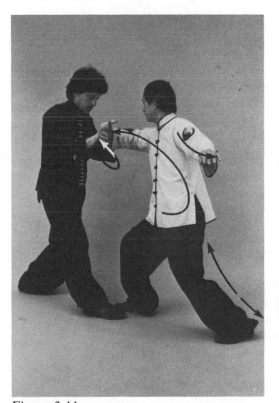

Figure 3-44.

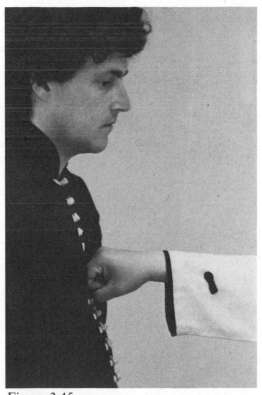

Figure 3-45.

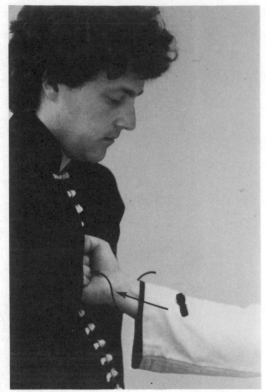

Figure 3-46.

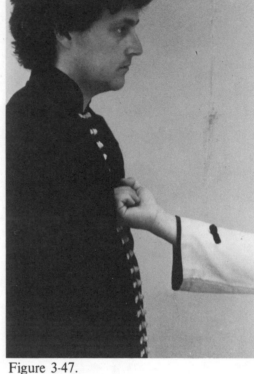

Figure 3-47.

many training methods have been developed. One of the common ways used in external styles is to drill your fist or knuckle into a bucket of mung beans. (Mung beans are used because of their medicinal properties.) With practice you will be able to drill deeper and deeper. Later, sand can be used in place of beans. Punching bags are also popularly used for drilling training. Start with your fist or knuckles touching the bag lightly (Figure 3-49). Suddenly generate the Jing from the waist and shoulder and drill your hand forward to bounce the bag away (Figure 3-50). Tai Chi uses less muscle than external styles, so the training approach is different. One method uses a thick layer of soft material, for example tissue paper, on a table (Figure 3-51). The fist is pushed down with a screwing motion (Figure 3-52). The muscles should be relaxed as the Yi strives to extend the Jing to the surface of the table. When you can bounce the Jing off the table, increase the thickness of the material. The thicker the material is, the greater the drilling power required. It is important to also do this exercise horizontally.

3. DUAN JING (Breaking Jing)

Breaking Jing is used for breaking the opponent's bones or joints. Forward Breaking Jing is commonly used to break ribs, and sideward or downward Breaking Jing is used to break limbs. The Yi is concentrated slightly beyond the target (see Figure 3-53). This is different from the penetrating Drilling Jing, where the Yi is concentrated deep

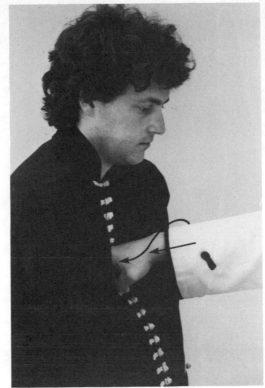

Figure 3-48.

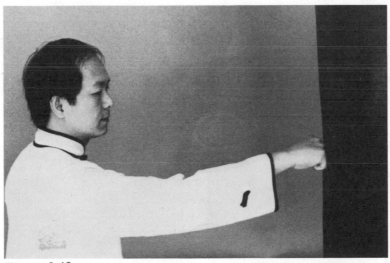

Figure 3-49.

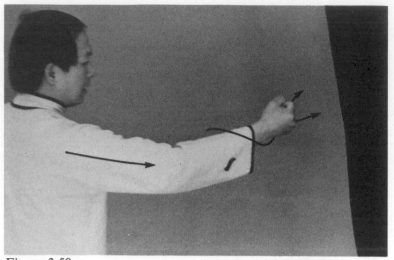

Figure 3-50.

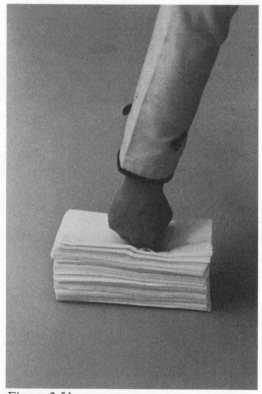

Figure 3-51.

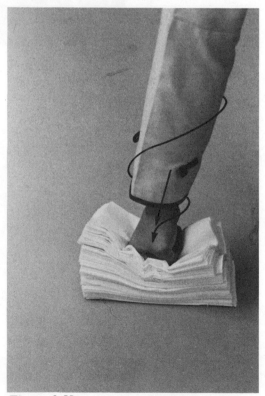

Figure 3-52.

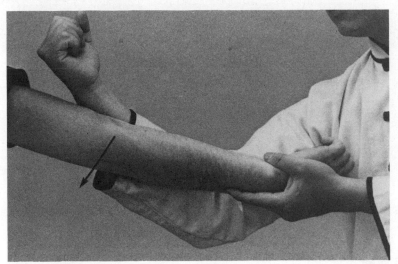

Figure 3-53.

in the organ being attacked. If you have ever chopped wood you should understand how to use this Jing. When you are chopping a branch, if you concentrate and aim a bit beyond the branch you should have little trouble chopping through it. Also, if just before the axe reaches the wood you suddenly increase your speed and jerk the power out, you will find that you can cut the branch without using much power.

In breaking, when the Chi and Jing reach the target the muscles must be tensed so that all the power is expended in the target. In Tai Chi Chuan, the time that you are tensed is kept as short as possible. This allows you to remain relaxed and make your breaking Jing sharper and more concentrated. A great deal of speed must be developed. Once the target is hit, the speed stops, but the Yi continues on through. It is important that the Yi be focused only slightly beyond the target. If you focus too far beyond the target, your Jing will pass uselessly through it. There is also a danger of injuring yourself. Because you normally tense your muscles only a short distance before the focus point, if the focus is too far beyond the target you will be relaxed when you hit. This will allow the power to bounce back to you and injure your arm or fist.

Many training methods are used both in the external and the internal styles. The most common way to train sideward Breaking Jing for use on the opponent's elbow is with a wooden rod about an inch and a half in diameter. Hold one end in one hand, fix the other end so that it cannot move, and hit it with your hand or forearm (Figure 3-54). Some people train with branches on trees. In the beginning, wrap the rod or branch with cloth to avoid injuring your arm. When applying Jing, the root must be firm. The power is generated from the legs, and guided by the waist onto the target. (See also the section on Sideward Hooking Jing.) Punching bags are also used, especially for training forward breaking Jing. To break ribs your Yi must be centered a little past the ribs, so aim your techniques a few inches inside the bag. Remember, Yi is the most important factor in breaking.

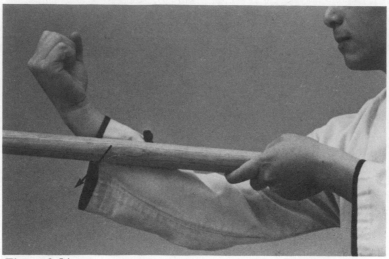

Figure 3-54.

4. HEN JING (Sideward Hooking Jing)

Hen Jing, which is called Kua Jing in external styles, is a hooking strike. A typical example in the Tai Chi sequence is Strike the Tiger. The Jing which is generated in the leg goes up the spine and coils outward, swinging the fist or elbow to strike the enemy from the side. This Jing is similar to Turning Jing (Joan Jing). Both use the same principles of coiling and Chi generation, but Hooking Jing is used for striking, whereas Turning Jing is used for defense. Also, Sideward Hooking Jing is done in a more explosive and destructive fashion, with your fist snapping back after striking. Your body is relaxed while you approach the target, and then suddenly all of your force penetrates the opponent's body. Turning Jing is used to turn the opponent's offensive Jing, therefore its motion is extended and continuous. A typical example of Turning Jing in the Tai Chi sequence is Wave Hands in Clouds. To train Hen Jing, first work on the coordination of your whole body, using a minimum of force and no target. Generate Jing in your legs, direct it with your waist, and express it through your fist or elbow (Figure 3-55). Stay very relaxed until just before the end of the swing, then tense your body and arm slightly and drop your weight into your feet, mentally balancing the force and counterforce in your fist and feet. Right after you strike, the fist should be snapped back so that all the energy goes into the opponent. When you can swing or coil your Jing out naturally, you should then start training on a punching bag (Figure 3-56). Hen Jing is a soft-hard Jing. It is first relaxed, and then sharp and penetrating. Its focus point is inside the opponent's body, so your arm and body stay relaxed until the surface of your target, or just before it. Once you hit the target, your body tenses slightly--just enough to put all your force into the target and prevent any force from bouncing back to you. Remember, the motion comes from the legs and the rotation of the body, not from the arms.

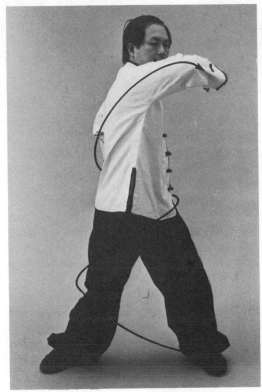

Figure 3-55.

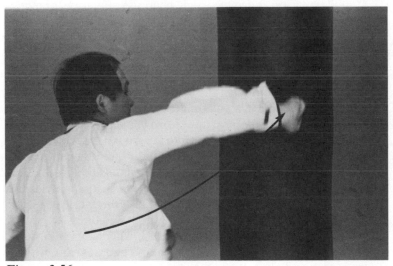

Figure 3-56.

5. CHARNG JING (Growing Jing)

Growing Jing is a soft, slow, and extended offensive Jing. It is actually a mixture of many Jings--Controlling, Neutralizing, Resisting, Drilling, and Coiling. Even though it is a mixture of many Jings, both Yin and Yang, Growing Jing is considered purely Yang because your Yi is concentrated on approaching and attacking the opponent. Once you have control of your opponent with Controlling Jing, but cannot yet attack because his defense is still strong, you can use Growing Jing to work your way through his defense. You should "grow" continually toward your opponent, evading his defenses, moving around resistance, inexorably overcoming all obstacles. Any offensive move he attempts must be immediately neutralized to the side to open him up, or else turned back on itself. When you encounter Resisting or Neutralizing Jings you must change your growing path until you reach your target. It is like passing a thread through a pearl whose hole has nine curves. Once your growing has reached your opponent's body, then you can attack suddenly with a fast, short Jing like Inch Jing or Centimeter Jing.

It should be clear from the discussion that Growing Jing is not completely soft. The muscles are tensed and relaxed repeatedly as you shift from one Jing to another. Because you are doing many techniques in a row, the Yi and Chi are long and extended. For Growing Jing to be effective, you must be skilled at Listening and Understanding. You must understand the opponent's Jing in order to control, neutralize, and overcome it.

Since this Jing is a mixture of several other Jings, the best way to master it is through pushing hands. When you do Growing Jing, your hands relentlessly and insidiously keep approaching the opponent. If you are thwarted, don't try to force your way in. Evade and coil around obstacles, and immediately neutralize any forward motion of the opponent. Keep your Yi on the opponent, adapt to circumstances, and keep moving toward him so that "when (the opponent) retreats, it becomes more and more urgent" (Appendix A-2).

6. CHEN JING (Sinking Jing)

In Sinking Jing you sink the body to escape from a grab, or to exert downward force in a pull or attack. When you strike downward, you cannot balance the force upward, so you must carefully drop your weight to direct the counterforce into the ground. As with other Jings, the mind must lead the motion. First the Yi sinks, then the Chi sinks, and the body will naturally follow. Sinking should be alive and responsive. Many people think that Sinking Jing uses the muscles to pull or hold down the opponent. As matter of fact, this is called "weighting". You should understand that sinking and weighting are different. Weighting has shape and is slow like Li, while sinking is shapeless and can be fast. Weighting power is clumsy and stagnant, while sinking is agile and alive. When Sinking Jing is used it looks relaxed but it is not relaxed, it seems tight and restricted but is not.

Sinking Jing can be used for either a direct or strategic attack. When a direct attack is used, the Jing is downward and forward, usually toward the opponent's stomach area (Figure 3-57). When the muscles on the stomach area are struck or pressed downward, they tense im-

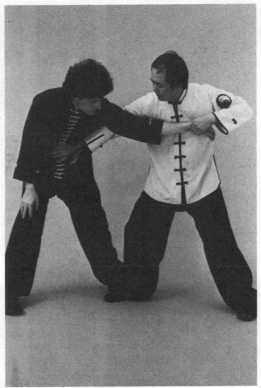

Figure 3-57.

mediately. Some of these muscles extend upward and surround the lungs. When they are struck, they constrict the lung, causing difficulty breathing and sometimes unconsciousness. This is called Sealing the Breath (Bi Chi). Sinking Jing is also used to provide power when you use Rollback to attack the opponent's arm.

To use Sinking Jing for a strategic attack, your hand first adheres and sticks to the opponent's arm. If you sink downward and apply this force to his arm, you can immobilize it and restrict further action. Usually, in order to prevent you from attacking after you have restricted his arm, your enemy will automatically raise his arm to resist your sinking. When this happens, you should then follow his upward power and use Lifting Jing to increase his upward motion. You may be able to unbalance and push him, or else raise his arm and attack underneath.

Sinking Jing is also involved in other Jings, such as Prying Jing, or downward Pluck Jing. When Sinking Jing is used to coordinate with Prying Jing, the body and elbow are dropped to escape from the opponent's Controlling Jing (see Prying Jing). When Sinking Jing is applied in downward Pluck Jing, it is used to thwart the opponent's kick or to trick the opponent into resisting you. When he starts to pull away, immediately add your forward Jing to his backward Jing and bounce him away. An example of this from the Tai Chi sequence is Pick Up the Needle from Sea Bottom followed immediately by Fan Back.

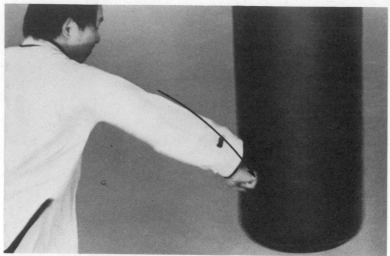

Figure 3-58.

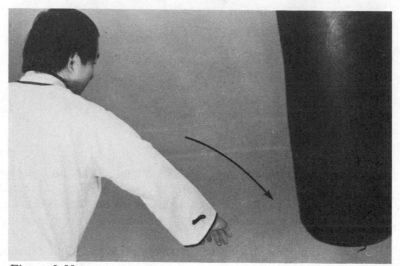

Figure 3-59.

Sinking Jing can be practiced as a downward punch or palm strike on the bag (Figures 3-58 and 3-59). The other applications need to be practiced with a partner.

7. TSUENN JING (Inch Jing)

Inch Jing is the generation and emission of Jing in a short distance. Most of the offensive Jings can be done this way. This Jing is hard to learn, but once learned, it gives a great advantage in a fight. When your attack takes place in a very short space and time, it is very hard for your opponent to sense it, understand it, and react. Drilling Jing is commonly done this way. However, unless your Chi is strong and you are very skilled, this short range attack will not be as powerful as the longer range attacks.

There are many possible applications for Inch Jing. It is often used after you have approached the enemy by using Growing Jing. When you have worked your way through the opponent's defenses and see an opening, you can strike effectively with no warning. Inch Jing is also often used for a second attack. When the opponent neutralizes your first attack, he will try to lead and control you, and then counterattack. When your opponent has neutralized your attack and thinks you can do nothing more, he will shift from Leading Jing to Controlling Jing. If you attack right at this time, you may be able to catch his Jing just as it is about to be emitted, and use it to knock him a great distance.

Inch Jing is also used when you have neutralized the opponent's attack and have led him into an unbalanced position. A sudden short attack will knock him down before he has a chance to recover his balance. Another common use of Inch Jing is when you control one of the opponent's joints through Controlling Jing. For example, if you control hiselbow with Rollback, you can suddenly apply Inch Jing and break or dislocate the joint.

To practice emitting Jing in a short distance, start with your fist one inch away from a punching bag. While the accumulation phase of the technique should be as short as the emission, you may want to start training with a longer accumulation phase. In this case, move your body as you normally would for a full sized punch, but have your fist move only a few inches. Once you get the motion, make the wind-up shorter and shorter, until there is no visible preparation for the punch. Keep your whole body relaxed when you throw the punch, and put all your power into the arm, but only bring the energy into the fist at the very end of the technique. The goal is to have the body and fist both move only a very short distance. It is desirable to also practice extending your Chi, for example by punching at a candle. Remember, the longer you practice, the stronger your power, and the more natural and smooth your power generation will be.

8. FEN JING (Centimeter Jing)

Compared with Inch Jing, Centimeter Jing is even shorter in both time and distance. Naturally, very strong Chi is required to make this Jing effective. This Jing can be used with the fingers, palm, fist, elbow, or shoulder. It is usually used right after the enemy's body is touched. For example, when your fingers touch the opponent's elbow, Centimeter Jing is used to grasp cavities to paralyze the elbow. If your fist or knuckle touches a vital cavity, for example the temple, Centimeter Jing can be applied suddenly to strike and rupture the artery.

The training methods of Centimeter Jing are the same as Inch Jing except that you often start the technique touching the target. This Jing takes even longer to train since Chi is needed more than muscle to make it effective.

9. LEENZ JING (Cold Jing)

Cold Jing is used for surprise attacks. The imagery of the name is that of a shiver from a cold wind which suddenly blows over you. It is a sudden attack from a "cold start", and there should be no visible preparation or other indication that you are going to attack. Cold Jing can be any technique--what characterizes it is the suddenness of its execution. This is one of the hardest Jings to learn and understand. It is said that Yang Ban-Huo specialized in Cold Jing and never met his match.

Since Cold Jing is a surprise attack, it is essential that the Jing storage time be as short as possible. If your opponent can sense that you are storing Jing, he can prepare for your attack. It is very important to psych out your opponent so that he doesn't suspect your attack. He attacks and you seem to retreat, but all of a sudden you attack him. Cold Jing is used while Yielding, Neutralizing, Controlling, or Adhere-Stick Jings are being used. For example, when you are neutralizing your opponent's Jing, he might sense it and prepare a strategy against your neutralization. When his Yi is on his new strategy and he is about to begin it, you suddenly change your strategy and attack. This sudden attack is called Cold Jing.

When you are about to use Cold Jing, you must be careful not to expose your intentions. You must be cool, calm, and steady. It seems like nothing is going to happen, then out of nowhere you attack.

Cold Jing depends upon faking out the opponent, and so you need a partner to practice it. You must first practice accumulating Jing as subtly as possible. Sometimes this may mean doing it in as short a time as possible. At other times it may mean accumulating Jing as inconspicuously as possible during your normal movement. The second part of Cold Jing is learning how to emit Jing instantly. This means that your body must be in the ideal position to do the particular technique, and when you attack your whole body moves as one unit. The third part of Cold Jing is patience. You must wait until you have your opponent in the right position before you do the technique. For example, if you want to push him, you must wait until he is unbalanced or almost unbalanced, and you must be in a position to instantly move his mass in an effective direction. If you wish to lock or break his arm, you must wait until his arm is in an exposed position and can be instantly incapacitated. If you pick the wrong time you may be countered, and if you try repeatedly to do a technique without being in a good position, the opponent will figure out what you are trying to do and will be on guard.

10. TYI JING (Lifting Jing)

Lifting Jing is the exertion of an upward force. It can be a pull or a push, and it is used to uproot the opponent. One example in the Tai Chi sequence is Embrace the Tiger and Return to the Mountain (Figures 3-60 and 3-61). Many techniques use some Lifting Jing. Wardoff has some lifting, and Push is often done upward. Sometimes a small lifting move is used to upset the opponent's root just before a major technique. Often a lifting technique is done right after a sinking move; a good example of this in the sequence is Fan Back (Figure 3-62). Sometimes you may lift before doing a sinking technique. For example, you may deflect an attack upward with Wardoff before using Rollback to lock the opponent's arm downward.

When you use Lifting Jing, you must have your root firmly grounded. The more Jing you apply downward, the more upward Lifting Jing can be generated from the legs. This Jing is not very fast but also not very slow. If you do it too fast, your own root will be affected, and if you do it too slowly, your opponent may sense your intention and change his strategy to thwart you.

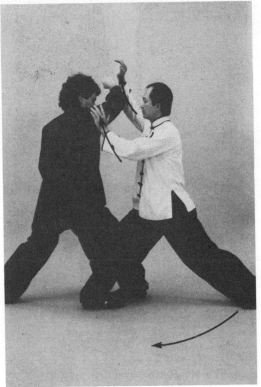

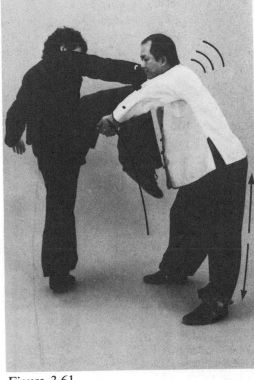

Figure 3-60.   Figure 3-61.

Lifting Jing can be practiced both on a bag and on a partner. A trick of lifting is, when you are in the right position and have found the center of mass of the bag or person, to think of sinking. This will help you to break his root. This works both when you are moving forward to a stationary opponent, as perhaps with Diagonal Flying, and when you are receiving an attack, as in Fair Lady Weaves Shuttle. With some techniques you may shift your weight forward and use the upward force that comes from sinking your weight into the front foot. Do this smoothly so that you "bounce" off the front foot.

b. Offense With Some Defense (Yang with some Yin) Jing:
1. AN JING (Push Jing):

Push Jing is applied by using one (Figures 3-63 and 3-64) or both hands (Figures 3-65 and 3-66) to push or strike the opponent's chest, arms, shoulders, or back. Frequently both hands will be on the opponent, but only one hand will do the actual pushing. Sometimes one hand will set the opponent up, and the other will push. Sometimes the opponent will react to your hands and evade you. In this case your two hands are alternately substantial and insubstantial as you follow his body. When you finally have him set up, one hand emits Jing.

The direction of the push can be forward, downward, or upward, and the attack can be long or short. Long Push Jing is used to push the opponent away, while short Push Jing is used to strike. Forward

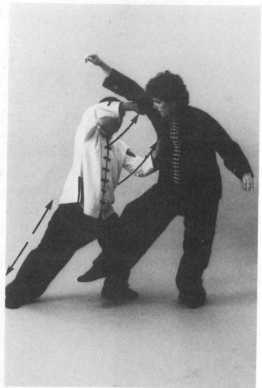

Figure 3-62.

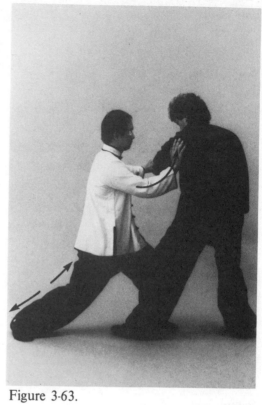

Figure 3-63.

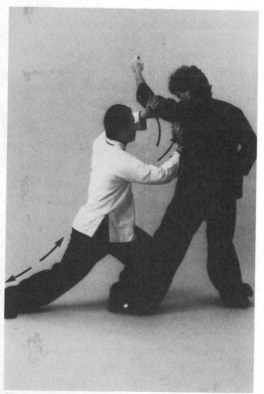

Figure 3-64.

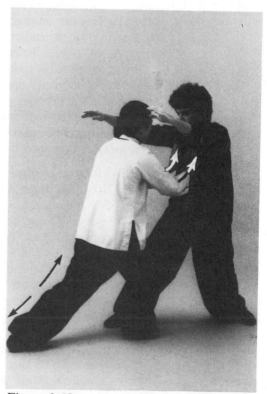

Figure 3-65.

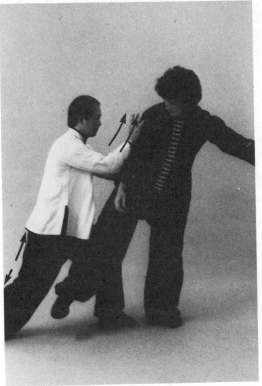

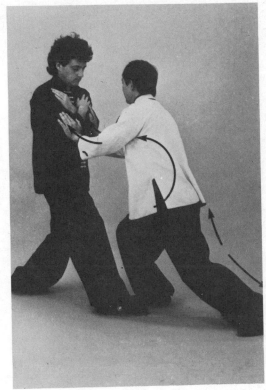

Figure 3-66.   Figure 3-67.

push is generally used to attack the chest or the shoulder blade. Downward Push Jing is often used to immobilize the opponent's arms and give you an opportunity for further attack. Upward Push can destroy the opponent's stability and balance. A major use of Push Jing occurs when you have neutralized an attack and have led the opponent into a bad position. If the opponent's balance is broken, or if he is in a position where it can be easily broken, you can send him flying if you push him from the correct angle.

The key to effective Push Jing is the legs. Your footwork adjusts the distance and sets up an advantageous angle of attack. Jing must be emitted from the legs and guided by the waist. Timing is also a decisive factor. The best time to use Push Jing is when the opponent is about to emit his Jing, but has not yet emitted it. When Push Jing is applied at this moment, the opponent can be bounced away with his own power. Remember, when using Push Jing, your body should not lean excessively in the direction of the push, otherwise your Jing may be used against you. Also, when pushing you should withhold some of your Jing. This will make it harder for your opponent to use your push against you.

Push Jing can be trained in a number of ways. For sandbag training, you must stand at the right distance, then use your leg to generate Jing and use your waist to guide the Jing to the bag. When the bag swings back to you at a different angle, adjust your position and push again, using either one hand or both hands. Treat the bag like a real

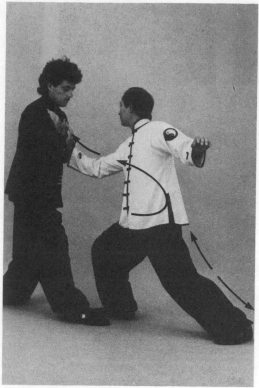

Figure 3-68.

opponent. If you continue the practice, you should be able to grasp the trick and the right timing of the push.

Of course you can also train Push Jing with a partner. Have the partner cross his arms on his chest to provide some cushioning (Figures 3-67 and 3-68). His hands should be flat on his chest so that you can feel his mass. Place your hand (hands) lightly on his forearms and try to feel any motion of his body. You may push him slightly to get him to move. A small push may also bring his center up so that you can push it. It is important to push his center of mass, because if you push anywhere else he will be able to yield and deflect you. Don't use a very hard Jing on your partner, as this may injure him. When you push him, try to catch his motion. If you catch him when he is moving slightly backward, you can add to his motion and send him flying. You can push him slightly and then withdraw a little bit. If he starts to resist your push he will move forward as you withdraw. Emit your Jing just as he is about to come forward, or else let him come forward a little bit and lift him slightly as he does so, and then continue his motion upward and away from you.

2. CHAI JING (Pluck Jing):

Pluck Jing is a pull used to upset the opponent's stability and set him up for an attack. It can be used to immobilize him, upset his balance, or stop his attack. To use Chai Jing, you usually have to first use Controlling Jing on one of the opponent's joints such as the

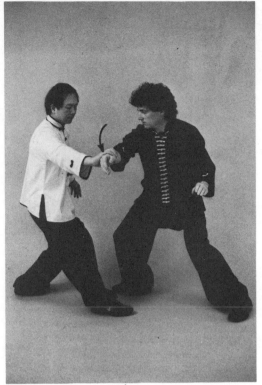

Figure 3-69.

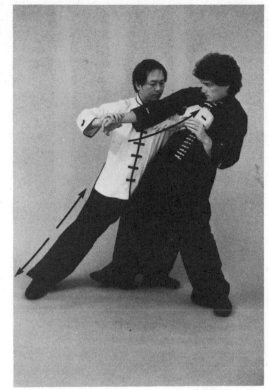

Figure 3-70.

wrist, elbow, or shoulder, and then pull his arm downward or sideward. In principle, when your opponent transmits Jing to his hand, the force must go through the shoulder, elbow, and wrist. If one of these joints is controlled and pulled, the Jing will be cut off and his root broken. The opponent will usually tense his muscles and use his Li to resist by pulling in the opposite direction. Once you sense his power, immediately follow the direction of his power and use your Press or Push Jing to attack. Once you grasp the trick of this, you will usually win.

When Pluck Jing is used to pull sideward, you usually pull the opponent's arm across his chest and downward. This prevents any further attack with his legs or other hand. Sideward Pluck is often used to set the opponent up for an attack, which may be Press, Push, Elbow-Stroke (Figures 3-69 and 3-70), or Shoulder-Stroke. When your opponent loses his balance you may also immediately kick his lower body (Figure 3-71) or sweep his leg to make him fall (Figure 3-72).

Pluck is also often used to pull downward. An example of downward Pluck in the Tai Chi Chuan sequence is Pick Up the Needle from the Sea Bottom. One of the applications of this form is to grasp the enemy's wrist and pull it down (Figure 3-73). When the opponent resists and pulls back and up, follow his motion and accelerate it with Fan Back (Figure 3-74). This is an example of "If there is a top, there is a bottom", and also of "To consider going upward implies considering downward" (Appendix A-1).

The sinking of the body in a downward Pluck is similar to Sinking

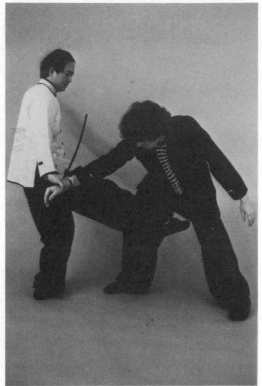

Figure 3-71.

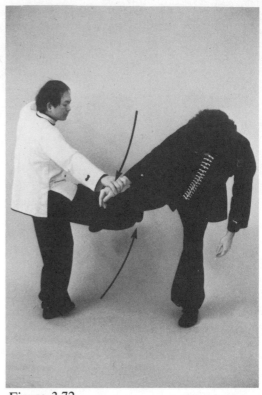

Figure 3-72.

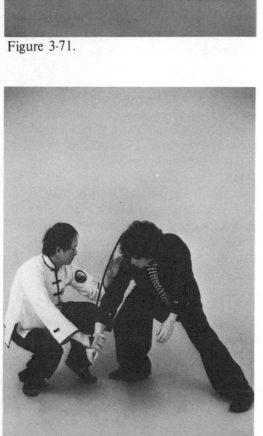

Figure 3-73.

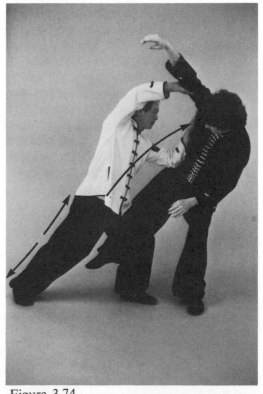

Figure 3-74.

Jing, but the application is different. Both Jings use a similar sinking movement of the body, but in Pluck Jing you are holding the opponent and pulling him downward. When you use downward Pluck Jing, you must be aware of your top. Your enemy might use the opportunity to strike your head or upper body.

In order for Pluck Jing to be effective, it must be strong and fast. If your pull is not strong enough to force your opponent into the defense, he might be able to use your power against you. If your pull is too slow, your opponent will have the opportunity to sense your intention and reset himself in a new position to your disadvantage. Most importantly, Pluck is an all-or-nothing technique. If you give up on it halfway through, you set yourself up to be countered, because your opponent's stability is still intact.

Learning to use Pluck is fairly easy, though it is harder to learn how to use it well. Be patient and wait for the right opportunity. If you have to struggle, you're doing it wrong. Work on correct timing, and be careful to avoid using Li. Since Pluck Jing must be used together with many other Jings such as Controlling Jing, Listening Jing, Understanding Jing, and Press Jing in order to be effective, a partner is necessary for the training. Experiment with different ways of using Pluck Jing to unbalance your partner, set him up for attacks, and stop his attacks.

3. ZOU JING (Elbow-Stroke Jing):

Elbow-Stroke Jing uses the elbow to strike or sometimes push the opponent. This is a short range attack, used when the opponent is too close for a hand technique. When an elbow attack is done properly with the correct timing it is very difficult to block, and can be more damaging than the hand. However, when used improperly it is easily defended against. Since the elbow is close to the center of your body, if your opponent can control your upper arm or shoulder he can easily use your Jing against you. It is important therefore to keep part of your force in reserve and not commit it all. Remember, Jing comes from your legs. Keep your stance stable and balanced, wait for the right opportunity, and control your technique through your waist.

Generally, there are two ways to Elbow-Stroke. The first is called Forward Elbow-Stroke (Tsen Zou Kau), and uses the elbow or forearm to strike forward (Figure 3-75) to attack the solar plexus or nipple area (Figure 3-76). Occasionally it is also used to attack the shoulder blade to numb the opponent's arm (Figure 3-77). When Forward Elbow-Stroke is used, it is destructive, powerful, and dangerous. The other Elbow-Stroke is called Sideward Elbow-Stroke (Tseh Zou Kau) and uses the upper arm near the elbow to push or strike (Figure 3-78). This technique is not as powerful and destructive as Forward Elbow-Stroke. A common way to use this technique is to first raise the opponent's arm to expose his underarm area (Figure 3-79). Next, step behind his front leg to keep him from withdrawing, and use your elbow to hit him or push him down (Figure 3-80).

In practice, you can use a bag to train both Forward and Sideward Elbow-Stroke. Treat the bag like your opponent's body for striking and pushing. Use your elbows as you would your fists, with the same relaxation and fluidity of application. You can also practice Elbow-

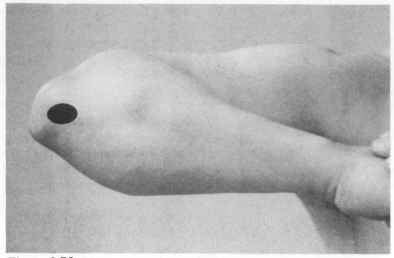

Figure 3-75.

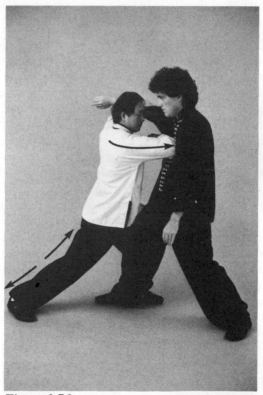

Figure 3-76.

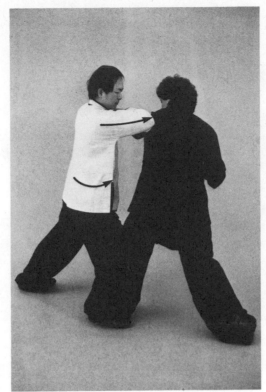

Figure 3-77.

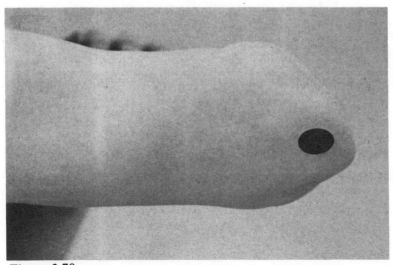

Figure 3-78.

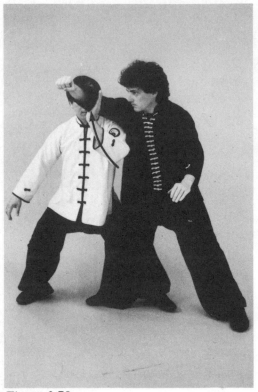

Figure 3-79.

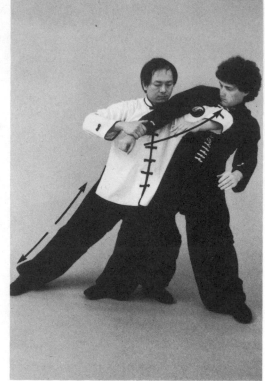

Figure 3-80.

Stroke on a partner if you do it as a push. The person being pushed should hold his arms on his chest to avoid injury (Figures 3-81 and 3-82). However, the best way to train Elbow-Stroke with a partner is to use a kicking pad (Figures 3-83 and 3-84). This allows you to train striking and pushing techniques realistically without worrying about hurting your partner.

4. NA JING (Controlling Jing, literally to grasp, seize, capture)

Controlling Jing is the controlling of a joint of the opponent. Na Jing is very important in Tai Chi Chuan because it is necessary to control the opponent before you can attack him. When you neutralize an opponent he is in a state of confusion and imbalance because he has lost his power. At this time you are already guiding him. If you can control him through his wrist, elbow, or shoulder you can attack with certainty.

When controlling the opponent, your movements and your touch must be light and agile. If your movements are heavy your opponent can easily sense them, and he will try to escape. If you wait for the right opportunity, when you do grasp him he will not be able to escape.

When two hands are used to control, one hand controls the elbow while the other controls either the wrist or the shoulder (Figures 3-85 and 3-86). When you use both hands to control, it is like using a balance scale to weigh something. When the opponent becomes heavy

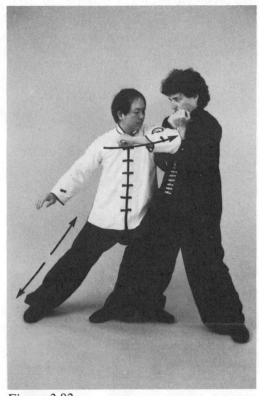

Figure 3-81.

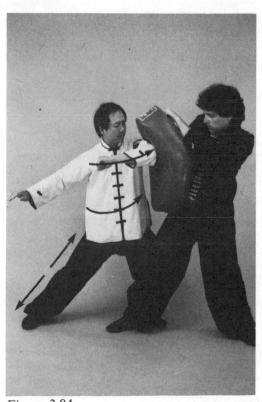

Figure 3-82.

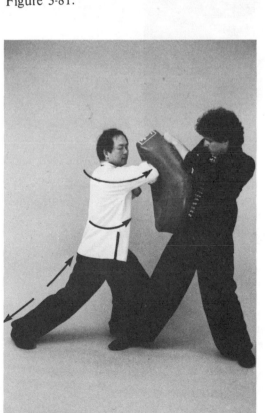

Figure 3-83.

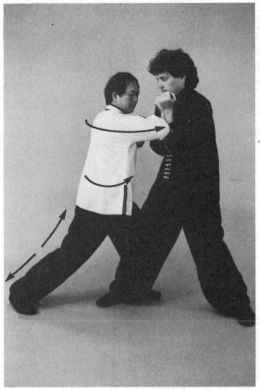

Figure 3-84.

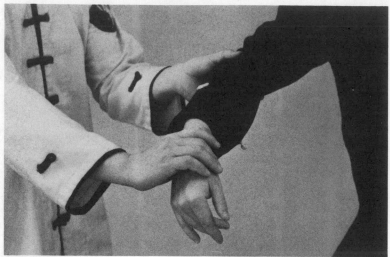

Figure 3-85.

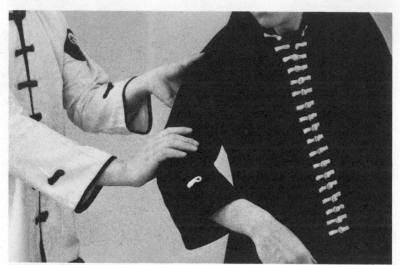

Figure 3-86.

at one point, you don't resist there, but instead maintain your control at the other point. Technically, your two hands alternate being substantial and insubstantial as they adapt to the opponent's movements. When using Controlling Jing, it is not only the hands but also the waist which controls the action. Do not use Li, but use your mind and Chi.

There are two kinds of Na. In the first kind, commonly called Chin Na, you actually grasp the opponent. The most basic Chin Na techniques are "dividing the muscle" and "misplacing the bone". In dividing the muscle techniques, the opponent's muscles in the joint area are twisted and overextended, tearing the muscle fiber and causing pain. Figures 3-87 and 3-88 show two examples in which the muscles in the wrist area are twisted and extended. In misplacing the bone techniques, the joint is twisted and bent in an abnormal direction to tear the ligament or dislocate the joint. Figure 3-89 shows an example in which the opponent's elbow is locked and overextended, and Figure

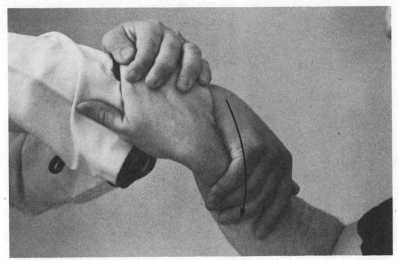

Figure 3-87.

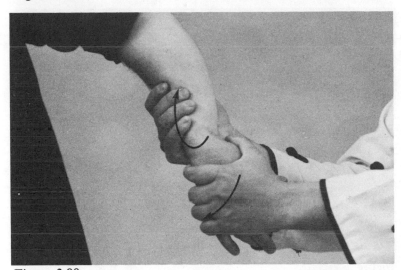

Figure 3-88.

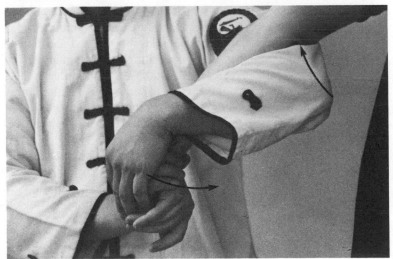

Figure 3-89.

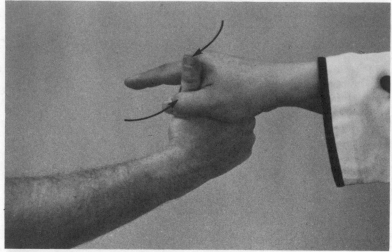

Figure 3-90.

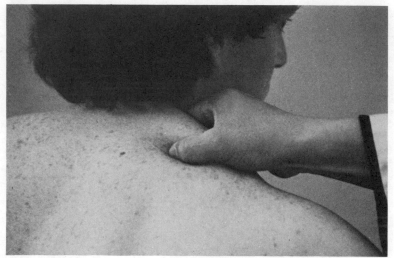

Figure 3-91.

3-90 shows an example in which the thumb is locked and bent.

There is another type of Chin Na technique called muscle and cavity grasp in which the opponent's muscles are grasped and pinched to cause pain and numbness. A typical example is shown in Figure 3-91 in which the shoulder muscles are controlled. Alternatively, the grasp can be used on acupuncture cavities to cause pain and numbness and immobilize the affected area. An example is shown in Figure 3-92 in which the cavities Quchi (Figure 3-93) and either Shaohai or Xiaohai (Figure 3-94) are pinched.

The second Na Jing controls the opponent without grasping or using any particular form. The techniques and theory of this Na Jing are higher than those of the Chin Na discussed above. In this Na Jing, you use your adhering and sticking ability on your opponent's joints to lead him and neutralize his slightest movement. When he attacks, you neutralize, when he withdraws you stick and follow. You do not actually grasp your opponent but you make him feel that he cannot

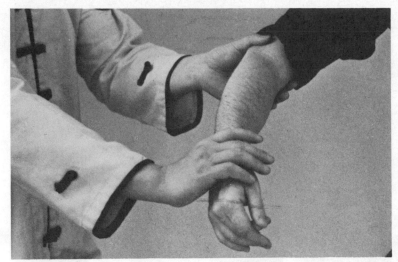

Figure 3-92.

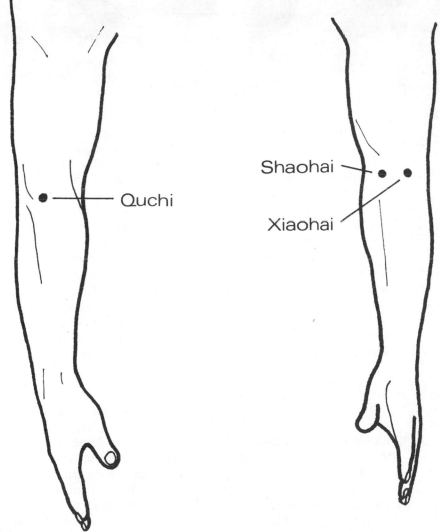

Quchi

Shaohai

Xiaohai

Figure 3-93.   Figure 3-94.

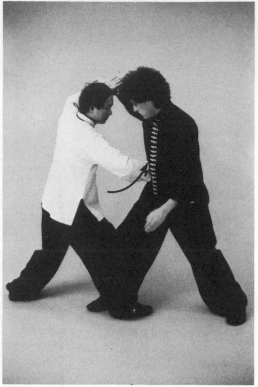

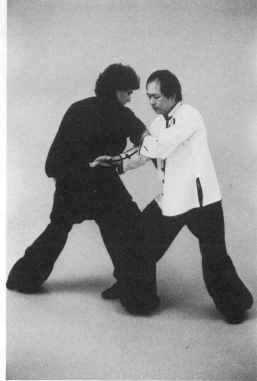

Figure 3-95.   Figure 3-96.

attack you and he cannot get away from you, as if you were a sheet
of flypaper that he can't shake off. When he tries to withdraw you
follow him, maneuvering him subtly into a bad position. When he
attacks, you evade and lead his attack further or in a different direction than he intended, and then apply subtle pressure to hold him in
an exposed position.

In order to make Na Jing effective, you must have good Listening,
Understanding, Neutralizing, and Leading Jings. You have to listen
to and understand his slightest motion, and then lead and neutralize
it so that he cannot free himself. Since there are so many Jings involved, it is impossible to practice without a partner. After several
years of practice, you should be able to coordinate your steps with
your Na Jing and maneuver your opponent into a completely passive
situation.

5. TSUO JING (Filing Jing)

Tsuo in Chinese means to rub or file. When Filing Jing is used,
you generally use the outside edge of your hand and forearm to "file"
forward, sideward, upward, or downward. This Jing can be used either
as a strike or as a pressing/rubbing action. It can be used against the
opponent's arm to stop a technique, or to either lock the arm for Chin
Na control or clear it out of your way just before you attack. When
Filing Jing is used against the body, the front or back of the waist
is the usual target (Figures 3-95 and 3-96). If the front side of the waist

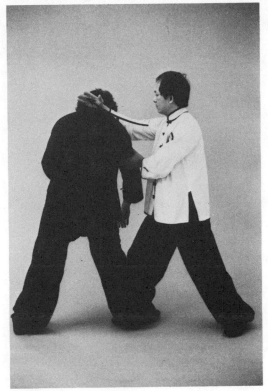

Figure 3-97.

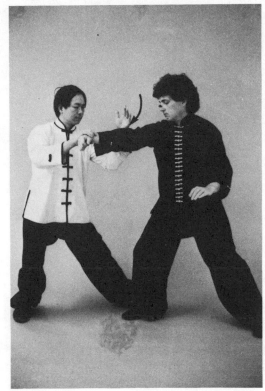

Figure 3-98.

is filed correctly, the muscle will contract and cause the lung to seal the breath (prevent breathing). If the back of the waist is filed, a direct or indirect injury to the kidney will result. It is also commonly used to attack the neck (Figure 3-97).

Filing Jing is commonly used to press or rub the arm down to seal and lock the opponent's attack. A typical example of filing down is shown in Figures 3-98 and 3-99 in which the opponent's attack is first intercepted and then filed down to open the neck for a filing attack (Figure 3-97). Upward filing is usually used to set up for striking or Chin Na control. An example of filing up is when you use your right hand to grasp the opponent's right wrist, and then file upward with your left arm on his upper arm (Figure 3-100). This lifts and twists his arm. You can then file downward, circling him down into a Chin Na control (Figure 3-101).

Both the bag and pushing hands can be used for Filing Jing practice. Figure 3-102 shows the direction in which the Jing is filed when a bag is used. When you file, keep your muscles relaxed, but suddenly tense them once the edge of the hand and forearm touch the target. The Jing is directed into the bag and sideward. When Filing Jing is practiced in pushing hands, you must neutralize your opponent's attack first. Once you are in the most advantageous position, apply your Filing Jing immediately. Figures 3-103 and 3-104 show the upward and downward filing training using a staff. You can also practice Filing Jing by yourself. Figures 3-105 and 3-106 show ways to practice filing up and down.

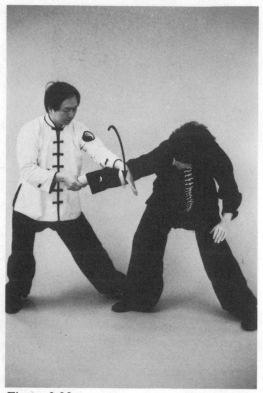

Figure 3-99.

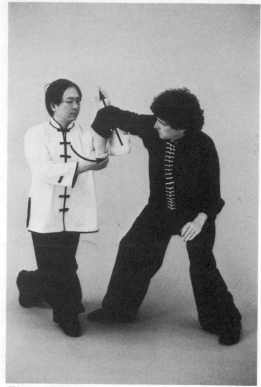

Figure 3-100.

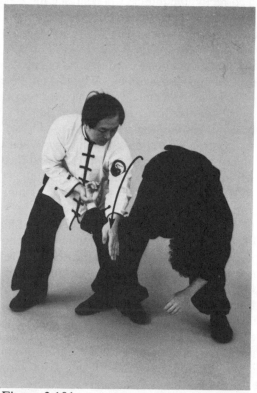

Figure 3-101.

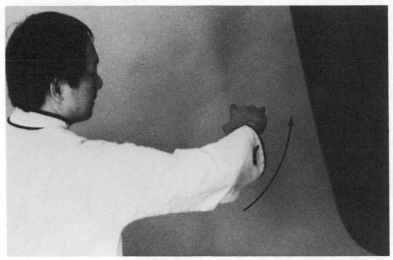

Figure 3-102.

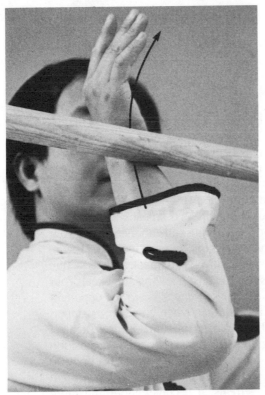

Figure 3-103.

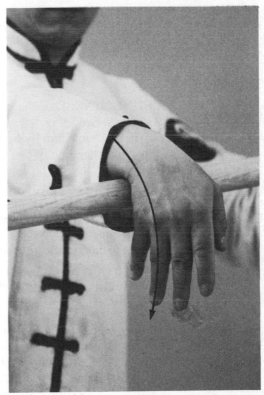

Figure 3-104.

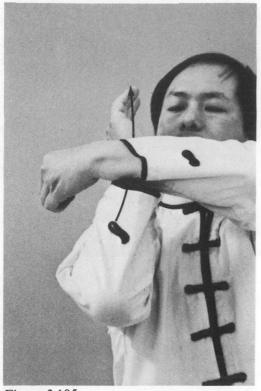

Figure 3-105.

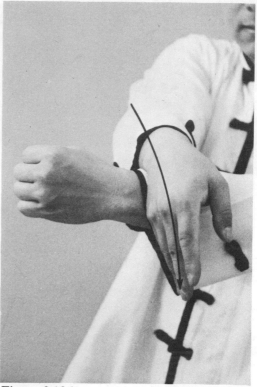

Figure 3-106.

6. SUNG JING (Send Jing)

To use Send Jing, follow the opponent's withdrawing motion, add to it, and "send" him flying away. This is a long Jing, but it is shorter than Growing Jing. When the opponent is using Yielding or Neutralizing Jing, you use the Jings of Adhere and Stick to take control of the situation, and then use Push. When it is used properly, the opponent will lose his root and be bounced away.

When the opponent is withdrawing, his Yi is on backing up. While this is happening, you should follow his Jing and enhance it with your forward motion and your own Jing to keep him passive. Take the initiative and keep him withdrawing until you can attack and "send" him flying away. When this Jing is used against Yielding Jing, keep your footwork alive as you adhere and stick. Keep close to the opponent so that his yielding strategy is useless, then when you have an opportunity, add your attacking Jing. When this Jing is used against Neutralizing Jing, you must step skillfully to reorient your position and redirect your opponent's Neutralizing Jing toward his body so you can control him. This is what is meant in the Tai Chi Chuan Classic: "when (the opponent) retreats, it becomes more and more urgent", (Appendix A-2).

This Jing is normally trained during Pushing Hands. Send Jing can be considered a strategic way of using other Jings. When pushing hands, be alert to opportunities for following the opponent as he withdraws. This Jing can also be trained with a sandbag. First push

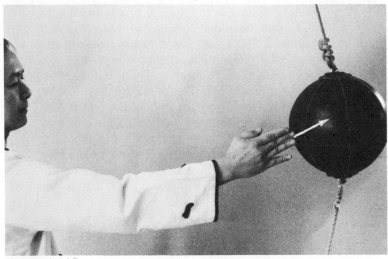

Figure 3-107.

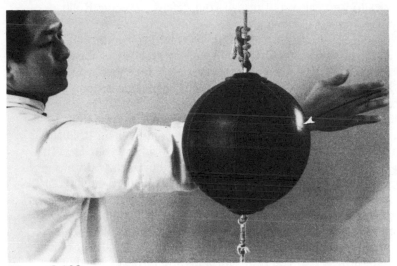

Figure 3-108.

the bag and start it swinging. When the bag comes within range, adhere lightly to it, and when it swings away follow and add your push. Remember that your push should be a sudden pulse so that the bag bounces away.

B. Defensive (Yin) Jing:
a. Purely Defensive (Yin) Jing:
1. LU JING (Rollback Jing)

Rollback Jing leads the opponent's attack past you after you have neutralized it. It is considered purely negative, or Yin, although in practice you will usually add a small amount of force. To understand the Yin nature of Rollback, consider what happens when you push a bag which is tethered top and bottom. If you do not push the bag directly in the center, it moves back just enough to avoid your force, and turns out of the way (Figures 3-107 and 108).

When you do Rollback, your hands are usually on the opponent's wrist and elbow. When he attacks, withdraw and turn your body to evade his attack, at the same time pulling him slightly to lead him past you. Rollback causes only a small change in the course of the opponent's attack--you let him go pretty much where he wants to go, but make sure that you aren't there. Pulling him slightly will lead him further than he intended so that he overextends himself and loses his root, or else it will guide him slightly off his intended course so that he loses his stability and becomes vulnerable to attack. Your Jing must **LEAD** him. This means that your force must be applied in about the same direction as the direction of his attack. If you apply force at too great an angle to his direction of attack, or try to change his course too radically, you are meeting force with force, and that is not Rollback.

In practice, it is sometimes necessary to wardoff the opponent's attack before doing Rollback. If the attack is fast and from short range, you may not be able to get control of his arm fast enough. In such a case, first deflect him with Wardoff, and if his attack continues or if he tries to force his way through your defense, execute Rollback in the direction he is moving.

Rollback is occasionally used offensively. Since you control the opponent's arm, it is often possible when you draw back to lock the elbow or break it with a quick turn. This application is very similar to Split Jing. You can also use Sinking Jing with this technique to apply sudden pressure downward.

There are two kinds of Rollback—large and small. In large Rollback (Da Lu) you step back as you lead him past you; in small Rollback (Shao Lu) you do not step, although you may adjust your feet. In small Rollback, for example, if he throws a right punch you ward it off upward and to your right (Figure 3-109). You then circle your right hand around his arm, and draw him to your left rear (Figure 3-110). This will open the right side of his body for a moment, allowing you to attack (Figure 3-111). Similarly, if he throws a left punch, ward it off upward (Figure 3-112). Curl your right hand clockwise around his arm so that you can control his arm at the elbow (Figure 3-113), and pull him off balance to your left rear. His left arm will probably be locked, allowing you to counter effectively with a press (Figure 3-114).

In large Rollback, step either directly backward or else turn 270 degrees and place your foot behind you. For example, if the opponent punches with his right, Stick and connect to his arm with your right arm (Figure 3-115). Follow his force and step back with your right leg. At the same time, control his arm at the wrist and above the elbow, and draw him to your right rear (Figure 3-116). The opponent should fall or lose his stability, giving you the opportunity to attack. The trick to making your opponent lose his stability is that right after you neutralize the attack, you suddenly add your Rollback Jing in a sharp pulse. If your neutralization is subtle and doesn't alarm him, a quick Rollback should catch him before he can resist.

Alternatively, instead of stepping directly back, step all the way around to your rear (Figures 3-117 and 3-118). This is done when the opponent is close and there is danger of his counterattacking with

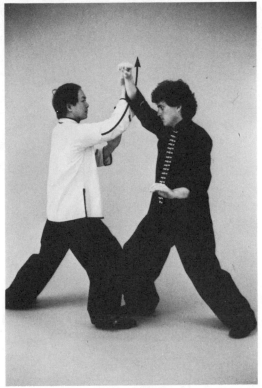

Figure 3-109.

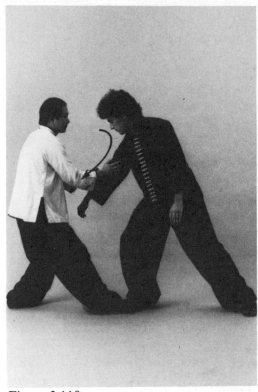

Figure 3-110.

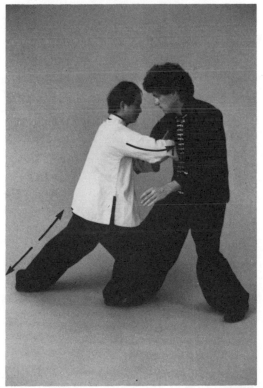

Figure 3-111.

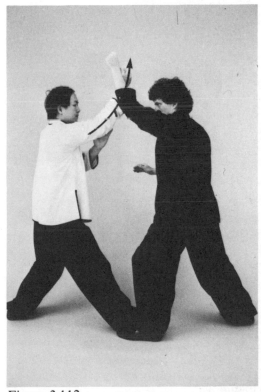

Figure 3-112.

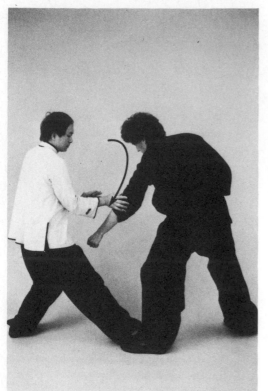

Figure 3-113.

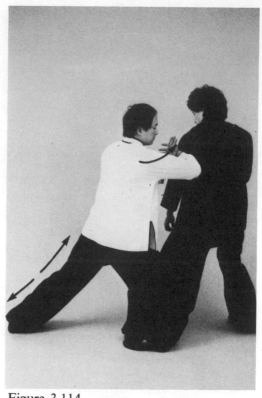

Figure 3-114.

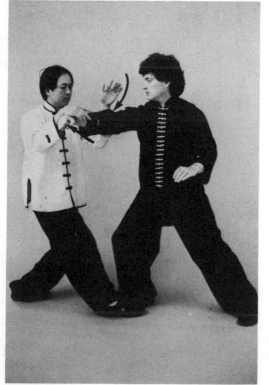

Figure 3-115.

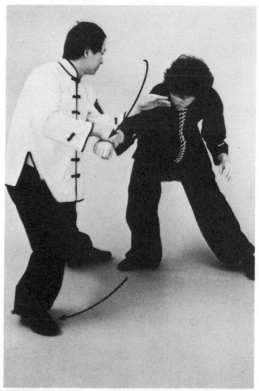

Figure 3-116.

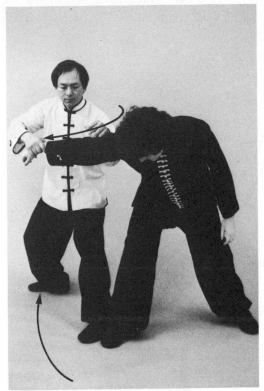

Figure 3-117.

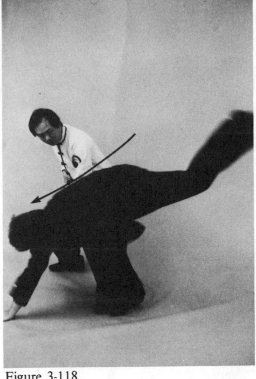

Figure 3-118.

Shoulder-Stroke if you don't get him completely past you. This application is a mixture of the motion of Rollback and Rend Jing.

Rollback is done in response to the opponent's attack, but in some cases you can provoke the attack. If you can push the opponent and cause him to push back, you may be able to extend his push enough to use Rollback, causing him to fall past you. However, if your Adhere-Stick Jing is not very good, this may be dangerous. Also, if you don't know how to use Leading Jing your Rollback will be ineffective because you will not be able to really control him. In this regard, when a beginner does Rollback, he should not draw the opponent in too close, but should curve the opponent away from him to avoid the chance of counterattack (Figure 3-119).

The key to Rollback is the waist and legs, not the arms. When using Rollback, first lead the opponent slightly upward, then sit back and sink, keeping the legs relaxed, and twist the waist to get the Rollback Jing out. In Pushing Hands you use Rollback continually to deflect and neutralize attacks. However, be careful not to try to use Rollback to lock or control the opponent when you cannot unbalance him, because he will counter or neutralize you.

Rollback must be trained with a partner. Any exercise which allows you to practice sticking, following, and yielding is preparing you for Rollback. See Chapter 3 of the second volume for Rollback pushing hands exercises.

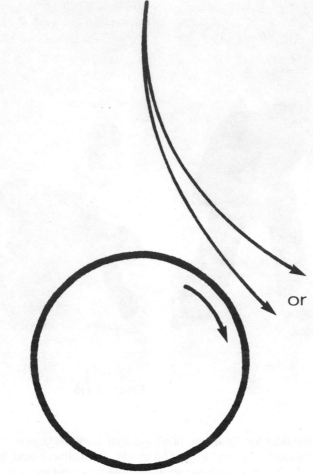

Figure 3-119.

or

2. TSAN NIEN JING (Adhere-Stick Jing)

This is the most fundamental and important Jing in Tai Chi Chuan. Tsan means adhere and Nien means stick. These are two different Jings, but they are always considered together because they cannot be separated. When you moisten your finger to pick up powder it is called Tsan. Nien means to stick and not come off. Basically, to adhere means to connect--you move to lightly attach your arm or hand to your opponent. Once attached, you stick with him and follow his movements, moving your body to evade his attacks, and following him as he retreats. Your opponent should feel that he can't get rid of you or shake you off. It is said:"When the opponent is hard, I am soft; this is called yielding. When I follow the opponent, this is called sticking. When the opponent moves fast, I move fast; when the opponent moves slowly, then I follow slowly. Although the variations are infinite, the principle remains the same" (Appendix A-2).

Adhere-Stick is the Jing of not losing the opponent. When you learn it properly the enemy is under your control. He cannot reach you because you are always in contact with him and can feel his attacks and avoid them, and he can't get away because you are right there ready to attack at his slightest error. It is said:"Guide (his power) to enter into emptiness, then immediately attack; Adhere-Connect, Stick-Follow, do not lose him"(Appendix A-7).

Tsan Nien Jing is developed initially on the hands and forearms, but once you develop a feeling for it, you can develop the same sensitivity and responsiveness in every part of your body. After a long period of training, if any part of your body is attacked, that part will automatically move just enough to avoid the attack, but not enough to break contact. Just as you move away to evade the attack, you will tend to move forward as he withdraws. There is flexibility in Tsan Nien Jing--you don't have to keep the same part of your body in contact with the opponent. You may meet his attack with a forearm, transfer the attack to the other arm, and then switch to a shoulder as you counter with Diagonal Flying.

It is said that this Jing is very subtle and has to be taught personally by a master. The master lets the student feel what Tsan Nien Jing is like, in a sense "charging his battery" with an understanding of the technique so that he can practice on his own and develop this Jing.

After a long period of study a layer of Chi is developed on the surface of the body. This is like a cloud on the skin, or like glue covering the whole body. The better the master, the thicker this layer is. It cannot be seen, but it can be felt by those who understand it. It is possible for two experts to evaluate each other just by sensing this layer of Chi.

This is the most important and basic Jing, and it is developed mainly through pushing hands, where you gradually build up a feeling for what it is. Relax and "listen" to your partner with all your attention. Keep your hands on your partner and concentrate on following him wherever he moves. Move your body to evade him as he attacks or advances, follow him when he withdraws, always keeping your hands lightly attached to him. Even when you move forward offensively or attack, emphasize listening so that you can adapt to whatever he does. If you get pushed or lose your balance, still stay attached to him if possible. Another way to train this Jing is through Tai Chi ball practice. This will be discussed in Chapter 3 of the second volume.

3. DSOU JING (Yielding Jing, literally "walking away Jing")

This is the Jing of no resistance. It is an insubstantial Jing, pure Yin in character. Dsou Jing comes from Understanding Jing, for if you don't understand the opponent's Jing, how can you walk away from it? In its purest form, Yielding Jing is simply moving away from the opponent's pressure. In Pushing Hands, when the opponent pushes against your arm, you become insubstantial where he is pushing. You may simply move directly away in the direction of his push, or you may empty the side of the body he is pushing against, turning your body to let his attack go past you. If you don't resist, the enemy will feel only emptiness wherever he advances. His power will also feel empty because it has nothing to push against. Beginners usually need a relatively heavy pressure applied to them before they yield, and if

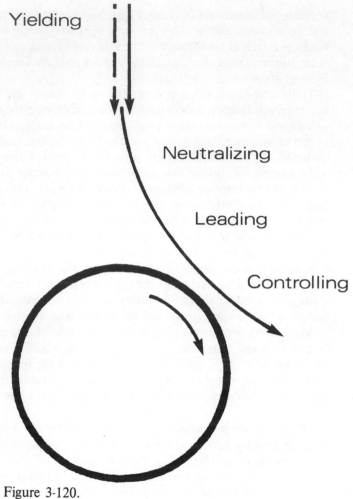

Yielding

Neutralizing

Leading

Controlling

Figure 3-120.

a light pressure is applied they tend to resist. This is because their sensitivity is still low, and they don't feel or understand the energy.

The key to Yielding Jing is the waist and legs. The footwork must be correct, and the waist must coordinate the body and legs when you move and turn to get out of the way. You must also understand Adhere-Connect and Stick-Follow, for if you cannot stay in contact with the opponent you cannot clearly know his motion.

In Tai Chi fighting strategy (see Chapter 5 of the second volume), Yielding and Adhere-Stick Jings are used to connect to the opponent when you are separate. When the opponent attacks, adhere to the attacking arm and yield completely without resisting or losing contact. In Figure 3-120, the enemy's attack is shown as a solid line, while your defensive action is shown as a dash line. Follow the opponent's direction and adhere to him without losing him. This is done through the skillful use of your legs, waist, and steps. Thus, it is said:"When the opponent is hard, I am soft; this is called yielding". Also, "When there is pressure on the left, the left becomes insubstantial; when there is pressure on the right, the right becomes insubstantial. Looking upward it seems to get higher and higher; looking downward it seems to get deeper and deeper. When (the opponent) advances, it seems longer and longer"(Appendix A-2).

The best way to practice Yielding Jing is through pushing hands. Listen to the opponent's attack carefully, readjusting your position smoothly and swiftly so that the attack meets only emptiness. This Jing can also be practiced with a bag. Start the bag swinging, and stay lightly attached to it. As the bag swings toward you, readjust your position to evade it.

A good exercise to train yielding is to have someone push you as you practice not resisting. Start in a bow and arrow stance with 60% of your weight on your front foot, and imagine that you are a molded rubber figure, glued to the floor. Wherever you are pushed—yield. Stick to the hand pushing you, and don't separate from it. This means when you are pushed you move back only as far as the hand moves, and no farther. When he pulls his hand back, adhere and follow it so that you come back to your starting position. This following back keeps your actions spring-like, and not just wet noodle-like. It also keeps you thinking offensively—you evade his attack and follow it back to attack him. Try to keep your stance as much as possible. Sometimes you will have to adjust your feet to keep your balance, but always come right back to your starting position. If you are pushed off balance, don't stop the exercise, just correct your stance.

There are three ways to yield. The first way is turning (Figures 3-121 and 3-122). This is the best way because you stay close to the opponent where you can attack him. As a general rule, when your right side is attacked, shift your weight to the left leg, and vice versa. You should generally move as little as possible, and only where you are pushed, i.e., when he pushes a shoulder you empty that shoulder and move it back while the rest of your body stays still. Remember to always follow his hand back until you reach your starting position.

The second way to yield is to simply move away from the attack. This is not quite as good as turning, because you lose the ability to counterattack. The third way to yield is to bend the body (Figure 3-123). There are times when you will have to do this to avoid resisting, especially in the beginning, but bending should always be the last choice. When you bend your lower body back you tend to expose your upper body, and vice versa. Yielding is just half of this exercise, the other half is the active side. Move your partner as if you are trying to loosen him up, for in fact you are. Don't use much Jing, especially with beginners, just move him around in ways he can usually deal with. Push mostly with one hand at a time, using single pushes and combinations as if you were boxing. Be rhythmic, but don't be like a machine. Do not try to knock your partner over too often, since this may prevent him from finding his root. This exercise is for helping him learn how to yield, so if you make him too tense or keep him off balance too much, he may start resisting and overreacting. Push and pull in every direction, all over his body, including legs, neck, and head. Alternate long and short pushes, straight and curved ones;

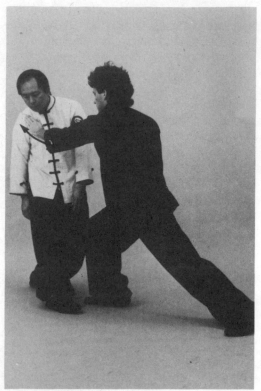

Figure 3-121.

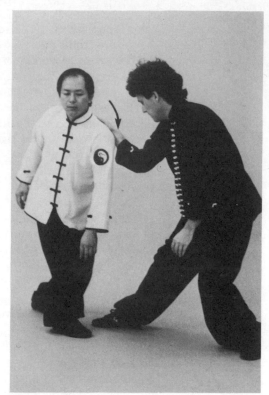

Figure 3-122.

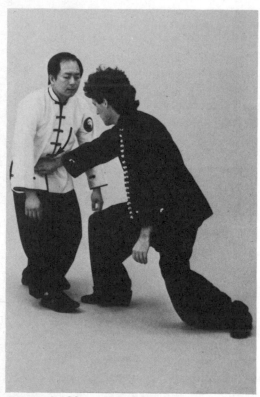

Figure 3-123.

vary the speed, and throw in some fakes to make sure he doesn't anticipate the push.

Pushing your partner around like this gives you an excellent opportunity to look at your body dynamics. Balance the force of your push with the counterforce going into your supporting foot. Make sure you move from the waist, coiling to accumulate energy, expanding slightly to emit energy. Don't throw your body forward when you push because you can be easily countered.

4. DIEN KAN JING (Resisting Jing)

This is the Jing of resistance. Even though you use force, this Jing is considered purely Yin because you do not initiate the action—you respond only when the opponent emits force onto you. Many people misunderstand Tai Chi and believe that only soft Jings are used, and that all resistance and hard Jings are avoided. This is an incomplete view of the art. Like any other Chinese martial art, Tai Chi uses a wide range of Jings. Soft Jings are emphasized, but the hard Jings are not given up.

There are three main uses for Resisting Jing. The first is as a training exercise to build up root and Chi support. Skilled Tai Chi practitioners who have trained their Chi to fully support their muscles will often train extending the duration of their Jing so that they will be able to resist long, powerful muscular attacks. Tai Chi masters will frequently demonstrate their Resisting Jing by standing in the War-doff position and having people push them. Sometimes Nei Kung masters will compare their Resisting Jings by pushing each other. As you extend the duration and increase the strength of Resisting Jing, the local Chi support must initially play a major role. Since the muscles tend to be tensed, Dan Tien Chi has difficulty reaching them. However, with sufficient training you will be able to relax and let the Dan Tien Chi circulate.

The second use of Resisting Jing is for Borrowing Jing. In this case you use Resisting Jing as the opponent starts his push so that he pushes himself away from you (see Borrowing Jing).

The third use is as a last resort when there is no other way to neutralize the opponent's attack. For example, if your wrist or arm is held tightly by a fighter from another style, you may have to use Resisting Jing to prevent him from doing anything more to control or hurt you. This is Jing against Jing, but it is not stiff or stagnant. You emit a pulse of force only when your opponent's Jing is applied onto you. Prevent him from continuing his action, and once his Jing is gone, immediately relax.

The easiest and most basic method of training Resisting Jing is to ask your partner to push your forearm (Figure 3-124). You can also train forearm against forearm with both side exerting force (Figure 3-125). A third way is to use either of the above two postures and have one person suddenly exert Push Jing, while the other uses Resisting Jing to resist the pulse of energy. Stay relaxed until the other person pushes, then use only enough force to stop his push, and then relax again.

When practicing, relax and transport Chi from your Dan Tien to your forearm, then lightly tense the forearm muscle to keep the Dan

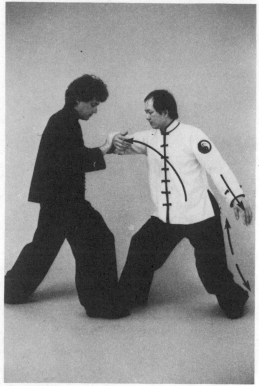

Figure 3-124.

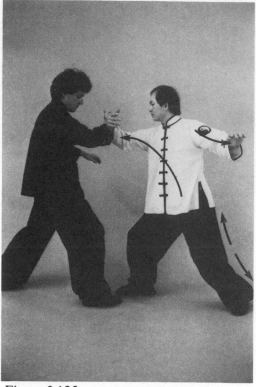

Figure 3-125.

Tien Chi there. This tensing will also generate local Chi, but if only local Chi is used, your Jing will be of a low level. Relax all the shoulder muscles as much as possible—the more you relax, the more your Dan Tien Chi can support the Jing. Remember, it is your Yi which leads and controls the Chi.

When doing these exercises, both practitioners must pay attention to their stability and central equilibrium. You can test each other occasionally by suddenly pulling your arm away. If the other person falls or loses his balance forward, it is because he has lost his center and is using his body's strength to push instead of Jing. When pushing or resisting, your Yi, Chi, and posture must be balanced, and your body should be upright.

5. GIEH JING (Intercepting Jing)

Intercepting Jing is used to intercept and control the opponent's attack. It is a mixture of visual "listening" with Understanding, Neutralizing, Yielding, Wardoff, and Adhere-Stick Jings. Normally during a fight your hands are not sticking to the opponent. When he attacks with a punch or kick, you use this Jing to meet his attack halfway. You must first direct some force into the side of his attacking arm so that you can adhere to it. You can then move the attack back toward him so that any further action is hindered, or use some other Jing such as Opening, Deflecting, or Rollback.

Intercepting Jing is usually the first Jing to be used when dealing with an attack. Both external and internal martial styles train it, however they use different approaches. Most external styles will intercept the opponent's attack first and counterattack as soon as possible. They will often use this Jing to block and bounce the attack away. The Tai Chi practitioner will make contact with the attacking arm and adhere to it, attempting to control the attacker through it. This is a refined technique which is much harder to do than the intercepting used by other styles. Unfortunately, the average person in Tai Chi nowadays emphasizes pushing hands and only trains the Jings which can be obtained from pushing hands. Consequently, when he encounters a punch, he does not know how to intercept it, and cannot apply the Jings he has learned.

To train Intercepting Jing you must first train your eyes to "listen", and then learn proper timing. Use your eyes to mentally "touch" the opponent. As with physical touching during pushing hands, your mind will eventually be able to understand the opponent's intentions. When your eyes listen and your mind understands, you will be able to effectively intercept attacks. Eye reaction training is the most important part of the training. This is best done with a partner, practicing with different types of attacks. This will be discussed in Chapter 5 of the second volume.

In addition to visual listening, and the technique of directing some force into the side of the attacking limb so that you can adhere to it, you must also learn how to use the fingers to connect to the attacking arm so that it cannot separate from you. When someone punches at you, first adhere to his forearm with your forearm (Figure 3-126). Neutralize his attack by leading it to the side, at the same time transferring contact from your forearm to your hand (Figure 3-127). Hook your hand lightly around his arm so that you can stick to it as it advances or withdraws. This is best learned with a partner. Start with slow punches, and gradually increase the speed. Initially use arranged routines, and gradually introduce variations.

6. HER JING (Closing Jing)

Closing Jing is a defense against a sudden attack to the chest. Your hands follow the opponent's arm or arms in and "smother" his attack. Your chest arcs in and rotates sideways slightly to avoid the attack as well as to accumulate energy for a counterattack (Figure 3-128). You may also find it necessary to step back. As you smother the attack, draw his hands together and control them, creating the opportunity for a counterattack. Typical examples in the sequence are the first parts of Lift Hands and Lean Forward, and Crane Opens Wings.

This Jing is developed in Pushing Hands. As you withdraw your chest from a sudden attack, if your hands are following the opponent you will find after a while that you start smothering the attack. With further practice, you will start accumulating energy while doing the motion, and eventually counterattacking.

7. JEUAN JING (Coiling Jing or Curling Jing)

Jeuan in Chinese means to roll up, curl, or wrap. It also has the sense of a snake curling around a branch. Because it can mean curling inward or curling outward, and also coiling like a spring, it is also

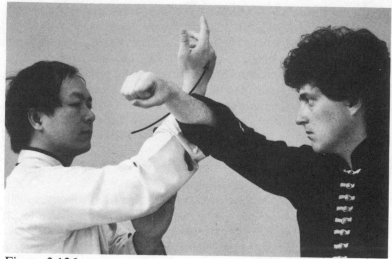

Figure 3-126.

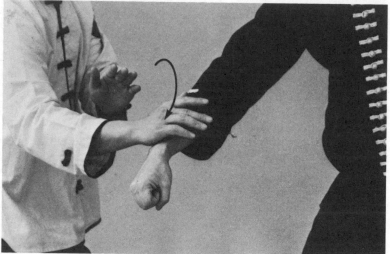

Figure 3-127.

translated coiling. In Tai Chi Chuan, Jeuan Jing refers to the clockwise or counterclockwise coiling of your arm around the opponent's arm. The body can also coil up and down to evade and neutralize the opponent. In addition to this coiling movement, the entire body, from lead hand to rear foot, also compresses and expands like a coiled spring. This springy, snakelike coiling accumulates energy in the posture, rather than in tensed muscles.

To train the hands and arms for Coiling Jing, practice wrapping and coiling your hands around a stick the way a snake coils around a branch (Figures 3-129 to 3-131). When you can wrap your hand and forearm back and forth, clockwise and counterclockwise around the stick without breaking contact, you will be able to control an opponent's arms.

8. CHAN SZU JING (Silk Reeling Jing)

Silk Reeling Jing is like Coiling Jing, except that it involves the whole

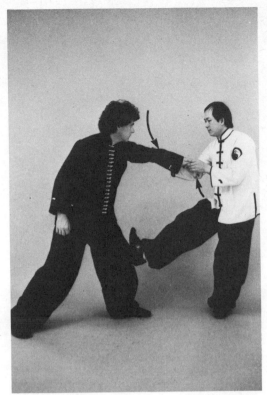

Figure 3-128.

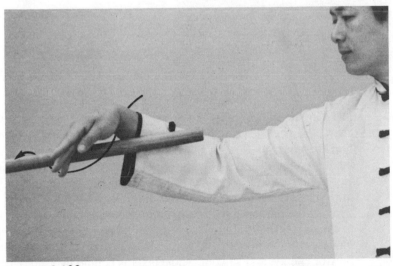

Figure 3-129.

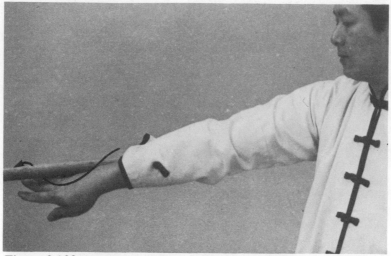

Figure 3-130.

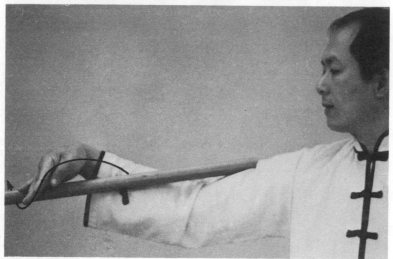

Figure 3-131.

body in the smooth back and forth coiling movements which are characteristic of Tai Chi. Whereas Coiling Jing is generally one direction at a time, Silk Reeling Jing can be an involved, continuous movement as you lead and follow the opponent, and adapt to his changes. It is a mixture Jing which contains Coiling, Prying, Drilling, Growing, Neutralizing, and Adhere-Stick Jings. When a silkworm spins its cocoon, the motion must be smooth and continuous, for any hitch in the movement will break the thread. When doing Tai Chi, your motion must be smooth and continuous so that you don't break the flow of energy, and so your whole body is behind every movement. When you pull thread from the cocoon, the cocoon spins. Chan Szu Jing also refers to this combination of linear and circular motion.

Silk Reeling Jing trains the body and hands in coiling, drilling, and growing, with both moving and fixed steps. More than this, it teaches the basic feeling of Jing—how the motion begins in the legs, and coils through the whole body and out the arms to the hands. The motion

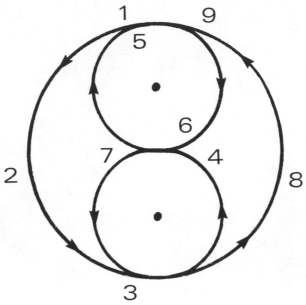

Figure 3-132.

of each part of the body comes from the motion of the part before it, e.g., the motion of the arms comes from the movement of the shoulders. Chan Szu Jing is also an excellent way to train listening, understanding, sticking and adhering, and not losing the opponent.

When using this Jing, follow the opponent's motion smoothly, whether you are evading and leading his forward motion, following his withdrawal, or controlling him as you move into an attack. While this Jing feels soft and smooth, it can be very aggressive strategically. When it is mixed with Growing, Coiling, and Drilling Jings it can be used to approach the opponent's body for further attack. When it is mixed with Neutralizing and Coiling Jings it can neutralize and control the opponent's attack and make his Jing seem to disappear into thin air. However, you must be skilled with the other Jings in order to use this Jing effectively.

To practice Silk Reeling Jing, follow the pattern of the Tai Chi symbol. There are several ways to do it, and once you learn one you can easily learn others and experiment on your own. For single person practice, as shown in Figure 3-132, start at 1 in the Bow and Arrow stance with your right palm facing out (Figure 3-133). Move your hand down to 2, rotating your hand to the right so the palm faces left (Figure 3-134). From 2 to 3, continue to rotate your hand until the palm faces up (Figure 3-135). From 3 to 4, sit back into the Four-Six stance and turn your body to the right, with the palm still facing up (Figure 3-136). From 4 to 5, turn your body to face forward, rotating your palm to

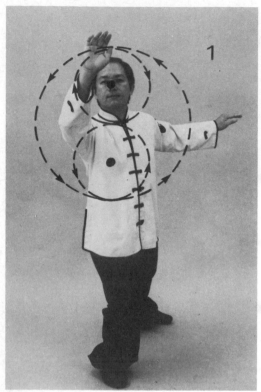

Figure 3-133.

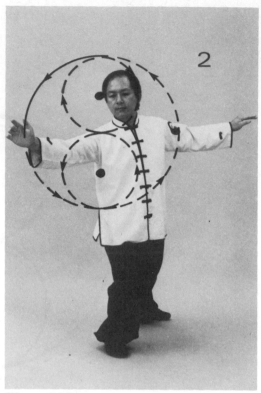

Figure 3-134.

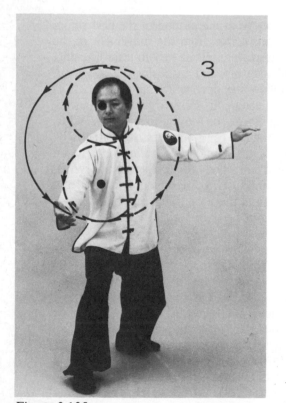

Figure 3-135.

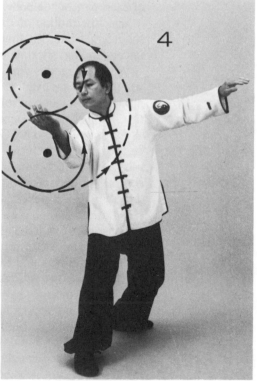

Figure 3-136.

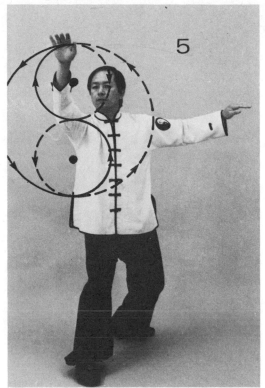

Figure 3-137.

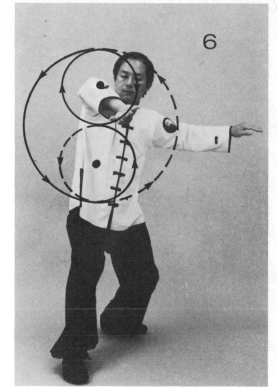

Figure 3-138.

face downward (Figure 3-137). From 5 to 6, turn your body again to the right and continue rotating your palm counterclockwise (Figure 3-138). From 6 to 7, turn your body forward and at the same time rotate your palm clockwise to face down (Figure 3-139). From 7 to 8, rotate your palm clockwise until it is facing up (Figure 3-140). Finally, from 8 to 9, change into the Bow and Arrow stance again and continue on to 1 (Figure 3-141), rotating your palm until it faces out. This pattern should be repeated continuously. The above description is only an example for the Tai Chi beginner. Once you are familiar with the above movements you can vary your stance or add stepping to coordinate the direction of the coiling with your strategy.

For two person Silk Reeling Jing training, the Tai Chi pattern is still used. However, you will complete only half of the cycle, and your partner will do the other half. As shown in Figure 3-142, one person is active and completes 1 to 4, then his partner becomes active and finishes from 4 to 7. When you are active, you neutralize, coil, drill, and grow. When you are passive, you listen, understand, stick and adhere. While practicing, your right forearm and wrist maintain contact with your partner's forearm and wrist (Figure 3-143). Starting at 1, circle down to 2 in the Bow and Arrow stance (Figure 3-144). Then shift your weight back into a Four-Six stance, turn your body to the right and at the same time rotate your palm until it faces up (Figure 3-145). At 4, your partner will take the active role, starting in the Bow and Arrow stance, repeating the same motions you made

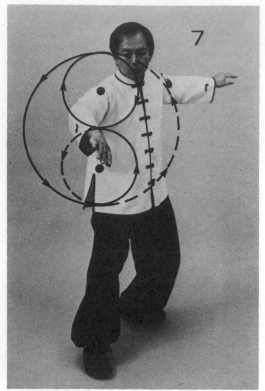

Figure 3-139.

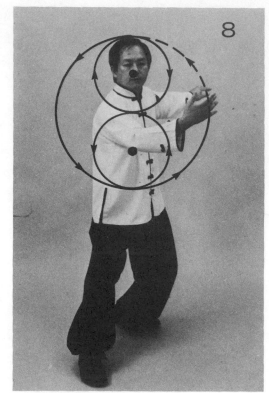

Figure 3-140.

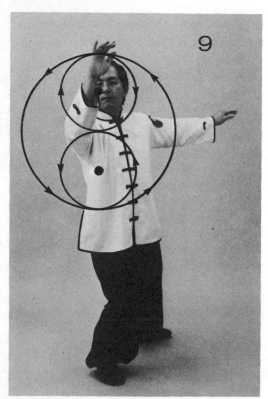

Figure 3-141.

Two Person

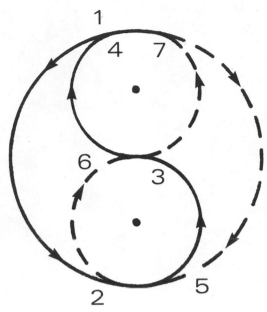

Figure 3-142.

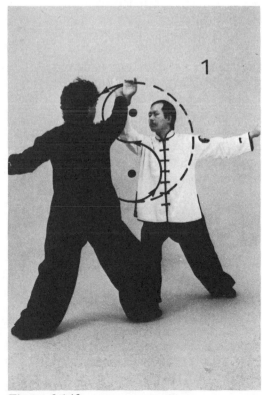

Figure 3-143.

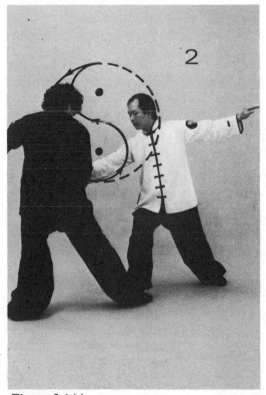

Figure 3-144.

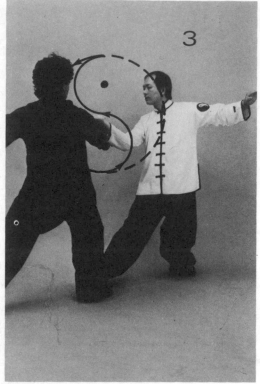

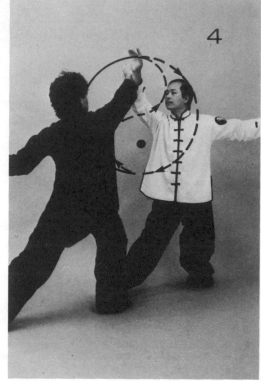

Figure 3-145.   Figure 3-146.

(Figures 3-146 to 3-149). First practice this exercise standing stationary, and when you are familiar with the techniques, practice coordinating stepping with the movements as you circle both to the right and to the left.

Two person Silk Reeling Jing training can also be done while you and your partner are stepping forward and backward. This allows you to switch from right hand to left hand practice and back. When you reach 1 during continuous practice you should neutralize your partner's power to the right. You can then use this opportunity to step forward and attack your partner's chest (Figures 3-150 and 3-151) or throat with your left hand (Figure 3-152). In order to prevent your attack, your partner must step back and use his left hand to intercept your attack (Figure 3-153). Once connected, he should continue the moving pattern. Alternately, you can attack your partner while your hand is up at 1. You can then step your left leg forward and attack your partner's chest under his right arm. Your partner should step backward and connect his left arm with yours.

9. JIUE JING (Prying Jing or Lever Jing)

Prying Jing is used when you twist your arm to escape from an opponent's grasp, or to free yourself from his sticking control. It is usually used when your techniques have been locked or sealed by your opponent's Controlling Jing, and you are in a bad position, or when you are held (Figure 3-154). When this happens, drop your elbow suddenly to reverse the situation (Figure 3-155). Do not try to move his

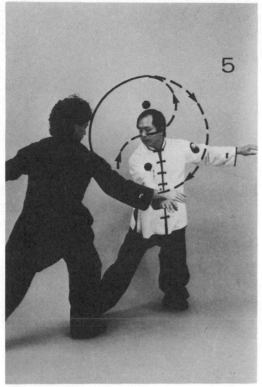

Figure 3-147.

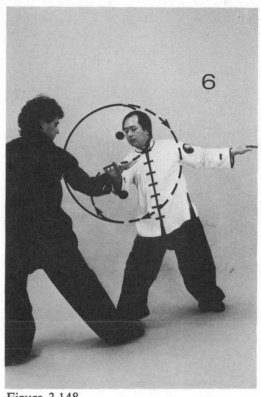

Figure 3-148.

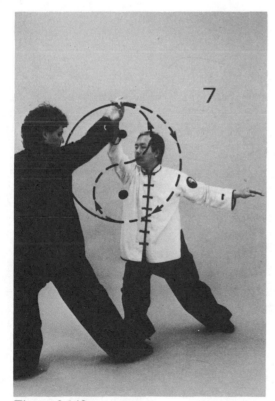

Figure 3-149.

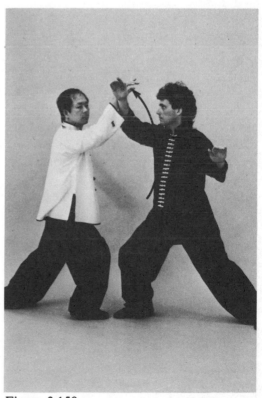

Figure 3-150.

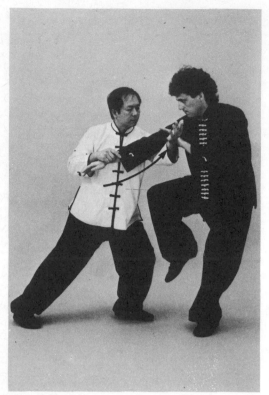

Figure 3-151.

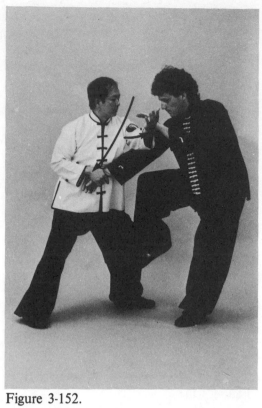

Figure 3-152.

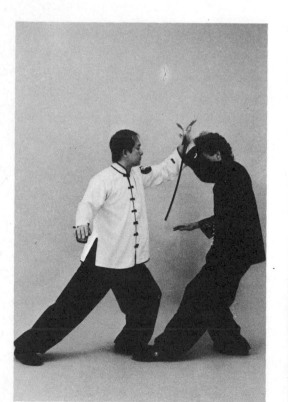

Figure 3-153.

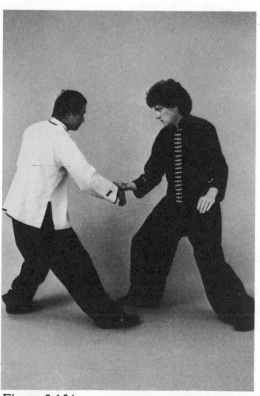

Figure 3-154.

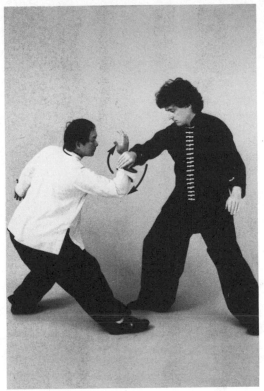

Figure 3-155.

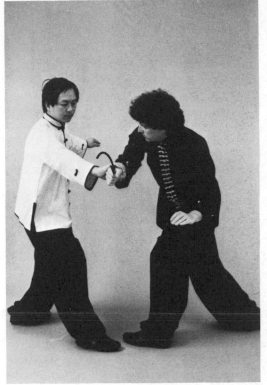

Figure 3-156.

hand, since this would be force against force. Instead use one part of his hand as a fulcrum, and lever your hand out of his grasp. Drop your body so that your whole weight is behind your arm motion, and adjust your stance as appropriate. As your hand is escaping, immediately rotate your hand and arm so that you now control him (Figure 3-156). This technique can be used even when the opponent is holding your arm with both his hands. Escapes such as this are usually done with Cold Jing so that the opponent has no warning or chance to change his technique.

To practice Prying Jing, have your partner grab your wrist or stick to and control your arm. Experiment with different ways to lever your arm free. Remember—don't fight his grasp. Use your weight to put all your force against one or two of his fingers.

b. Defense With Some Offense (Some Yang in Yin) Jing:

   1. HUAH JING (Neutralizing Jing. Literally, to smelt, change, influence.)

     Neutralizing Jing is using four ounces to repel one thousand pounds. It is an insubstantial Jing, but it is not purely Yin—there is also some Yang in it. This means that when you understand your opponent's Jing, you use a little power to neutralize and lead it to the side, upward, or downward. Figure 3-157 shows the direction of the opponent's Jing and your Jing as you neutralize the attack. This is different from Yielding Jing, which is purely yielding without any

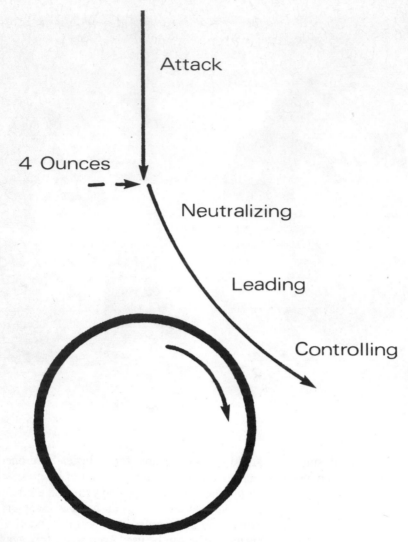

Attack

4 Ounces

Neutralizing

Leading

Controlling

Figure 3-157.

pressure on your part. Neutralizing Jing is a combination of Sticking, Yielding, and Leading Jings. It is somewhat active, whereas Yielding Jing is purely passive. Usually, as you are using Neutralizing Jing you are also storing part of your energy for a counterattack. It is said that "Huah has some Peng Jing (Wardoff)", because you sometimes bounce the opponent away as you neutralize his attack. This saying also implies that you often have to put a little force into the opponent's arm in order to connect to it (see Intercepting Jing).

The key to Neutralizing Jing is timing. This is the Jing of using the enemy's power against him, so when the enemy's Yi (mind) has already started to attack and he is about to emit Jing, you must immediately seize this opportunity to neutralize. If you wait until your opponent's Jing is almost all emitted, unless you are an expert, it will be too late to use four ounces to neutralize his one thousand pounds. Thus, it is said: "The opponent does not move, I do not move; the opponent moves slightly, I move first" (Appendix A-3).

Wherever you feel pressure, neutralize. Do not use the arms and shoulders, because that would be Li (muscular strength) and not good Tai Chi. You must rely totally on the waist and legs to neutralize the attack. Stick to the opponent and follow his posture, speed and height. As his attack comes in straight, your neutralization should be curved. Neutralization is a circle. When you are a beginner, your circle will be large, but as your skill increases the circle will get smaller and smaller. A large circle gives you more time to listen, understand, and then neutralize. However, when the circle is large your opponent has time to sense your intention and change his strategy. A Tai Chi expert whose circle is small will wait until the opponent's Jing is almost all out and his Yi is fully on the attack. Then, when he reacts, the opponent will not be able to change his motion. Of course, this small circle defense is dangerous because it lets the opponent's attack almost reach your body. You must be very quick and good at listening, understanding, and neutralizing, otherwise you will not succeed. This is why it is said :"First look to expanding, then look to compacting, then you approach perfection"(Appendix A-3).

Some beginners believe that yielding is neutralization, but this is not the case. Neutralization must use some force, because an attack may be very strong. It is wrong to believe that Tai Chi Chuan relies only on softness. The best Tai Chi masters look very soft on the outside, but on the inside they are as hard as steel. It is not only that their Yi (Mind) is strong, but their internal Jing is also strong. This strength does not show on the outside. It is also wrong to believe that the mind directly guides the Jing. If you use your mind to directly control the muscles, Chi support will be limited and muscular strength will predominate. Rather the mind should guide the Chi, which in turn guides the Jing. This is how to use the truly internal energy called Jing. If you use this Jing to neutralize, using the correct timing and a correct understanding of the opponent, then you can truly neutralize a force of one thousand pounds with four ounces.

Neutralization begins with Adhere-Connect and Stick-Follow. Once these are developed, you will begin to understand Jing, which means that you will be able to understand the opponent's intentions. Once you understand his intentions you will be able to neutralize effectively, and then you will be light and agile.

You must neutralize correctly before you can counterattack effectively. If you cannot neutralize effectively to gain an advantage, how can your own attack succeed? If a martial artist's skill is high, he may move forward as he neutralizes, perhaps counterattacking at the same time. In this case the upper body looks like it is withdrawing, but the legs are already moving forward. The best way to learn Neutralizing Jing is through pushing hands practice. You can also stand with your arm in the Wardoff position, and have your partner apply Push Jing. The moment you feel his energy, withdraw slightly and turn your body. Adhere to his arm. Do not push his arm away, instead lead it to the side. This is done by turning your body, not by moving your arm independently of your body. In the beginning you may deflect his attack at a 45 degree angle, but as you gain in skill, the angle will get smaller.

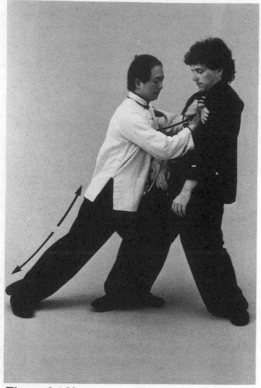

Figure 3-158.

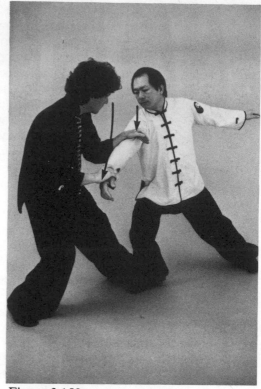

Figure 3-159.

2. GHI JING (Press Jing, literally to squeeze or compress)

Press Jing is a push which is often applied at an angle to the original line of motion. A hand is held against the forearm or wrist (Figure 3-158) to press against the opponent's arms, shoulder, or body in order to knock him down or push him away. The technique may also be used as a strike.

Press is often used to counter the opponent's Rollback Jing. For example, if you push and the opponent uses Rollback on your right arm (Figure 3-159), first adjust your waist and legs to put yourself in a good position and the opponent in a bad position. Place your left hand on your right forearm where you intend to apply force, and use Press in the correct direction to make the opponent lose his balance (Figure 3-160). Press Jing is also commonly used to counter Shoulder-Stroke (Figure 3-161) or Elbow-Stroke (Figure 3-162). Again, you must first adjust your position, and then press the opponent either from inside (Figure 3-163) or from the back (Figure 3-164) to make him lose his balance.

When Press is used as a strike, it is sharp and short. The striking zones are usually on the chest or shoulder blade. When certain targets such as the solar plexus or the cavities near the nipples (Yingchuang, Rugen, and Jiuwei)(Figure 3-165) are struck, the opponent's breath can be sealed. When the center of the shoulder blade (Tianzong)(Figure 3-166) is attacked, it can make the opponent's entire arm and shoulder numb. In order to strike the chest, you usually use Small Rollback

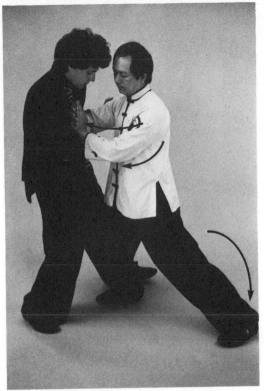

Figure 3-160.

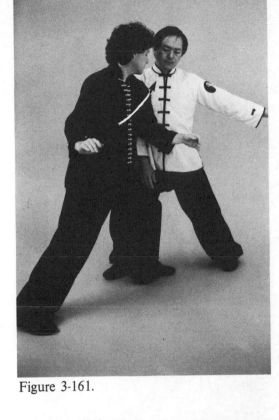

Figure 3-161.

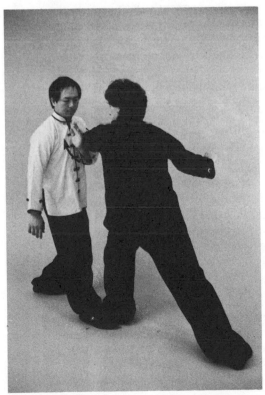

Figure 3-162.

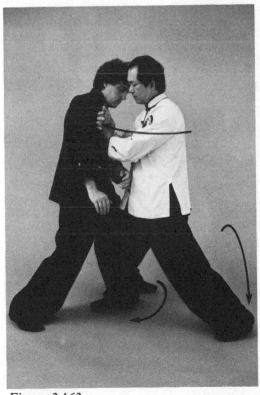

Figure 3-163.

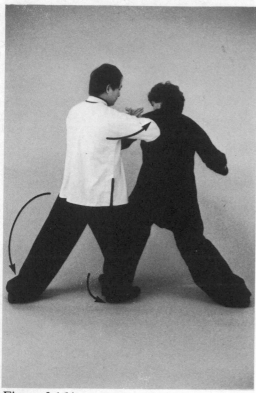

Figure 3-164.

(see Rollback Jing) first to open up the opponent's chest area. Right after the Rollback is applied, immediately use Press Jing to strike his solar plexus or nipple area to seal his breath. When you want to attack the shoulder blade, first use Large Rollback to break the opponent's root and expose his shoulder blade (see Rollback Jing). You may then use Press Jing to strike his shoulder to numb his arm.

When using Press Jing, do not use Li from the arm, because the opponent will be able to use his Li against it. Use the Jing from the legs and control it with your waist. When pressing the opponent, your body should be centered and stable—it should not lean in the direction you are pressing. When you are executing an upward Press, your Yi should be on breaking the opponent's root. Sometimes a small amount of Lifting Jing is used just before the Press to make the opponent float. Press can also be applied downward. This is used to seal the opponent's arms and open him up for a second attack.

Press can be trained on a bag or partner in the same way Wardoff is trained. It is often practiced on a partner in combination with Rollback (see Volume 2, Chapter 3 for Rollback and Press training).

3. LIE JING (Rend Jing)

When you rend or tear something, you pull it in two directions at once. When you use Rend Jing, you use your two hands or your hands and a foot to tear the opponent off his stance. This often has a whirlpool effect, as you twist him down.

When Rend Jing is used for attack, it is frequently used right after

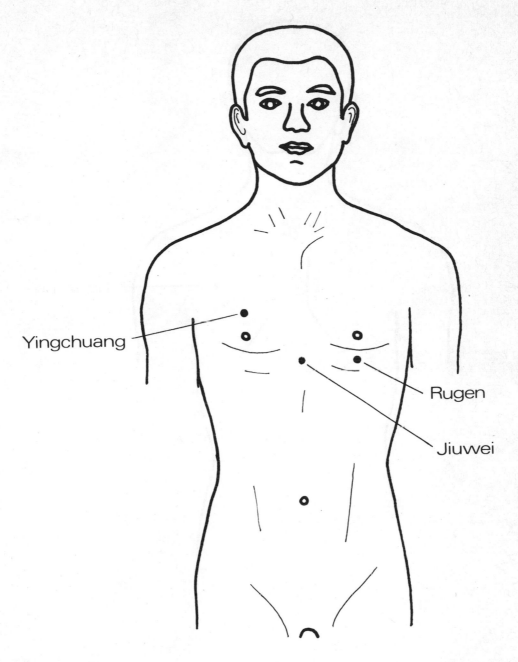

Yingchuang

Rugen

Jiuwei

Figure 3-165.

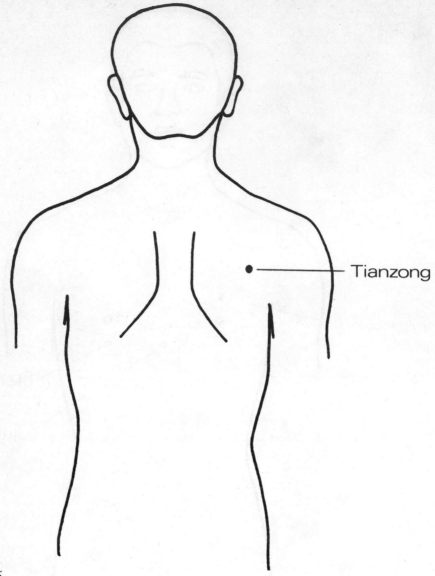

Tianzong

Figure 3-166.

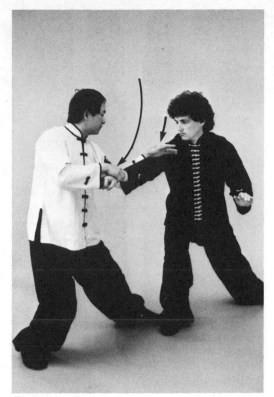

Figure 3-167.

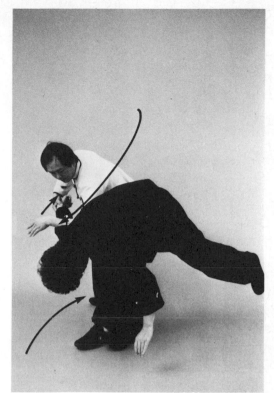

Figure 3-168.

Rollback Jing or Pluck Jing. For example, when you use Rollback and have your opponent in an unstable position, twist your body to change the direction of your pull (Figures 3-167 and 3-168). Before your opponent can regain his balance, your Rend Jing pulls him off his feet. The same principle applies when Rend Jing is used after Pluck Jing. If you have pulled your opponent's lead arm to his left and have unbalanced him, you can block his front leg with your left leg and take him down (Figures 3-169 and 3-170). Alternatively, if your Pluck causes the opponent to resist, you may be able to step behind his leg and use Rend in the direction of his movement, taking him down to his rear (Figures 3-171 and 3-172).

When Rend Jing is used for defense, first change the direction of your opponent's attack and make him miss his target, then use Rend Jing to make him lose his balance. For example, when your opponent uses Rollback Jing, do not resist, but instead calm yourself and follow his Jing. Change the direction of his Jing by rotating your body, lock one of his legs with your leg, and pull him off his feet (Figures 3-173 to 3-175). In this case you have used your enemy's Rollback Jing against him.

To use Rend Jing effectively you must have a firm root, otherwise when you try to move your opponent you will lose your own root and be controlled by him. As with any other technique, you must use the correct timing and choose the right opportunity. If you can sense your opponent's intention just before his Jing is completely out,

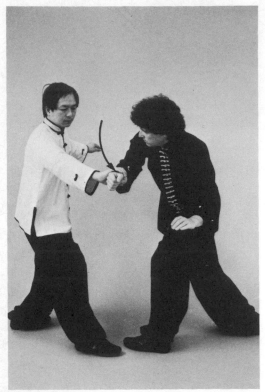

Figure 3-169.

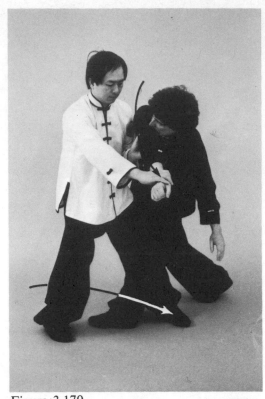

Figure 3-170.

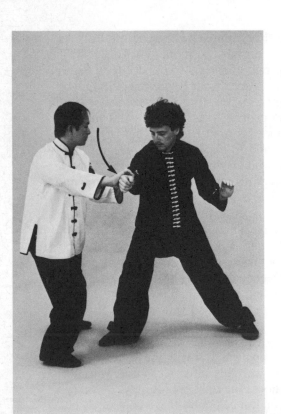

Figure 3-171.

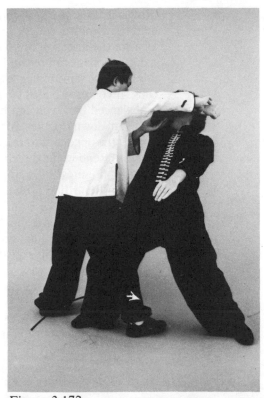

Figure 3-172.

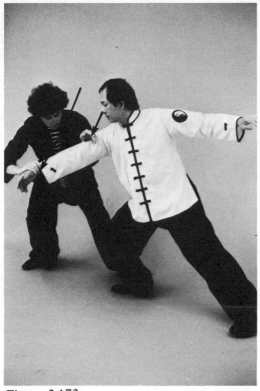

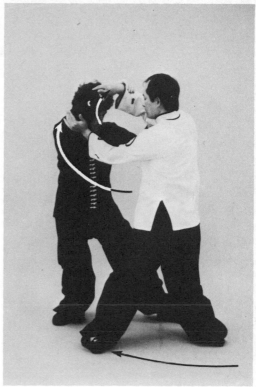

Figure 3-173.　　　　　　　　　Figure 3-174.

you will have the best chance for success. When you are using Rend as a takedown, don't use Jing until you have the opponent either un-balanced or overextended, so that he will lose his balance the moment you apply Jing.

Rend Jing can be trained through pushing hands and by practicing individual applications with a partner.

4. KAU JING (Shoulder-Stroke Jing)

Shoulder-Stroke Jing uses the shoulder to attack the opponent. This Jing can be long or short—long to bounce or throw the opponent, short to strike, particularly to the solar plexus or shoulder blade cavi-ty. The outside of the shoulder is especially used for striking, while the front and back are often used for throwing the opponent. Shoulder techniques can be applied in any direction.

Shoulder-Stroke is frequently used when your opponent uses Rollback against you (Figure 3-176). Follow the direction of his Rollback, then redirect the force toward him and use your shoulder to bounce him away or strike him (Figure 3-177). This Jing can be used anytime your enemy's chest, shoulder blade, or armpit are ex-posed to attack. When used as a strike, Shoulder-Stroke is similar to Elbow-Stroke, except that it is done from a shorter range.

Shoulder-Stroke Jing is also used in throwing or takedown techni-ques. The opponent can be thrown with the same motion you use to throw a shovelful of snow over your shoulder (Figure 3-178), or

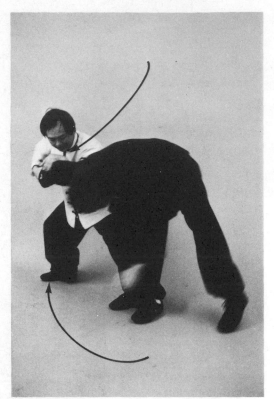

Figure 3-175.

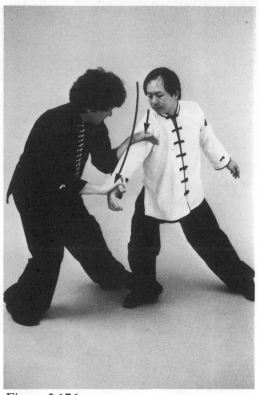

Figure 3-176.

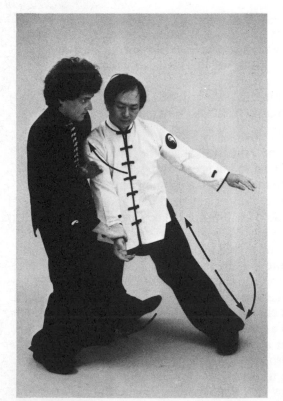

Figure 3-177.

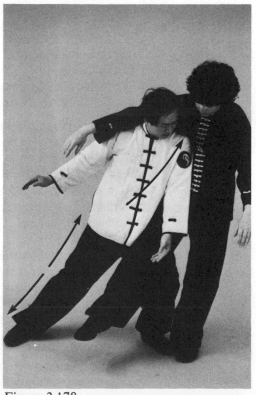

Figure 3-178.

taken down over your leg with a shrug of your shoulder (Figures 3-179 and 3-180).

Shoulder-Stroke Jing can be practiced on a bag. Be sure to step in close enough so that you don't have to lean. Practice sharp strikes and slower pushes. You can also catch the bag on your arm, roll it toward your shoulder as you withdraw slightly and coil to accumulate energy, and then bounce the bag away.

When you practice with a partner, a kicking bag or other type of padding (Figure 3-181) will let you use full power without hurting him. You can practice pushes and light strikes without cushioning if your partner holds his arms across his body for protection (Figure 3-182). His arms should be touching his chest so that they don't absorb the force of your technique. Diagonal Flying and similar techniques also use the shoulder, and can be practiced with a partner.

5. YINN JING (Leading Jing)

Leading Jing moves with the opponent's force to lead him into a disadvantageous position. It is usually used between Neutralizing Jing and Controlling Jing. When the opponent attacks, neutralize his attack until most of his Jing has been expended. Lead his remaining Jing so that he becomes overextended, unbalanced, or otherwise vulnerable to attack. Leading Jing uses the other person's Jing, adds to it, and either redirects it or leads it further than he had intended.

This Jing is usually easy to apply to beginning Tai Chi students and to people who throw their weight forward when they attack. It is harder to use against the more experienced fighter. When your opponent keeps some of his Jing in reserve and is wary of being led, you have to use false Leading Jings to confuse him. You may have to lead him high and attack low, or lead him straight and attack laterally.

Since Leading Jing works together with Listening, Understanding, and Neutralizing Jings, the only way to learn it is through pushing hands. To learn Leading Jing, after you have neutralized your partner's attack, lead it a little further. Only experience can teach you how to lead his Jing, and how to put him into positions that allow you to attack. This is a subtle Jing, so be careful not to get into the habit of hauling on the other person's arms. If you can't lead him, don't force it. Wait for another opportunity when you can smoothly lead him a little further than he had intended.

6. JIEH JING (Borrowing Jing)

Borrowing Jing is the trick of using the opponent's Jing so that he is bounced out by his own power. It is one of the hardest Jings to understand and apply, but once you understand it you will have a great advantage in a fight. It is a high art which, when mastered, may even be done without your conscious attention.

Many Tai Chi practitioners misunderstand this Jing, thinking it is like Neutralizing Jing or Yielding Jing. Others may think that to apply Borrowing Jing you follow the opponent's Jing and add your own Jing to his to make him fall. In fact, that would be a combination of yielding and leading—the real Borrowing Jing is more aggressive. If the opponent attacks, you bounce him, if he is about to attack but

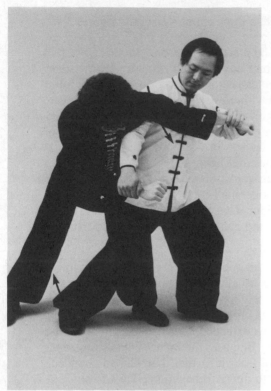

Figure 3-179.

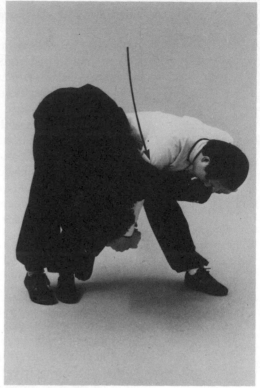

Figure 3-180.

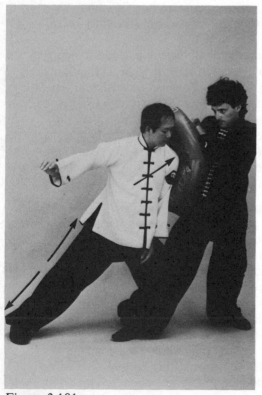

Figure 3-181.

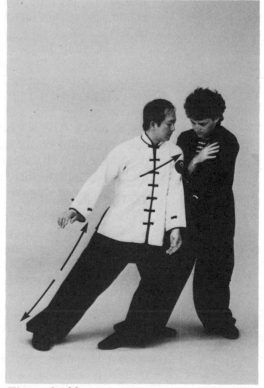

Figure 3-182.

hasn't yet attacked, you still bounce him. With Borrowing Jing you give back just what you were given—if the opponent's Jing is hard, so is yours; if his is soft, so is yours. Usually you need to use only a small amount of Jing, which can be applied through almost any part of your body.

Stability is extremely important, as is the coordination of the waist and legs. However, the most important factor is timing. There are two timings that can be used. The first is when your opponent is just about to emit his Jing, but has not yet emitted it. This is the same timing that is used with Neutralizing Jing. It is easier than the second timing and is usually learned first. When the opponent is about to emit his Jing, his Yi is already on moving forward. Use your Resisting Jing to catch him just as he emits his Jing. Since you prevent his forward motion, he will push himself away. If you add some of your Jing to his momentum, you can bounce him far away. The classics say:"The opponent does not move, I do not move; the opponent moves slightly, I move first"(Appendix A-3). We can use an example to explain this. When a person is about to step through a door, and has lifted his foot and started to move forward, if the door is suddenly shut, the person will usually be bounced backward. If the timing is right, you do not need much energy to do this.

The second timing is just before your opponent's Jing is completely out. When someone is striking you, his Yi is on the striking, and this Yi is focusing his Jing so that it reaches its maximum at a point inside your body. If you stop his forward motion just before his Jing reaches its maximum, his Yi will be interrupted, but he will not be able to stop his forward energy. As with the previous timing, since he cannot go forward, his energy will bounce back to him. If his arms have any stiffness he will bounce backward, especially if you add your own energy to the motion. In order to understand this, imagine that someone is punching you, and you are holding a strong, resilient balloon in front of you. If you move the balloon forward into his punch just before the punch reaches the balloon, you will find that his power will not just be stopped, it will be bounced back into him. You can see that this Borrowing Jing is higher than the one mentioned above.

In order to use either timing, you must be skilled in Resisting Jing, and must have your Chi developed throughout your body so that your body is resilient like a balloon, yet strong enough to bounce back the opponent's power. A strong root is also necessary to absorb the other person's power and send it back to him. Your opponent should have the feeling that he is pushing a wall which pushes back at him at the same time, so that he only succeeds in pushing himself away from it. Borrowing Jing requires a high level of Understanding Jing, and great subtlety. If your opponent sees that you are alert and ready for him, he will be very careful. If he thinks you are vulnerable, then he will attack with a lot of force. There are stories of Tai Chi masters bouncing opponents several yards away. The harder the opponent attacks, the further he bounces.

When you have mastered the basic Jings and wish to practice Borrowing Jing, have a partner push you and work on the first timing. Try to catch him just as he is about to emit his Jing. When you

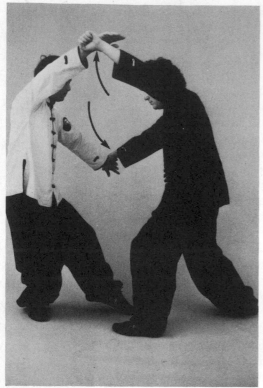

Figure 3-183.

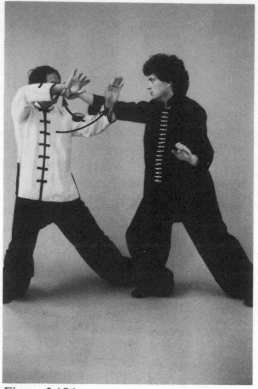

Figure 3-184.

perceive his Jing, direct it into your root and let it bounce directly back into him. Add a small amount of your own Jing, but not too much. Rather than trying to push him as he is pushing you, guide him so that he pushes himself away from you. To practice the second timing, yield before your partner's attack, and when his energy is three quarters expended, direct the rest of it into your root and let him bounce off your root.

7. KAI JING or **JANN JING** (Opening Jing or Spreading Jing)

Opening (or Spreading) Jing is one of the most basic Jings in the martial arts. When your opponent's Jing is coming toward you, connect to his arm and "open" your arms to lead him to the side. This is a long Jing, so the muscles are used more than with other Jings. When the opponent attacks, connect to his arm and neutralize, then lead him further. Grasp his wrist or other joint as necessary, then "open" or "spread" your arms, pulling him into an exposed position so you can strike him. In the Tai Chi sequence, many forms belong to this Jing such as Crane Opens Wings (Figure 3-183) and Seal Tightly (Figure 3-184).

Train this Jing during Pushing Hands the way you would train Leading Jing. As you neutralize your partner's attack, "close" your body (arc your back and draw in your arms near your body). Then "open" your body to extend his motion.

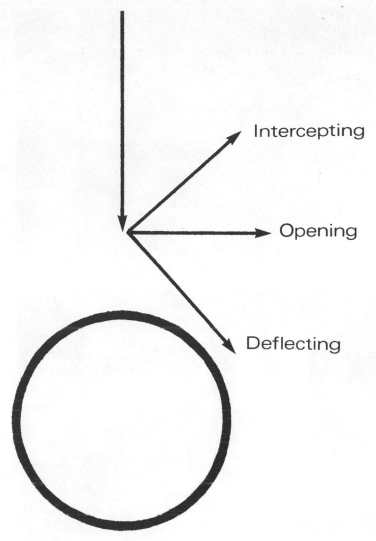

Intercepting

Opening

Deflecting

Figure 3-185.

8. BO JING (Deflecting Jing)

Deflecting Jing is similar to Opening Jing, except that you deflect the attack past you and to your rear. Since you are changing the course of the opponent's attack only slightly, your arms do not extend out very far. Figure 3-185 shows the difference between Deflecting, Opening and Intercepting Jings. With Deflecting Jing you are only in contact with the opponent's arm for a short time. You do not try to adhere to his arm, rather you deflect it past you so that you can counterattack.

To train this Jing, have your partner punch your chest (Figure 3-186), and use your arm to deflect it to the side (Figure 3-187). Your main action is to turn your body so that the waist does the work and not your arm. Your body must withdraw somewhat so that you do not deflect the attack too sharply to the side.

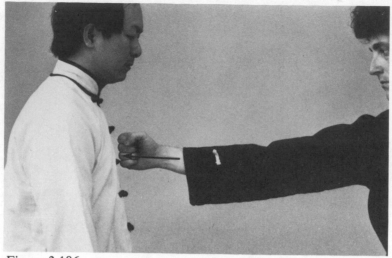

Figure 3-186.

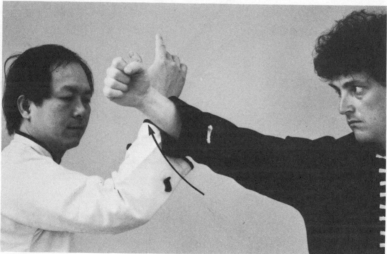

Figure 3-187.

9. JOAN JING (Turning Jing or Twisting Jing)

Turning Jing is a turning movement generated by the waist and expressed through any part of the body. Sometimes when you are grabbed or controlled you can reverse the situation and gain the advantage just by turning or twisting part of your body such as the wrist, arm, or waist. Many offensive Chin Na moves uses this Jing. Offensive or defensive, the motion is generated by the waist. This allows you to get your whole body behind the move so that it is strong without needing much force.

When your opponent grabs your right wrist with his right hand and pulls down (Figure 3-188), first use Prying Jing to drop your elbow and loosen his grip. At the same time, use Turning Jing to turn your wrist so that your palm faces him and can grasp and control his wrist (Figure 3-189). Another example is Wave Hands in Clouds. Assume your opponent has grasped your right wrist with his right hand (Figure 3-190). Rotate your body to the right and rotate your palm to face

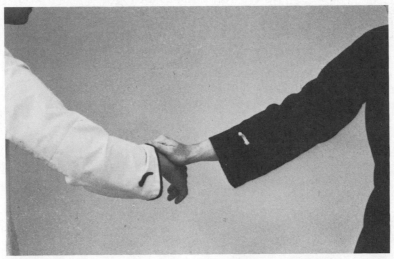

Figure 3-188.

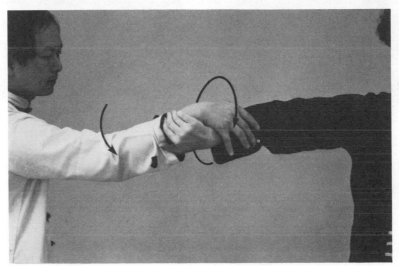

Figure 3-189.

out (Figure 3-191), putting the opponent into a defending position. This turning is done with the whole body so that he cannot easily resist it.

Turning Jing is also used in Chin Na to control the opponent. For example, once you have grasped your opponent's wrist, put your forearm on his elbow (Figure 3-192), and then rotate your whole body downward to control him (Figure 3-193). If you also turn to the side you will spiral the opponent down and pull him off his root. This application is similar to Rend, only longer.

Practice Turning Jing with a partner. Consult the Chin Na applications discussed in Volume 2.

10. JER DYE JING (Folding and Entwining Jing)

Folding and Entwining Jing is the use of small turning and leading movements of the hands and arms to evade, redirect, and control the opponent's arms. Folding is when one part of the body bends to escape

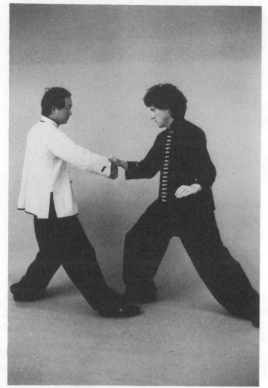

Figure 3-190.

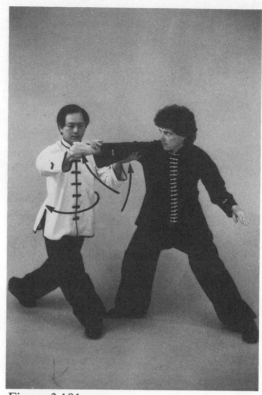

Figure 3-191.

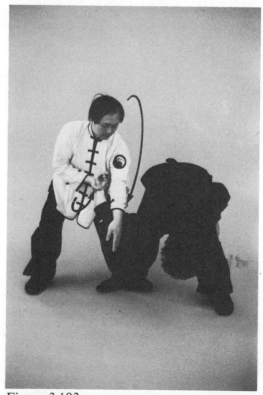

Figure 3-192.

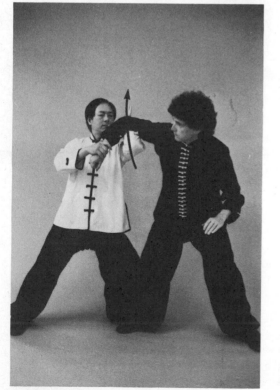

Figure 3-193.

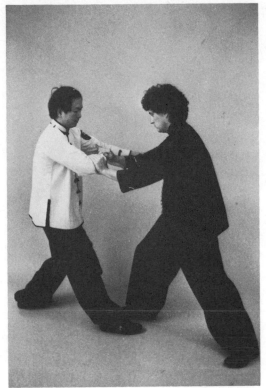

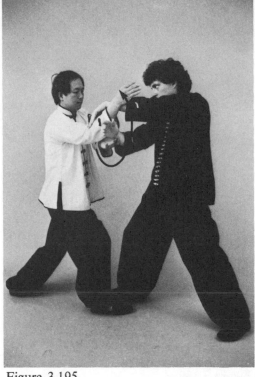

Figure 3-194.   Figure 3-195.

being controlled. This motion is easily continued into a spiralling movement through which your hands entwine or wrap around the opponent's arms and control them. This Jing is a combination of Leading,
Controlling, Prying and Coiling Jings. It is frequently used in Chin
Na and pushing hands. For example, when the opponent controls one
of your arms, that arm evades or escapes while your other arm leads
the opponent's hand away or controls it (Figures 3-194 to 3-198).
Although there is relatively little body motion in this Jing, the waist
must still guide the motion so that the whole body can support it.
This Jing is very common in southern martial styles such as tiger,
snake, and crane, which, like Tai Chi, emphasize close-range fighting.

    To practice this Jing during Pushing Hands, lead your partner's
Jing and wrap your hands around his arms. Keep alert for opportunities to continue the spiralling of his arms into Chin Na techniques. See the smear training in the Pushing Hands chapter in Volume
2.

C. Neutral (Neither Offense nor Defense) Jing:

1. DOU SOU JING (Trembling Jing or Shaking Jing)

    This Jing is a sudden trembling or shaking of the body which is
used primarily as a training method for generating and transmitting
Jing. You can also use it when you are held tightly, as in a bear hug,
to escape or even cause serious internal injury to your attacker. It
is sometimes used to raise the Spirit of Vitality.

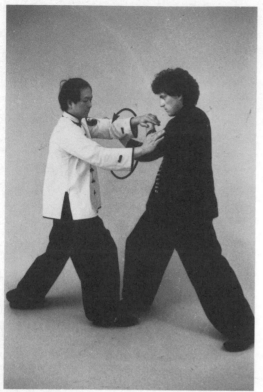

Figure 3-196.

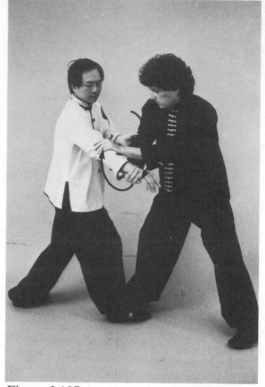

Figure 3-197.

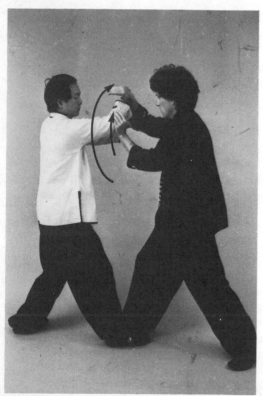

Figure 3-198.

To get an idea of this Jing, watch a dog or bird shake water off its body. You will notice that the motion is like a shiver in that it is a sudden, almost compulsive explosion of motion and energy. There is a lot of energy expended in a small space, and the water can fly quite a ways. The animal's stance is very stable, and the power is generated from the inside out. These are very important principles in the generation of Jing. Chang San-Feng's Tai Chi Classic states that:"The root is in the feet, (power is) generated from the legs, controlled by the waist and expressed by the fingers. From the feet to the legs to the waist must be integrated, and one unified Chi"(Appendix A-1). The Tai Chi beginner must learn these principles before he can apply his Jing to anything else.

To practice this Jing, stand in a stable stance and relax. Imagine that you are shaking water off your whole body. First twist your body to one side, then twist back and forth in a quick, shiver-like motion. Generate the Jing in your legs, and use your waist to lead it to your shoulders and arms. Do not try to control the movement too much, or you will be stiff and the energy will not reach your limbs.

2. DING JING (Upright Jing)

Upright Jing is a Jing which can be felt but not seen. It is the Jing which a fighter uses to hold his body upright and centered, and at the same time raise his Spirit of Vitality. It is said:"An insubstantial energy leads the head upward. The Chi is sunk to the Dan Tien"(Appendix A-2). This is an example of the division of substantial and insubstantial in the body. Let the Chi sink to your abdomen so that it becomes substantial, and your upper body and head become insubstantial. As the Chi sinks, there is a corresponding rising of energy and a lifting of the head from inside. You can also imagine that you are suspended like a puppet from a string on the top of your head. Since the top of your head is being lifted, the rest of your body sinks and the substantial settles in your abdomen.

In this Jing, Yi is more important and critical than the form. When your Yi is balanced up and down, your body will be upright, the root will be firm, and your spirit will be raised. Ding Jing training is closely related to rooting training since the downward Rooting Jing will enhance and help to balance the Upright Jing.

3. PAN JING (Rooting Jing)

Rooting Jing is the energy of sinking your root deep into the ground. A good root is necessary for stability as well as for the generation and transmission of energy. Rooting Jing can also be used defensively when your opponent tries to move you or knock you down. This Jing training is very popular among Chinese martial styles. It is commonly called Chian Gin Juey (Thousand Pound Sinking). In this training, your Yi is the key to success—you must imagine that you weigh a thousand pounds and your opponent can't move you even slightly. Your entire Yi is straight down and the Chi is directed a few inches beneath your feet.

A good way to train this Jing is by standing in a horse stance on bricks (Figure 3-199). Your Yi must be directed straight downward—if your Yi is scattered your feet will move sideward and the bricks will fall. This training can also be done on ice or marbles.

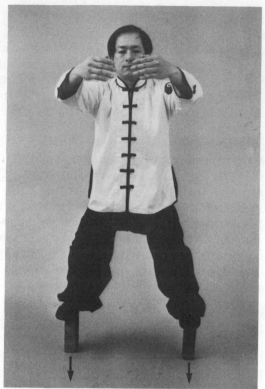

Figure 3-199.

4. LIN KORN JING (Aloft Jing)

Aloft Jing is the energy generated in the waist, legs, and feet for jumping. This Jing is used whenever a Tai Chi fighter needs to jump up for kicking or withdrawing. As with the Jing in the arms, the use of Li is cut to a minimum. In Aloft Jing, the waist starts the motion, then the legs contribute their energy, and finally the feet push off the ground. The Chi sinks down to support the action. This Jing is harder than any of the Jings applied through the hands. In ancient times good Tai Chi masters were said to be able to jump several yards into the air. Because this Jing is hard to understand and train, it has been gradually ignored.

D. Leg Jing (Twe Jing):

The Jings discussed above are expressed primarily through the hands, arms, and shoulders. When Jing is expressed through the legs, the principles of generation and expression are somewhat different. The Jing which is expressed by the upper body is rooted in the feet, generated by the legs, and controlled by the waist. When you kick you are on only one foot, and so your root and your ability to generate Jing are weakened significantly. Since it is more difficult to maintain your center and balance, it is harder for your waist to control and direct the Jing. When your body's balance is off, it is also more difficult to balance your Jing and Chi, and your power is cut down considerably.

Although there are many difficulties in the training, the legs can still be very powerful and effective tools in combat. They are longer than the arms, and can therefore attack sooner and from a greater range. There is a saying in Chinese martial society "One centimeter longer, one centimeter of advantage" (Yi fen charng, yi fen li). This means that if your weapon is longer than your opponent's, you have an advantage. Furthermore, because the legs are well below eye level, it is harder to sense their attacks. To remedy this, Chinese martial artists train to watch and sense the opponent's shoulder movement. Whenever someone attacks with either hands or legs, his shoulders must move first. If you have enough experience, you should be able to sense your opponent's intention just before his attack starts.

Because the legs have stronger muscles, they can still generate a great deal of power even if Chi is not used. If you know how to use your Chi to express Jing through your legs, your legs will be more powerful than your hands and they will be undefeatable. Some kicks, particularly low kicks, can be done without sacrificing too many of the conditions necessary for the generation of Jing.

Chinese martial artists have researched different ways of kicking to minimize the reduction of Jing. They have divided the kicks into four categories: Low Kicks, Middle Kicks, High Kicks, and Spinning Kicks. Each of these four groups has advantages and disadvantages. There are at least 40 different kicking techniques trained in the different styles of Chinese martial arts. Tai Chi Chuan uses only a few kicking techniques, most of them low, to assist the hand techniques. The hands remain the main weapons in Tai Chi Chuan.

a. Low Kicks:

Of all the kicking techniques, low kicks are probably the fastest, safest, and most effective. These kicks specialize in attacking the knee and below. The most common targets are the knee, leg (Tiaokou and Zhongdu cavities), ankle (Jiexi cavity), and foot (Taichong cavity)(Figures 3-200 and 3-201). Most of the southern martial styles emphasize low kicks. There is a proverb that says: "Tzwu bu guoh shi" (foot not higher than the knee). This is because whenever you kick higher than the knee, you start losing your center and stability. Not only that, you open the door to the groin area which your opponent can take advantage of. Furthermore, a kick higher than the knee is easier to block.

When kicking low, it is still usually possible to maintain enough of your center, balance, and stability to generate Jing. Even though your waist control is limited, you can train your legs to develop a high level of destructive power. The disadvantage of low kicks is that they are short range. In order to use them for middle and long range, it is necessary to hop or jump to approach the opponent. However, whenever you do this, you lose your root, stability, and balance. For this reason, the middle, high, and spinning kicks usually predominate in long range fighting.

Because of these reasons, and because of the adhere-stick principle, Tai Chi emphasizes mostly short range fighting and low kicks. The common kicks in Tai Chi Chuan are Tsae, Chuay, Di Chie, Di Chiau, and Di Shaou. The general principles for generating Jing are the same for all of the low kicks, most of the middle kicks, and some of the high kicks. The Jing is first generated from the leg on the ground. Before the Jing passes out the kicking leg, the waist jerks so that the Jing reaches the foot in a powerful, short pulse (Figure 3-202). This is difficult to learn, but if you persevere you will grasp the trick and suddenly understand it.

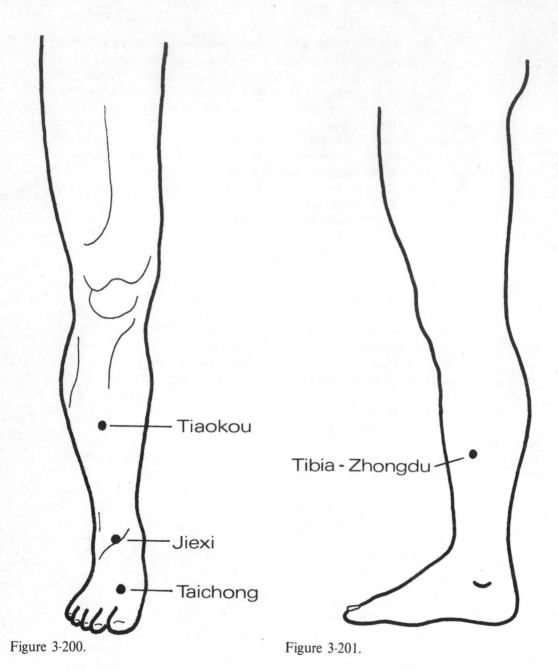

Figure 3-200.

Figure 3-201.

Remember that balancing Yi and Chi is as important with kicks as it is with hand techniques. In order to get the maximum energy out to your kicking leg you must put your Yi into your supporting foot.

Next, we will discuss the low kicking Jings which are commonly used in Tai Chi Chuan.

1. TSAE JING (Forward Stepping Jing):

Tsae Jing uses the bottom of the foot to attack primarily the knees and the top of the feet. It is fast and sharp, concentrated and precisely directed. In short range fighting, you can sometimes use the rear foot to attack the opponent's knee (Figure 3-203). If you use the right angle,

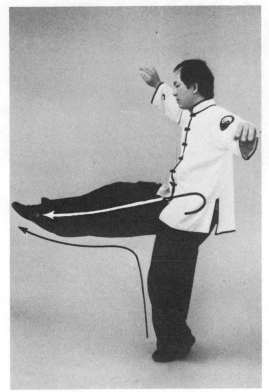

Figure 3-202.

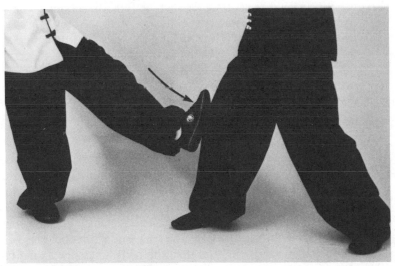

Figure 3-203.

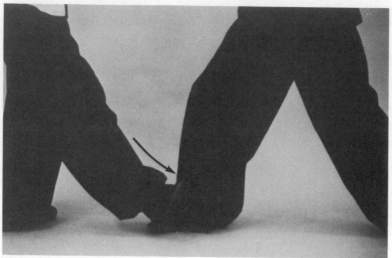

Figure 3-204.

the knee can be broken. The front foot is frequently used to attack the opponent's front foot by hopping forward (Figure 3-204). If you step on the right spot you will numb the leg and limit his ability to kick and move. To do this kick, lift the foot up to cock the leg, and snap it forward and down. Jing is generated by the supporting leg and directed to the target by the waist's jerking motion. The kick is relaxed until just before the target.

2. CHUAY JING (Stamping Jing):

Chuay Jing uses the heel to stamp on the knee, shin, ankle, and back of the foot. Chuay Jing is similar to Tsae Jing, but it is more penetrating and destructive. With Tsae Jing, the jerking of the waist matches the Jing generated from the leg. With this Jing however, the jerking of the waist is a little behind the leg's Jing. In other words, the leg first leads the foot to the target, and just before the foot hits, the waist jerks forward to enhance the Jing. Chuay Jing is usually used to attack the opponent's front leg with your own front leg or rear leg, usually at a downward angle (Figure 3-205). It can also be used to attack the back of the foot (Figure 3-206).

3. DI CHIE JING (Low Snap Cut Jing):

Di Chie Jing is a snap kick which uses the outside of the foot to attack the opponent's leg (Figure 3-207). Common targets are the ankles, shins, and knees. When attacking the ankle, the Jing is directed forward and downward. The waist leads the leg's Jing, and the body sinks to increase downward power. The sequence of movements is as follows: the waist first leads the knee out as the foot lags behind, the foot then snaps out, and then the body sinks just as the foot is about to strike the target. When Di Chie is used to attack the shin, the Jing generated from the other leg is directed forward and slightly downward to the target (Figure 3-208). The body does not usually sink in this attack. When this kick is used for a knee attack, the Jing is directed forward to the opponent's knee.

Generally speaking, Chie Jing is sharper and more penetrating than

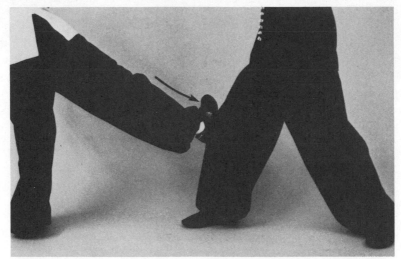

Figure 3-205.

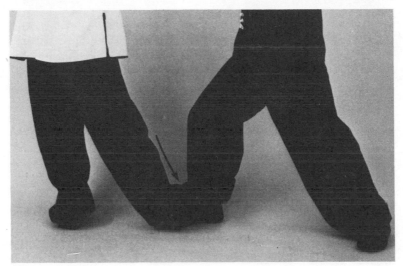

Figure 3-206.

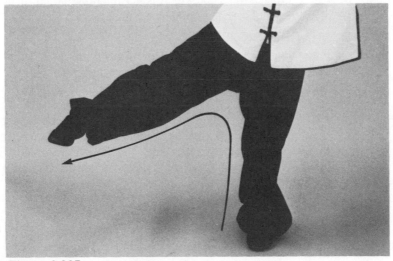

Figure 3-207.

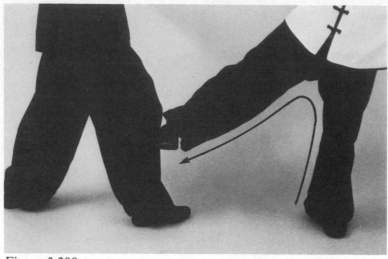

Figure 3-208.

Tsae Jing and Chuay Jing. However, its power is weaker, and so its breaking capability is less. Chie Jing is used in many martial styles. Its shin and knee attacks are fast and can usually forestall the opponent's attack. If the body is not dropped for the ankle attack, it too can be fast, although in this case its power would be reduced.

4. DI CHIAU JING (Low Lift-Hook Jing):

Di Chiau Jing specializes in attacking the shin. It is sometimes called Sarn Ding (Upward Press Kick) or Lieu Twe (Strolling Kick) by other styles. To use this kicking Jing, hop forward on the rear leg and kick upward with the ball of the front foot (Figure 3-209). To hop, rock your weight onto the front foot, and let your rear leg come forward. Just before the rear foot touches the ground, start the kick with the front foot. The kicking leg stays relatively straight as it rises to strike the shin (Figure 3-210). Hopping is usually necessary to set up the right range and to generate forward power. This kick is generally not very powerful. However, because it is applied suddenly, and because it attacks the shin, which is a vulnerable target, it may be possible to immobilize the opponent with just one kick.

5. DI SHAOU JING (Low Sweep Jing):

Di Shaou Jing uses the bottom of the foot (Figure 3-211) to strike the side of the ankle, shin (Figure 3-212), or knee. Though not very destructive, this kick is very useful. It can break your opponent's root and upset his stability, opening the way for another attack. If done accurately to the side of the shin or knee it can numb your opponent's leg and limit his fighting capacity. When using this Jing, the root in the other leg is extremely important. The Jing is generated mainly by turning the waist and is directed down to move the kicking leg.

b. Middle Kicks:

Most of the middle kicks are used for mid-range fighting. Common targets are the stomach (Zhongwan cavity), waist (Zhangmen cavity), abdomen (Dan Tien or Qihai), groin (Shayin cavity)(Figure 3-213), and

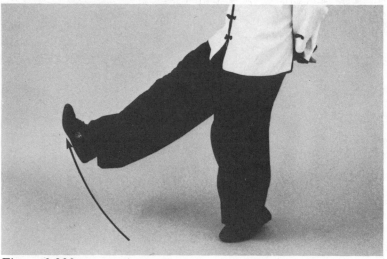

Figure 3-209.

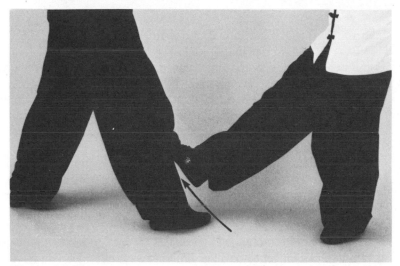

Figure 3-210.

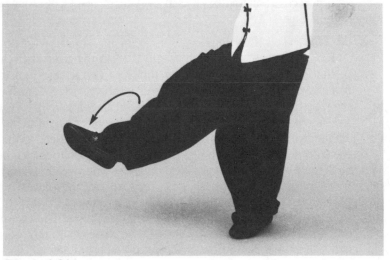

Figure 3-211.

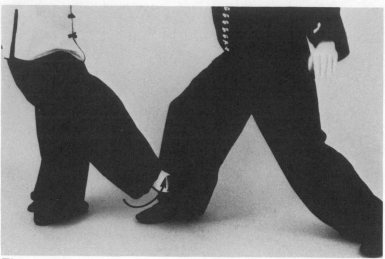

Figure 3-212.

thigh (Jimen, Xuehai, and Futu cavities)(Figures 3-214 and 3-215). Whenever you use the middle kicks you lose a portion of your stability, and weaken your Chi and Jing balance. You also expose your abdomen and groin to attack. To minimize this vulnerability it is important to kick fast. In addition, because your stability and balance are minimal, it is much harder to generate Jing from the supporting leg than it is with the low kicks. However, if you practice perseveringly it is still possible to reach a high level of power.

To generate a more powerful Jing, some styles twist the waist and hips. However, this significantly weakens your root. When a person who uses this hip and waist twisting is blocked or misses his target, he frequently is so off balance that he is vulnerable to a quick counterattack. The Chinese consider the root supremely important. Jing must be generated by the rooted leg and guided by the jerking of the waist. It will take you longer to develop Jing this way, but once you have done it, you will be able to kick from a more advantageous position.

The most common middle kicks in Tai Chi are: Ti, Deng, Jong Chiau, and Jong Chie.

1. TI JING (Toe Kick Jing):

Ti Jing is a "toe" kick which usually attacks the groin with the top of the foot (Figure 3-216). Either the front or the rear foot can be used. Usually when the front leg is used, the rear leg hops forward to set up the range and increase the forward Jing (Figure 3-217). While this hopping is taking place, the waist jerks to enhance the kicking Jing and direct it to the target. When the rear leg is used for the kick, the front leg should be rooted firmly first. Then the rear leg pushes back to generate the forward kicking power, your weight shifts to the front foot, and the rear leg kicks forward. As the power is being generated, the waist also jerks and directs the Jing to the target. Your kicking leg should be snapped out like a flexible spring. The knee moves out first and then the foot follows. When done accurately, this kick can kill, so you should be very careful when practicing.

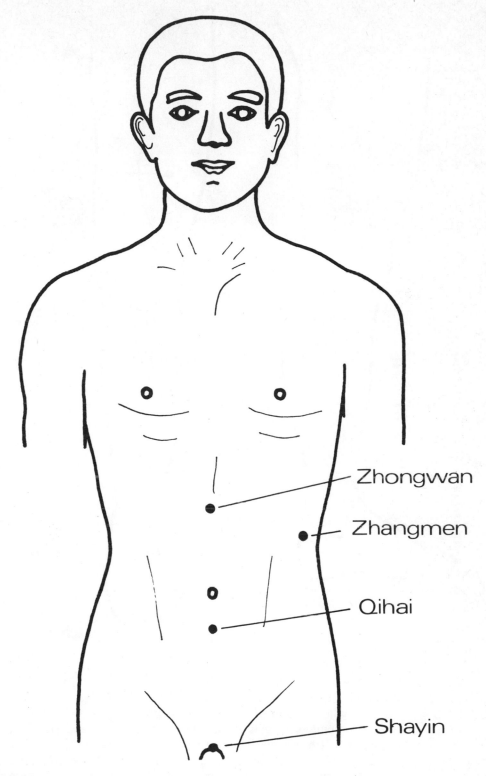

Zhongwan

Zhangmen

Qihai

Shayin

Figure 3-213.

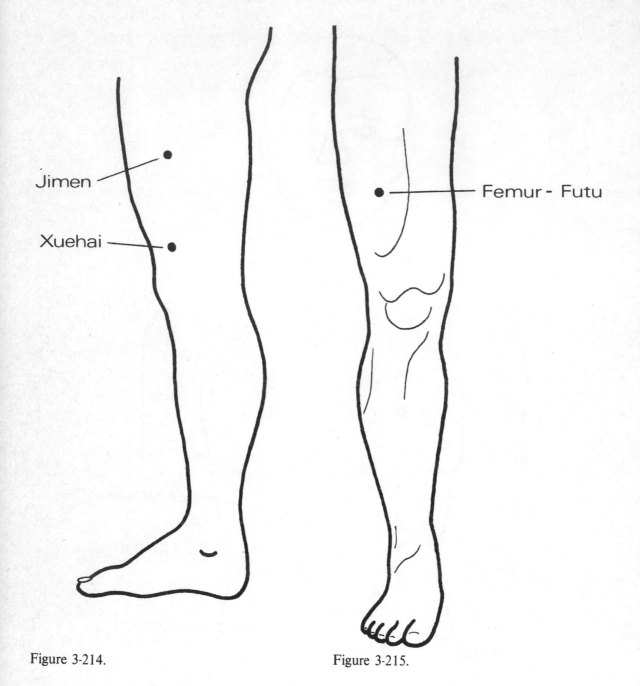

Jimen

Xuehai

Femur - Futu

Figure 3-214.

Figure 3-215.

2. DENG JING (Heel Kick Jing):

Deng Jing snaps the heel out to the opponent's midsection (Figure 3-218). Common targets are the groin, solar plexus, and Dan Tien (Figure 3-219). The technique is similar to Ti Jing except that the heel is used instead of the toe. Again, the knee lifts first and the foot curves in toward you and then snaps out to the opponent. This kick is usually more powerful than the toe kick, and because the heel is used, it is more effective against some targets.

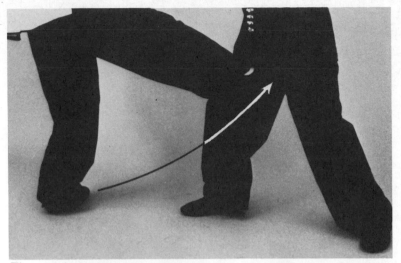

Figure 3-216.

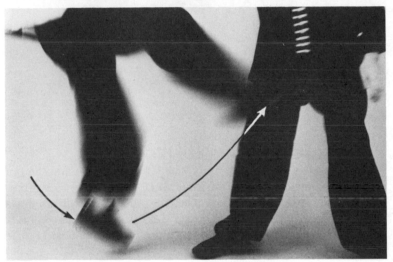

Figure 3-217.

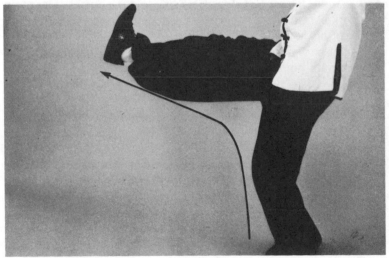

Figure 3-218.

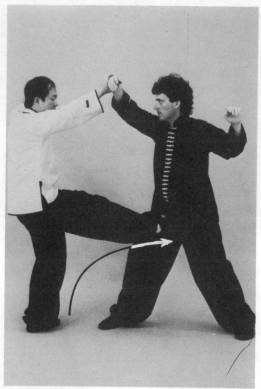

Figure 3-219.

3. JONG CHIAU JING (Middle Lift-Hook Jing):

This is a straight-leg rising kick. The technique and the principle of Jing generation are the same as Di Chiau Jing. However, it is a longer range kick than Di Chiau Jing, and it is usually used to attack the cavity behind the groin (Figure 3-220). Because the power is hooked and directed upward, it can reach this cavity more easily than most other kicks. When done accurately, this attack will cause death.

4. JONG CHIE JING (Middle Snap Cut Jing):

Like Di Chie Jing, Jong Chie Jing uses the outside edge of the foot to kick. Common targets are the abdomen, stomach, waist, and the side of the waist (Figure 3-221). Jong Chie Jing can be done either in place or hopping. Hopping is used to shorten the range and generate forward power.

c. High Kicks:

Chinese martial artists seldom use single-foot high kicks because they sacrifice root, stability, and balance. Also, in order to avoid counterattack, high kicks must be extremely fast, and recovery time must be short. As with middle kicks, some non-Chinese martial styles use the hip and waist to generate Jing, and sacrifice the root entirely.

Because high kicks can be effective in long range fighting, Chinese martial artists will use them, but in a different way. The Chinese martial artist generally uses double kicks—in other words, one leg leaps up and forward, and then pulls back to move the other leg out. This mo-

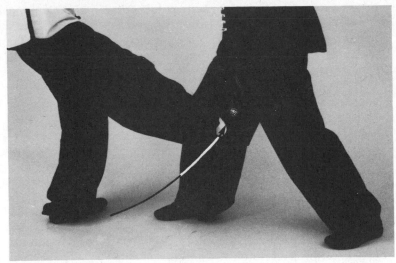

Figure 3-220.

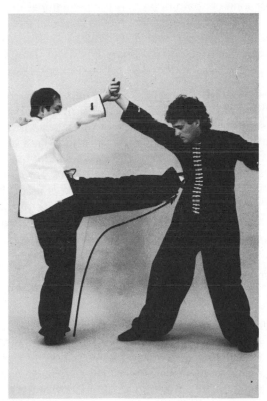

Figure 3-221.

tion generates Jing. The waist also jerks to speed up the kick and enhance the kicking power. Therefore, when the high kicks are used, you don't have any root at all—your body is completely in the air. While one leg is attacking, the other leg is curved up to protect vital areas such as the abdomen and groin. When you land, drop immediately into a low stance to regain your stability. This kicking strategy allows you to be mobile and agile. The semi-stable state should be avoided—it is probably the worst situation to be in when you are fighting.

In Tai Chi Chuan, high kicks are seldom used. The main use for such kicks is to cover the distance to the opponent, and to increase forward Jing. Even when double jump kicks are used, it is only to attack the middle and lower body.

d. Spinning Kicks:

Most of the spinning kicks are classified as high kicks. The difference is that spinning kicks use the waist to spin the whole body and thereby generate Jing. There are two kinds of spinning kicks—stable spinning and jump spinning. In stable spinning kicks, one leg stays rooted and supports the waist as it generates jerking power and leads the kicking leg in a circular motion to strike the target. These kicks use the motion of only part of the body to generate power. Typical examples of the stable spinning kick are external sweep (Wai Bai) and internal sweep (Nei Bai). The other kind of spinning kick is jump spinning, in which the body completely leaves the ground and moves in a complete circle. The waist generates spinning power and leads it out to the leg. A typical example of this kick is the tornado kick (Shain Fon Twe). Tai Chi uses only two stable spinning kicks: external sweep and internal sweep.

1. WAI BAI JING (External Sweep Jing):

Wai Bai Jing uses the outside edge of the foot to attack. Common targets are the kidneys and the back of the head (Figure 3-222). One leg stays firmly rooted while the waist jerks in a curved motion to generate the power and move the attacking foot in a circular motion (Figure 3-223). This kick is also used to kick a weapon out of a person's hand (Figure 3-224). When this Jing is used, the circular motion is first generated by a quick, circular jerk of the waist. If you are kicking with your right leg, it starts out moving to the left before it cuts over to the right. Once the kick reaches the highest point, the waist twists suddenly to pull the leg abruptly down. When the foot hits the target it is just past the highest point in its arc, and moving downward. Striking the target downward this way generates the most force.

2. NEI BAI JING (Internal Sweep Jing):

Nei Bai Jing is similar to Wai Bai Jing, except that it circles in the opposite direction. In Nei Bai Jing the bottom of the foot is used to strike. Common targets are the kidneys, stomach, and head (Figures 3-225 and 3-226). It may also be used to strike the opponent's hand to force him to release his weapon. The principle of Jing generation is the same as Wai Bai Jing, however the timing of the strike is different. With Nei Bai Jing you usually strike when the foot reaches the highest point, although on occasion this kick will be used to strike downward to the back of the head. The waist generates power as with

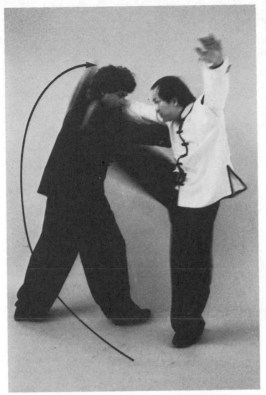

Figure 3-222.

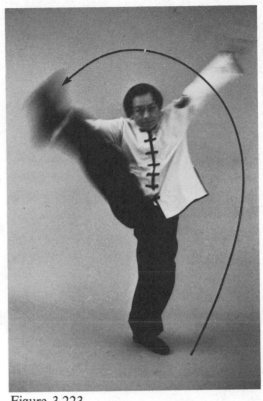

Figure 3-223.

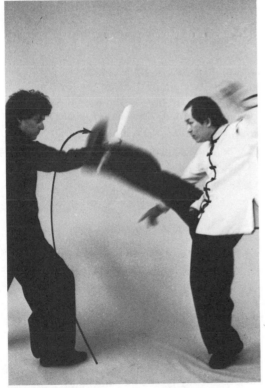

Figure 3-224.

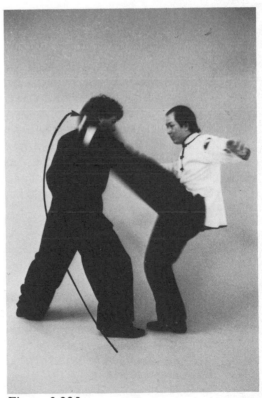

Figure 3-225.

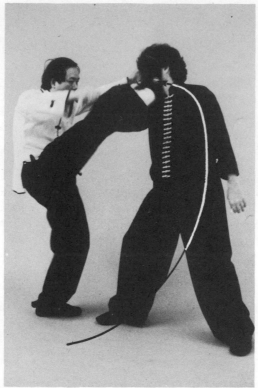

Figure 3-226.

Wai Bai, although the motion is harder to learn and takes more practice.

3-7. Summary of Jing Training

After reading about Jing theory and the different types of Jing, you are probably wondering how to start training. As matter of fact, all of the training principles and methods have been discussed in the last section. In this section we would like to review and highlight the important points for the benefit of those who have not had experience in Jing training before. Hopefully this section will lead you to the entrance of this secret. Since Tai Chi Chuan specializes in hand applications, we will discuss only hand Jings. Once you have grasped the trick of generating hand Jings, you should have no problem in figuring out the leg Jing training by yourself.

Sensing Jing:

Sensing Jings are much harder to train than the manifested Jings. They take a lot of patience, and especially a lot of time. This is because the higher levels of Sensing Jing require well-developed Chi circulation. Even if you do not practice any Chi Kung exercises other than the Tai Chi sequence, you can still train your Sensing Jings by using your natural sensing ability.

Since you are developing your sensitivity to another person's motion and intention, it is generally necessary to have a partner to train sensing Jing. If no partner is available, the Tai Chi ball can provide some training, but it can only take you to a certain level. Pushing hands is the most important way to train. The more you practice, and the greater the variety of body types and personalities you encounter, the more you will progress. Listening Jing is the first step. After much listening, you develop a feel for what is happening, and can tell from a touch or a slight motion what the opponent is doing, or even what he is planning to do. When you have reached this level, you have entered the gate of Understanding Jing. How well you progress with these Jings depends upon two factors. The first, sensitivity of feeling, depends to a large degree on how well developed the Chi circulation to your skin is. The second factor is calmness of the mind. When your mind is calm, you can concentrate to feel and sense. Without a calm and concentrated mind, your attention is scattered and your sensitivity is reduced.

When you have practiced for many years, you may then reach a level where you can sense the opponent's Jing even before it is emitted. It is said: "After you have mastered techniques, then you can gradually grasp what 'Understanding Jing' (Dong Jing) means. From 'Understanding Jing' you gradually approach enlightenment (intuitive understanding) of your opponent's intention. However, without a great deal of study over a long time, you cannot suddenly grasp this intuitive understanding of your opponent". It is also said: "After understanding Jing, the more practice, the more refinement. Silently learn, then ponder; gradually you will approach your heart's desire" (Appendix A-2).

Yin (Passive) sensing Jing training will be discussed in the pushing hands chapter in volume 2. Yang (Active) sensing Jing is trained through your Yi. First you build up your Chi either in the Dan Tien or in a particular part of the body, usually the arms. This Chi is then passed into the opponent's body, in coordination with your exhalation, to disturb his Chi pattern. If you coordinate the technique with an inhalation, you can withdraw Chi from his body. This subject is discussed more fully in the author's Chi Kung book.

Manifested Jing:

Manifested Jings are easier to understand and train than sensing Jings. Yin (Passive) manifested Jing, because it is a response to an attack, needs a partner for training. It will be discussed in the pushing hands training in the second volume and will not be repeated here. In this section we will focus on the Yang (Active) manifested Jing training, since it is the most basic and easiest to approach of all the Jings. You can train Yang manifested Jing without a partner because it is generated within your body. Once you understand the key points you can develop a fair level of skill by training with a punching bag, sand bag, or candle. It is useful to select individual techniques from the sequence and practice them repeatedly, practicing rooting, balancing energy, and getting the Jing out to the hand or arm being used. It is also very helpful to do the solo sequence at medium and fast speeds. The most important factor is understanding the theory and principles. Naturally, a good instructor can save you a lot of time and confusion.

Active manifested Jing is also called Emitting Jing (Fa Jing). You must firm your root, generate your preliminary Jing with your leg and pass it up to meet the Jing generated by the waist. This waist Jing is important in directing the leg Jing to the right place. The combined Jing is then passed to the shoulder to join with the Jing generated there, and the total Jing is expressed through your hands. These different parts must be coordinated and timed precisely so that the Jing is integrated, for only then can it reach a high level. Your Yi must lead the Chi to flow naturally in support of the relaxed muscles for the Jing to be expressed at maximum power. From this point, the stronger your Chi support, the stronger your Jing will be. The ultimate goal is to cut muscle usage down to a minimum and have the Chi predominate.

From this theory review, you can understand that in order for you to emit your

Jing, you must know: 1. How to generate Jing from the rooted legs. 2. How to generate Jing from the waist and connect it with the Jing from the legs. This also includes knowing how to lead Jing to the desired place. 3. How to combine this Jing with the Jing generated by the shoulders, and express it through the hands. 4. How to refine the unified Jing and enhance it through hip and thigh relaxation, arcing the chest, and storing Jing in the elbow. We will now discuss these four items in detail.

1. Generation of Jing from the legs:

Generally, there are three ways to generate Jing with the legs: forward and backward, sideways, and upward. For all three ways of Jing generation, the root is critical—without a firm root it is like trying to push a car while you are standing on ice. In order to generate Jing, you must lead your Yi and Chi down first, and at the same time push down through your bent legs. This pushing down will cause the reaction force, which is the source of the Jing, to bounce back from your leg.

When you push backward to generate forward Jing (or push forward for backward Jing), the direction of the push must be accurate. The leg muscles should be tensed for as short a time as possible. Treat your legs like springs—when you compress them they push in the opposite direction. The push must be done in a short time in order to generate the pulse-like spring power. If the push is done too slowly, your leg muscles will be tensed and the power generated will be Li instead of Jing. When you want to generate upward Jing, follow the same principle as that of forward and backward Jing generation except that you push straight down.

For sideways Jing generation, twist your legs as if winding a spring, and then twist back with a jerk. The Jing is generated from the twisting. You must follow the same key points as described above. Remember to tense the leg muscles for only a very short time, and to keep them loose and relaxed the rest of the time.

2. Generation of Jing from the Waist:

Once you have generated the Jing with your legs, your waist plays the major role in its application. As it passes the Jing on, it directs, controls, and enhances it with it's own Jing. The timing is extremely important—if it is off, the Jing from the legs will be broken or weakened, and become useless. The waist should start to generate its Jing just before the Jing from the legs reaches it. This is like a relay race—the second runner starts running before the first runner reaches him. In this case, the waist Jing leads and directs the leg Jing to the target.

Generally, there are two ways to generate Jing with the waist: laterally and forward. Lateral Jing is commonly used to direct the Jing to the arm for forward striking if only a single hand is used, or to direct the Jing to the side for a sideward strike. In order to generate lateral Jing, the waist is twisted and then jerked back. A single forward jerk can direct Jing to the hand for a forward strike, and a complete back and forth jerk can generate spinning and rotating Jing for a sideward strike. The forward waist Jing is usually used for a double hand push or strike. To generate it, the waist (abdomen) is caved in slightly to accumulate Jing, and then straightened out suddenly to emit.

Here, the author would like to point out two things. First, since when you generate Jing with your legs you push downward in order to project the force away from the legs, the force is actually going toward your head. If you do not direct this leg Jing completely into the arms, part of the force will go to your head and make it jerk, which will cause headaches. Second, if you fail to direct the leg and waist Jing out to your arms, part of the Jing will remain in the waist area and cause the intestines to jerk and vibrate, causing pain or even injury. Beginners frequently have either or both of these problems. When you feel pain you should stop practicing. When the pain goes away, resume practice, but cut down the strength of the Jing. The more tense you are, the worse it will be. Remember, relaxation is the medicine.

3. Generation of Jing from the Shoulder:

Like the waist, the shoulder can generate both sideward and lateral Jing. Lateral Jing is usually used to direct and enhance the Jing coming from the waist for a sideward strike, while the forward Jing is generally used for striking forward. The trick of timing for the shoulder Jing is the same as for the waist, i.e., slightly ahead of the incoming Jing from the waist.

4. Other Posture Coordination:

Once you grasp the above keys to Jing generation, you have entered the door to Jing training. However, your Jing may still not reach a high level because the connections from the legs to the waist, the waist to the shoulders, and from the shoulders to the hands may be incomplete. If these places are not connected continuously, the Jing will be weakened or even broken. The main culprit is tenseness, which bottlenecks the energy and hinders the smooth flow of your body. Also, in order for these three areas to contribute their Jing, your posture must be correct. You must be able to store and emit Jing from the various parts of your body. You must be relaxed so that the Jing can flow, and you must find your Jing storage in curves.

A common way to test your Jing is with a candle. Stand in a stable stance so that your extended hand is about a foot away from the candle. Try to put out the flame using either a punch or an open hand strike (Figure 3-227). Use Jing in a relaxed, whip-like motion. If your Jing is powerful, accurate, and concentrated, you should be able to extinguish the flame with the wind generated from your motion. Once you can extinguish the flame from a distance of one foot, increase the distance. Naturally, your mind and Chi must be more concentrated and the Jing more powerful in order to do this.

You can reach a fairly high level of Jing expression using this method and emphasizing Yi and posture. However, you will find that further progress is limited unless you develop your Chi. If you strengthen and train your Chi, it will eventually become the main factor in your Jing, and your level of energy will continue to rise.

Here the author would like to bring up a very important point. Most of this discussion has been based on your being in a stable situation. As matter of fact, in a fight, both you and your opponent are moving. Therefore, even if you can emit very strong Jing when you are standing steady, this does not mean that you will be able to generate the same kind of Jing while you are moving. This is because

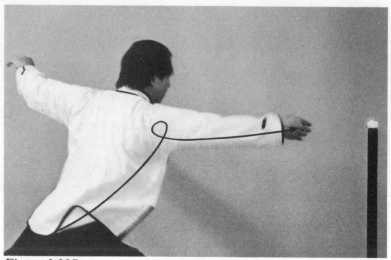

Figure 3-227.

when you are moving your root is very weak. You have probably experienced that, although you can hit a bag with a certain amount of power from a stable stance, if you are moving while you are punching you lose at least half your power. If you want to fight effectively, you must train emitting the various Jings while moving, and develop fighting strategies and tactics which take this into account. Doing the Tai Chi sequence fast will greatly help to train this. Simply put, the trick to using Jing effectively while moving lies in timing. You should emit Jing while your feet are rooted. Once the Jing is generated and transmitted to your extremities (substantial hand and supporting foot), you can step or change your stance. Naturally, you will still lose part of the Jing, since you have lost the root which balances the energy in the hand. However, if you keep practicing, you can learn how to root and emit Jing in an instant, and then quickly continue your movement. It is clear then that a large part of strategy consists of setting up your footwork most advantageously, so that you can be mobile, and then, when you strike, be rooted so that your opponent cannot escape from you. Volume 2 of this book will discuss the strategies of footwork and Jing.

As mentioned in the beginning of this chapter, the author's knowledge of and experience with Jing is limited. Because of this, some Jings are discussed in only a limited way. Also, because the various Jings are explained according to the author's background and understanding, it is possible that the reader may not agree with his ideas completely. It is the author's desire to encourage martial artists to research this side of the art which has been so neglected for so many years.

第四章
結論
CHAPTER 4
CONCLUSION

Hopefully this volume has given you a better concept of Tai Chi theory and principles. You no doubt have a number of questions, especially about Jing, since it has been kept secret for centuries. This volume is the first major discussion of Jing in the English language. You should study and practice, experiment and research. Discuss and share your ideas with others. Most important of all, you should be humble enough to ask others. In China, it is said: "Maan jau soen, chian show yi", which means "Satisfaction causes damage and humility gains benefit". You should understand that as long as you are humble, you will continue to learn until one day you become a real Tai Chi master. When you feel full, you are satisfied and naturally not humble enough to ask and research. Like most of Chinese culture and the martial arts, Tai Chi is an accomplishment of art, culture, skill, morality, and self-discipline. The more you know the less you feel you know. Every time you reach a higher level of Tai Chi Chuan, your ability to understand will also increase. Therefore, you should study this volume again and again, especially Appendix A which contains the translation of ancient poetry and songs and commentary. These works are the creations of many experienced masters through hundreds of years of research and study.

Reading this volume and understanding the theory and principles of Tai Chi Chuan is still not enough to become a proficient Tai Chi martial artist. You must also know the other part of the Tai Chi secret: Tai Chi fighting techniques. Tai Chi was created for fighting, and every form which has been passed down from generation to generation contains many secret fighting techniques concealed inside. Usually, these techniques remain secret unless you have earned the trust of a teacher or have been chosen as the successor of a style. There are more than 250 Tai Chi techniques known today. There are more which are still hidden in the forms and waiting for you to discover them. To help you in this, the author will publish a second volume of advanced Yang Style Tai Chi Chuan which will specialize in the fighting techniques which are hidden in the forms, pushing hands, and the fighting set.

Theory and practical experience are mutually related. The deeper you understand the theory, the better you can put it to work. In the same way, the more experience you have, the greater your ability will be to analyze the theory.

Tai Chi theory and principles are so deep and profound that it is impossible to cover them completely in a single volume. The author hopes that this volume will lead you to the right path and help you to avoid straying too far off the path. Even if you master the material in this book, you should not be satisfied, but should continue to research the art.

APPENDIX A

TAI CHI POETRY AND SONGS

INTRODUCTION

In the last seven centuries many songs and poems have been composed about Tai Chi Chuan. These have played a major role in preserving the knowledge and wisdom of the masters, although in most cases the identity of the authors and the dates of origin have been lost. Since most Chinese of previous centuries were illiterate, the key points of the art were put into poems and songs, which are easier to remember than prose, and passed down orally from teacher to student. The poems were regarded as secret and have only been revealed to the general public in this century. We have chosen fifteen which are the most popular and are considered the most accurate.

It is very difficult to translate these ancient Chinese writings. Because of the cultural differences, many expressions would not make sense to the Westerner if translated literally. Often a knowledge of the historical background is necessary. Furthermore, since every sound has several possible meanings, when anyone tried to understand a poem or write it down he had to choose from among these meanings. For this reason, many of the poems have several variations. The same problem occurs when the poems are read. Many Chinese characters have several possible meanings, so reading involves interpretation of the text even for the Chinese. Also, the meaning of many words has changed over the course of time. When you add to this the grammatical differences (generally no tenses, articles, singular or plural, or differentiation between parts of speech) you find that it is almost impossible to translate Chinese literally into English. In addition to all this, the translator must have much the same experience and understanding, as well as similar intuitive feelings as the original author, in order to convey the same meaning.

With these difficulties in mind, the author has attempted to convey as much of the original meaning of the Chinese as possible, based on his own Tai Chi experience and understanding. Although it is impossible to totally translate the original meaning, the author feels he has managed to express the majority of the important points. The translation has been made as close to the original Chinese as possible, including such things as double negatives and, sometimes, idiosyncratic sentence structure. Words which are understood but not actually written in the Chinese text have been included in parentheses. Also, some Chinese words are followed by the English in parentheses, e.g. Shen (Spirit). To further assist the reader, the author has included commentary with each poem and song. For reference, the original Chinese of each song has been included after the translations.

1. TAI CHI CHUAN TREATISE
by Chang San-Feng

太極拳論 張三丰

Once in motion, every part of the body is light and agile and must be threaded together.

一舉動 ，週身俱要輕靈 ，尤須
貫串 。

Ching Ling, the Chinese words which are translated "light and agile", are used to describe the movement of monkeys: responsive, controlled, and able to move quickly. The body should be a coherent whole, with all of its parts connected and unified by the energy (Chi) moving within them, like ancient Chinese coins connected by a string.

Chi should be full and stimulated, Shen (Spirit) should be retained internally.

氣宜鼓盪 ，神宜內斂 。

The Chi which is generated in the Dan Tien should fill the entire body like air fills a balloon or a drum. Doing the Tai Chi Chuan sequence with a controlled mind circulates the Chi and strengthens it, which leads to a healthy body. Although the Chi is full and stimulated, your mind is centered so that the Chi isn't scattered. Retaining the Spirit of Vitality internally means to be calm and patient, and restrained in your actions. This helps to avoid giving away your intentions to the opponent, and conserves your Chi.

No part should be defective, no part should be deficient or excessive, no part should be disconnected.

無使有缺陷處 ，無使有凸凹處 ，
無使有斷續處 。

Tai Chi Chuan emphasizes balance, efficiency, and precision. No posture or part of the body should stretch out too far or be pulled in too much. Every motion should be smooth, always just right; every force just enough to do the job. Each posture should be rounded and should involve the whole body in a smooth, continuous, flowing motion.

The root is at the feet, (Jing is) generated from the legs, controlled by the waist and expressed by the fingers. From the feet to the legs to the waist must be integrated, and one unified Chi. When moving forward or backward, you can then catch the opportunity and gain the superior position.

其根在脚 ，發於腿 ，主宰於腰 ，
形於手指 。由脚而腿而腰 ，總須

完整一氣。向前退後，乃能得機
得勢。

If you are firmly connected to the ground, and if, from the feet to the waist, you move as a coherent unit, then your Jing will be strong and you will be agile and responsive enough to gain an advantageous position. The Chi of the entire body must be unified in the technique. It is important to balance the force and Chi of the substantial (active) hand with the root in the feet, and to balance the insubstantial force suspending the head with the Chi sunken to the Dan Tien.

If you fail to catch the opportunity and gain the superior position, your mind is scattered and your body is disordered. To solve this problem, you must look to the waist and legs.

有不得機得勢處，身便散亂。其
病必於腰腿求之。

If you fail in an attempt to attack your opponent, or defend poorly against an attack, it is probably because your mind and body were unbalanced and disorganized. When this is the case, your mind is scattered and your root is loose. When your root is not firm, you lose the foundation through which the legs generate power, and your waist consequently loses control and its actions become meaningless. To remedy the situation you must readjust your waist and legs into the most advantageous position, enabling you to rebuild your root and stabilize yourself.

Up and down, forward and backward, left and right, it's all the same. All of this is done with the Yi (mind), not externally.

上下前後左右皆然。凡此皆是意
，不在外面。

For any direction, with any motion, it always comes down to adjusting the waist and legs. You do not rely on quick, forceful motions of the body or arms. Instead, the mind perceives the situation and the most effective solution, and it directs the body.

If there is a top, there is a bottom; if there is a front, there is a back; if there is a left, there is a right.

有上即有下，有前即有後，有左
即有右。

Tai Chi Chuan emphasizes completeness and balance. When attacking high, you must defend low. When moving in one direction, you must balance Jing and Chi in the opposite direction. When attacking or defending on one side, you must be aware of the other side.

If Yi (mind) wants to go upward, this implies considering downward. (This means) if (you) want to lift and defeat an opponent, you must first consider his root. When the opponent's root is broken, he will inevitably be defeated quickly and certainly.

如意要向上，即寓下意．若將物
掀起，而加以挫之之意．斯其根
自斷，乃壞之速而無疑。

    Your enemy's root is his foundation. When his root is broken, he will lose his foundation and his Jing will not be generated from the legs and controlled by the waist. This will greatly limit his fighting ability. If you wish to knock him down or push him away, you must first break his root so that he is unstable and can be easily defeated.

Substantial and insubstantial must be clearly distinguished. Every part (of the body) has a substantial and an insubstantial aspect. The entire body and all the joints should be threaded together without the slightest break.

虛實宜分清楚，一處有一處虛實
，處處總此皆如是．周身節節貫
串，無令絲毫間斷耳。

    It is very important to distinguish between substantial and insubstantial in your body and in the opponent's. The hand which is acting upon the opponent is substantial, while the other hand is insubstantial. The leg with more weight on it is usually substantial, but an insubstantial leg (such as the front leg in the false stance) becomes substantial upon kicking. When pushing, the front of the hand is substantial, while the back of the hand is insubstantial. You must also clearly distinguish and respond to the opponent's substantial and insubstantial. When the opponent attacks your right side, that side should become insubstantial, and your left side should become substantial and attack him. In order to do all this effectively, your entire body from the feet, legs and waist to the fingers must work like a unit and move as if threaded together.

ADDITIONAL SENTENCES FROM CHANG SAN-FENG

What is Long Fist? (It is) like a long river and a large ocean, rolling ceaselessly.

長拳者如長江大海滔滔不絕也．

There are two styles of martial arts called Long Fist (Chang Chuan) in China. One is Tai Chi Chuan, in which case Chang Chuan is translated "Long Sequence". This is because the Tai Chi sequence is long and the movements are performed smoothly and continuously like a flowing river. The other Chang Chuan is translated as "Long Fist" and refers to a Northern Shaolin style which emphasizes long range fighting strategies.

What are the thirteen postures? Peng (Wardoff), Lu (Rollback), Ghi (Press), An (Push), Chai (Pluck), Lie (Split), Zou (Elbow-Stroke), Kau (Shoulder-Stroke), these are the eight trigrams. Jinn Bu (Forward), Twe Bu (Backward), Dsao Gu (Beware of the Left), Yu Pan (Look to the Right), Dsung Dien (Central Equilibrium), these are the five elements. Wardoff, Rollback, Press, and Push are Chyan (Heaven), Kuen (Earth), Kann (Water), Lii (Fire), the four main sides. Pluck, Split, Elbow-Stroke, Shoulder-Stroke are Shiunn (Wind), Jenn (Thunder), Duey (Lake), and Genn (Mountain), the four diagonal corners. Forward, Backward, Beware of the Left, Look to the Right, and Central Equilibrium are Gin (Metal), Moo (Wood), Sui (Water), For (Fire), and Tu (Earth). All together they are the thirteen postures.

十三勢者，掤、擭、擠、按、採
、捌、肘、靠，此八卦也．進步
、退步、左顧、右盼、中定，此
五行也．掤、擭、擠、按，即乾
、坤、坎、離，四正方也．採、
捌、肘、靠，即巽、震、兌、艮
，四斜角也．進、退、顧、盼、
定，即金、木、水、火、土也．
合之則為十三勢也．

This paragraph lists Tai Chi's basic postures and their correlates. This is discussed in Chapter 1, section 4.

2. TAI CHI CHUAN CLASSIC
by Wang Dsung-Yueh

太極拳經 王宗岳

What is Tai Chi? It is generated from Wu Chi. It is the mother of Yin and Yang. When it moves, it divides. At rest it reunites.

太極者，無極而生，陰陽之母也
。動之則分，靜之則合。

Tai Chi can be translated as "Grand Ultimate", or "Grand Extremity", and Wu Chi is translated as "Without Ultimate", "Without Limit", or "No Extremity". Wu Chi can also mean "No Opposition". That means Wu Chi is uniform and undifferentiated. For example, at the beginning of the universe, there was no differentiation, and this state is called Wu Chi. With the first motion things separated into complimentary opposites, called Yin and Yang, and this state is called Tai Chi. From the interaction of Yin and Yang, all things are generated and grow. All objects, ideas, spirits, etc. can be identified as either Yin or Yang. Tai Chi Chuan was created according to this theory. In the beginning posture of the Tai Chi sequence, the mind is calm and empty, and the weight is evenly distributed on both feet. This state is Wu Chi. As soon as your mind leads the body into Grasp Sparrow's Tail, the hands and feet differentiate into substantial and insubstantial. The interaction of substantial (Yang) and insubstantial (Yin) generates all of Tai Chi Chuan's fighting strategy and technique.

No excess, no deficiency. Following the opponent, bend, then extend.

無過不及，隨屈就伸。

No part of your posture should be exaggerated or constricted, nothing should be too concave or too convex. When you stick to and follow the opponent, do only what is appropriate—no more, no less. In pushing hands, when your opponent pushes your arm, yield. Adhere lightly to his arm, following his motion with no separation or resistance. When he attacks, give way elastically, and when he withdraws, extend to follow him. This also implies that when he pushes your right side, the right side withdraws and the left side extends to attack him.

When the opponent is hard, I am soft; this is called yielding. When I follow the opponent, this is called sticking.

人剛我柔謂之走，我順人背謂之
黏。

When the opponent attacks you, do not resist him, but instead give way so that his attack misses you. The Chinese term translated as "yielding" literally means "walk away". Sticking to the opponent means to maintain contact with him and follow his motions so that when the right time comes you can make the appropriate move.

When the opponent moves fast, I move fast; when the opponent moves slowly, then I follow slowly. Although the variations are infinite, the principle remains the same.

動急則急應 ， 動緩則緩隨 ， 雖變化萬端 ， 而理為一貫 。

The principle here, as in the previous two sections, is to stick to the opponent and follow his motions. You can then respond appropriately no matter what he does. Although there are many techniques, they are all variations on the one basic principle of stick and follow.

After you have mastered techniques, then you can gradually grasp what "Understanding Jing (Dong Jing)" means. From "Understanding Jing" you gradually approach enlightenment (intuitive understanding) of your opponent's intention. However, without a great deal of study over a long time, you cannot suddenly grasp this intuitive understanding of your opponent.

由着熟而漸悟懂勁 ， 由懂勁而階及神明 。 然非功力之久 ， 不能豁然貫通焉 。

When you can stick and follow, and have mastered the various techniques, then you will gradually begin to understand the opponent's Jing and be able to interpret his intentions. The more you practice, the more sensitive you will become. Only then can you enlighten yourself and interpret the opponent's intentions with just a touch, or even without touching him at all.

An insubstantial energy leads the head upward. The Chi is sunk to the Dan Tien.

虛領頂勁 ， 氣沉丹田 。

An insubstantial energy lifts the head upward so that it feels like the head and body are suspended by a string attached to the top of the head. This energy is balanced by the Chi sunk to the Dan Tien and the bottom of the feet. When the head is upright, the Spirit of Vitality will be raised, alertness will increase, and the body will be straight and erect from the tailbone to the top of the head. When Chi is sunk to the Dan Tien, the mind is calm, and the root is strengthened.

No tilting, no leaning. Suddenly disappear, suddenly appear.

不偏不倚 ， 忽隱忽現 。

The head and body are balanced upright. Do not tilt your body in any direction. If you maintain a relaxed, centered, and balanced posture, and stick and follow, you will be able to respond easily and lightly to your opponent. You will then be able to "disappear" in front of the opponent's attack, and "appear" with your own attack where he doesn't expect you.

When there is pressure on the left, the left becomes insubstantial; when there is pressure on the right, the right becomes insubstantial. Looking upward it seems to get higher and higher; looking downward it seems to get deeper and deeper. When (the opponent) advances, it seems longer and longer; when (the opponent) retreats, it becomes more and more urgent. A feather cannot be added and a fly cannot land. The opponent does not know me, but I know the opponent. A hero has no equal because of all of this.

左重則左虛，右重則右杳。仰之則彌高，俯之則彌深，進之則愈長，退之則愈促，一羽不能加，蠅蟲不能落，人不知我，我獨知人，英雄所向無敵，蓋由此而及也。

Wherever the opponent attacks, that part of you withdraws. When he tries to reach you, you fade away, just out of range of his power. When he tries to withdraw, you stick to him like glue. He feels that you are right there pushing him, and he can't get away. No matter what he does, you stick and follow. After much practice you can be so sensitive and accurate in your response that a feather can't touch you without setting you in motion. The opponent can never catch hold of you to figure you out, but you always know him. If you reach this level, no one will be able to match you.

There are many martial art styles. Although the postures are distinguishable from one another, after all, it is nothing more than the strong beating the weak, the slow yielding to the fast. The one with power beats the one without power, the slow hands yield to the fast hands. All this is natural born ability. It is not related to the power that has to be learned.

斯技旁門甚多，雖勢有區別，概不外壯欺弱，慢讓快耳。有力打無力，手慢讓手快。是皆先天自然之能，非關學力而有為也。

Tai Chi Chuan is different from most other Kung Fu styles in which one uses his natural born abilities of strength and speed to defend himself. Tai Chi's applications are much deeper than one would expect. It not only takes time, patience, and perseverance to learn the skills and techniques, but also requires talent and a comprehending mind to understand the theory, strategy, and approach.

Consider the saying: "four ounces repel one thousand pounds". It is apparent that this cannot be accomplished by strength. Look, if an eighty or ninety year old man can still defend himself against multiple opponents, it cannot be a matter of speed.

察四兩撥千斤之句，顯非力勝．
觀耄耋能禦眾之形，快何能為．

Tai Chi Chuan teaches you to rely on technique and understanding the opponent, rather than mere strength or speed. After doing the sequence correctly for many years, your body will be healthy and you will have built up an internal energy which is quite different from external strength. If you understand the principles of neutralization, adhering and sticking, and if you have practiced Tai Chi pushing hands and applications for many years, you will be able to fight effectively even when you are old.

Stand like a balanced scale, (move) lively like a cartwheel.

立如平準，活似車輪．

The body stands upright, centered and in equilibrium, just like a scale balancing two weights. Neutralize incoming forces by moving your whole body as a unit, with the center line of your body acting as the axle.

(When the opponent presses) sideward (or) downward, then follow. (When there is) double heaviness (mutual resistance), then (there is) stagnation. Often after several years of dedicated training, one still cannot apply this neutralization and is controlled by the opponent. (The reason for this is that the) fault of double heaviness is not understood.

偏沉則隨，雙重則滯。每見數年
純功，不能運化者，率為人制，
雙重之病未能悟耳．

Whether the opponent attacks high or low, left or right, you do not resist him. Instead you yield and follow, adhering to him patiently until you have the opportunity to attack. If you struggle against him, the liveliness of the interaction stagnates, and victory will go to the one with the most external strength. In Tai Chi, the attacking hand is considered "heavy" because it is putting weight or pressure on the opponent. The Chinese character "Jong" can be translated as weight and "Shuang" as pair or double. Therefore, some authors translated "Shuang Jong" as "double weighting". However, the same character "Jong" can also be pronounced "Chung" and translated as "repeated overlapping". Therefore, "Shuang Chung" can be translated as "double overlapping". This means "mutual covering and resistance" and has the sense of two forces struggling against each other, each striving for the upper hand. If you study for many years, but never grasp the importance of avoiding this "mutual resistance", then you will never learn the knack of neutralizing the opponent's force.

To avoid this fault you must know Yin and Yang. To adhere means to yield. To yield means to adhere. Yin not separate from Yang. Yang not separate from Yin. Yin and Yang mutually cooperate, (understanding this) is "Understanding Jing (Dong Jing)".

欲避此病須知陰陽。粘即是走，
走即是粘。陰不離陽，陽不離陰
，陰陽相濟，方為懂勁。

You must thoroughly internalize the principle of always yielding to the opponent's attack while remaining lightly attached to him. Your Yin defense is dependent upon his Yang attack, and one with it. When you have neutralized his attack, your Yin becomes Yang as you attack. If you always stay in contact with your opponent and carefully pay attention (listen) to his motion and Jing (energy), you will gradually develop the ability to understand his intention. Once you learn how extreme Yin becomes Yang and extreme Yang becomes Yin, you will learn the knack of timing your attacks and defense, and will gain the ability to "borrow" your opponent's force. When you know these things you know Understanding Jing.

After Understanding Jing, the more practice, the more refinement. Silently learn, then ponder; gradually you will approach your heart's desire.

懂勁後愈練愈精，默識揣摩，漸
至從心所欲。

Once you understand Jing, the more you practice, the more you will progress. Your own study and experience, which you ponder silently in your own mind, is your main source of improvement. If you follow this method you can eventually reach the highest levels of achievement, where whatever you wish is done naturally.

Fundamentally, give up yourself and follow the opponent. Many misunderstand and give up the near for the far. This means a slight error can cause a thousand mile divergence. The learner, therefore, must discriminate precisely.

本是捨己從人，多誤捨近圖遠。
斯謂差之毫釐，謬以千里，學者
不可不詳辨焉。

The most important principle is to give up yourself and follow the other person. This does not mean becoming totally passive and just meekly following him, giving up counterattacking in the hope of someday suddenly becoming a master. When one side of a wheel or the Tai Chi diagram moves backward, the other side moves forward. Attack and counterattack, like Yin and Yang, are inseparably linked. Pay attention to the enemy in front of you. Stick and follow patiently and conscientiously, and when an opportunity presents itself, attack. If instead you try this and that to attack your enemy, or actively try to get him in a defective position, this is called "giving up the near for the far".

It is important for the student to be very discriminating in determining what is right and wrong, because a small error of principle in the beginning of training will have greater and greater consequences as time goes on.

Every sentence in this thesis is important. Not a single word has been added carelessly, or for decoration. Without a high degree of wisdom you won't be able to understand. The past teachers were not willing to teach indiscriminately, not just because of (the difficulty of) choosing people, but also because they were afraid of wasting their time and energy.

此論句句切要，並無一字敷衍陪襯，非有夙慧不能悟也。先師不肯妄傳，非獨擇人，亦恐枉費功夫耳。

The Tai Chi classics describe a very high level of awareness and understanding. Each description is an attempt to bring the reader closer to the principles of Tai Chi and to the experiences of the author. No part can be separated from the others, and nothing can be omitted. The author arrived at his understanding through long and arduous effort, and anyone wishing to learn his art must be willing and able to match this effort.

3. THIRTEEN POSTURES: COMPREHENDING EXTERNAL AND INTERNAL TRAINING
by Wang Dsung-Yueh

十三勢行功心解 王宗岳

Use the Hsin (heart, mind) to transport the Chi, (the mind) must be sunk (steady) and calm, then (the Chi) can condense (deep) into the bones. Circulate the Chi throughout the body, it (Chi) must be smooth and fluid, then it can easily follow the mind.

以心行氣，務令沉着，乃能收歛
入骨。以氣運身，務令順遂，乃
能便利從心。

When the Hsin (heart, mind) wants to do something, the Yi (will) mobilizes the Chi. In Tai Chi Chuan practice, where the mind goes, the Chi goes. When transporting (guiding) the Chi through your body, the mind must be clear, steady, and calm. Then, the Chi can be circulated deep into the bones.

The power used in Tai Chi applications is called Jing. If the Jing is united with and supported by Chi, it can reach its highest level. However, if it is not coordinated with and supported by Chi, the Jing will come from only the posture's dynamic force. The Jing which is supported by Chi has many variations. It can range from Jings which function on the skin such as Listening Jing (Tien Jing), Understanding Jing (Dong Jing), and Adhering Jing (Jian Jing), to Jings which come from deep within the bones, where offensive Jings such as Wardoff Jing (Peng Jing) are generated. If the Chi cannot reach deep into the bones, the Jing will lose its internal Chi support and become merely external dynamic force.

When Chi circulates throughout the body in Tai Chi practice and meditation, it must not be stagnant or discontinuous. In time the Chi will flow smoothly and quickly to the place where it is required. In the beginning, this will be difficult. After years of correct practice, Chi can be used to support Jing whenever the mind wishes.

(If) the Spirit of Vitality (Jieng-Shen) can be raised, then (there is) no delay or heaviness (clumsiness). That means the head is suspended. Yi (Mind) and Chi must exchange skillfully, then you have gained the marvelous trick of roundness and aliveness. This means the substantial and the insubstantial can vary and exchange.

精神能提得起，則無遲重之虞。
所謂頂頭懸也。意氣須換得靈，
乃有圓活之妙。所謂變轉虛實也

The "Tai Chi Chuan Classic" by Wang Dsung-Yueh states "An insubstantial energy leads the head upward". If you cultivate this feeling, which is like having the head and body suspended by a thread from above, and balance this with the Chi sunk deeply into the Dan Tien, then the postures will be erect and straight, and the Spirit of Vitality (Jieng-Shen) will be able to rise up to the top of the head. The Spirit of Vitality is the basic vital energy of your body. When you lift this energy to the top of your head, your postures will be firmly rooted and you will be alert and responsive; therefore there will be no delay or clumsiness.

When the mind and Chi are coordinated, then your skill and techniques can be round, smooth, and alive. Therefore, you can easily move yourself to exchange substantial and insubstantial in response to your opponent's actions.

When emitting Jing, be calm and relaxed, concentrated in one direction. When standing, the body must be centered, calm and comfortable, so you can handle the eight directions.

發勁須沉着鬆淨，專注一方。立身須中正安舒支撐八面。

When using Jing to attack, your mind must be calm and your body relaxed, i.e., your movement and circulation must be unhindered and unrestrained. Your attention and your energy must be concentrated in the direction of attack.

Your body should be erect, centered, and stable, and should not lean to any side. If you are calm and relaxed, and your postures natural and comfortable, you will be able to deal with attacks from any direction without resistance or stagnation.

Transport Chi as though through a pearl with a "nine-curved hole", not even the tiniest place won't be reached. When using Jing, (it is) just like steel refined 100 times, no solid (strong opposition) cannot be destroyed.

行氣如九曲珠，無微不到。運勁如百鍊鋼，無堅不摧。

When you build up your Chi and have achieved "Small Circulation", you must accomplish "Grand Circulation" and fill the entire body with Chi. When you use Jing, it must be supported by Chi. Jing and Chi should not be separated. A Chinese emperor had a large pearl that he wanted to put on a string. However, the hole through the pearl was not straight, but instead had nine curves. It was impossible to push a string through it. A wise man finally tied a very fine thread to an ant, and caused the ant to walk through this nine-curved channel pulling the thread. In the same fashion, your mind must lead the Chi throughout your body from the skin to deep inside the bones until it reaches every last part. When you cultivate your Chi, you can develop an internal (Chi supported) energy called Jing which is far superior to external, or purely muscular, strength. This Jing will enable you to overcome and destroy any opposition, no matter how strong or hard.

The appearance is like an eagle catching a rabbit, the Spirit is like a cat catching a mouse.

形如搏兔之鶻，神似捕鼠之貓。

An eagle circles high in the air, watching for prey. When it sees a rabbit it suddenly plunges down, appearing out of nowhere to snatch its prey. When a cat sees a mouse it doesn't attack at once, but instead stalks it, biding its time till the right opportunity presents itself. While poised and watching, the cat is the very model of Spirit—alert, vital, centered, and controlled.

(Be) calm like a mountain, move like a river.

靜如山岳，動如江河．

Your spirit and posture must be calm and stable like a mountain. Any motion large or small should flow like a river—continuous and fluid.

Accumulate Jing like drawing a bow, emit Jing like (a bow) shooting an arrow.

蓄勁如張弓，發勁如放箭．

You accumulate energy by bending like a bow, and then snap straight, propelling your opponent away. Remember that you must draw the bow before you can shoot the arrow, and you must accumulate energy before you can emit it. Here "accumulate" implies two things: 1. Chi is generated and accumulated at the Dan Tien and condensed in the spine for supporting the Jing. 2. Jing is stored in the most advantageous posture to either neutralize or attack.

Find the straight in the curved; accumulate, then emit.

曲中求直，蓄而後發．

Store Jing in the curves and coils of your posture, but emit Jing in a straight line. When an opponent attacks, move your body to evade him and accumulate energy, and then snap straight to attack. Similarly, you can curve the opponent's attack away from your body, and then emit force to send him off on a tangent or right angle. Your counterattack comes out of the neutralization of his attack. You accumulate energy from his pressure, then release it.

Power is emitted from the spine; steps change following the body.

力由脊發，步隨身換．

"Power" here is "Nei Jing Li". Nei Jing means internal energy and Li means muscular strength. Any movement requires Li, and this is all that most people ever use. When you train your internal energy through meditation, Chi Kung, and the Tai Chi Chuan form, you can develop an energy in which the muscles are supported more and more by Chi. The spine is the major path of Chi. When Chi is built up in the Dan Tien it will pass through the Sea Bottom (Haidi) and tailbone (Wyelu), follow the spine up to the shoulders, and finally move into the arms and hands for defense and offense. Therefore, the Dan Tien is the source of Chi, but the spine is the distributor of the Chi from where it is extended to the arms.

When Tai Chi Chuan is to be used for fighting, you should not only acquire Jing with strong Chi support, but also develop a fighting strategy. This is extremely important, for a good Tai Chi fighter uses footwork to position his body most advantageously for each technique.

To collect is to release; to release is to collect; broken, then reconnected.

收即是放，放即是收。斷而復連
。

Just as you bend a bow and then release it, you accumulate energy and then emit it. When you neutralize an attack your counterattack should follow immediately. The one leads to the other as Yin leads to Yang. Immediately after emitting Jing, the Jing is said to be "broken". But your Yi (concentration) is not broken, and its continuity restores the Jing.

Back and forth (with the opponent) must have folding and mutual entwining. Advancing and withdrawing must have rotation and variation.

往復須有摺疊，進退須有轉換。

When you are pushing hands or sparring, you are exchanging techniques back and forth. You must be flexible and adaptable, folding and bending as appropriate. When you attack with the hand and the hand is deflected, you "fold" and attack with the elbow. If the elbow is blocked, you fold again and attack with the shoulder. "Folding" can also refer to the spiralling motion of Chan Szu Jing (silk reeling energy). The Chinese translated "mutual entwining" refers to when your arms are wrapping around your opponent's arms, and you are twisting and twining around, trying to gain an advantage. This is like the children's game where you put your hand out, palm down, and the other person puts his hand on top of yours. You then put your other hand on top of his, he puts a hand on top of yours, and on and on.

When you advance and withdraw during attack and neutralization, you must be rotating your waist and varying your steps. You move in different directions and change your techniques in infinite variation.

(First) extremely soft, then extremely hard. If able to breathe (properly), then (you) can be agile and alive.

極柔軟，然後極堅剛。能呼吸，
然後能靈活。

Before you can be hard, you must first cultivate softness. Only through complete relaxation can you develop your Chi and become supremely sensitive and responsive to your opponent's actions. Only by learning not to rely on external muscular strength (Li) can you develop your internal energy and achieve real strength. It is necessary to learn how to breathe properly, that is, to develop your Chi, and then coordinate your actions with your breathing and your Chi. Only then can you be truly agile, responsive, and alive.

Cultivate Chi straight (naturally), no harm; Jing can be coiled and accumulated, (and) still have surplus.

氣以直養而無害，勁以曲蓄而有
餘。

If you develop your Chi naturally, there will be no danger. You must procede slowly and patiently, step by step. Don't push too hard, or try to do advanced techniques before you have completed all the preceding steps. When you move correctly, your energy is alternately coiling up and expanding. It is possible to accumulate energy, and at the same time have enough to move around and attack.

The Hsin (heart, mind) is the order, the Chi is the message flag, and the waist is the banner.

心為令，氣為旂，腰為纛．

In ancient Chinese armies, when the general sent an order to a subordinate, the messenger carried a message flag so that the subordinate commander could be sure that the order came from the general. The banner refers to the flag that this sub-unit followed into battle. In Tai Chi Chuan the mind is the leader and directs the Chi. The waist leads the whole body into action.

First look to expanding, then look to compacting, then you approach perfection.

先求開展，後求緊湊，可臻於縝密矣．

When you begin practicing, first make the movements and postures large and open. As you progress, the movements and postures, and the circles they embody, become smaller and smaller until eventually you function with almost no motion at all. At this time your defense will have no gaps, and your attacks will be certain.

It is also said: the opponent does not move, I do not move; the opponent moves slightly, I move first. Seems relaxed, but not relaxed; seems extended, but not extended. Jing (can be) broken, mind not broken.

又曰：彼不動，己不動，彼微動己先動，似鬆非鬆，將展未展，勁斷意不斷．

Your actions are determined entirely by what the opponent does. If he doesn't move, you don't move either. However, all of your attention is concentrated on him, so that when he begins to move you can immediately act with certain effectiveness, because you are aware of his intention. In Tai Chi practice, you first build up Listening and Understanding Jings. Once you have mastered them, you will be able to sense and understand your opponent's intention even if he only moves slightly. Once you sense the opponent's intention, you should seize the opportunity, and move fast and first before the opponent's Jing is emitted. If you catch him when his mind is intent upon attacking, he will not be able to easily switch to a defensive mode of thought. This is how it is possible to deflect a force of one thousand pounds with a force of four ounces.

Both your Spirit and posture may look relaxed, but they are alert. Your Jing and postures look extended, but they are restrained. When you emit Jing, there is a momentary break until you recover, but the continuity of your attention is not disturbed.

It is also said: first in the Hsin (heart, mind), then in the body; the abdomen (is) relaxed and clear (sunken) so the Chi condenses into the bones; the Spirit is comfortable and the body is calm; remember this in the heart at all times. Do remember: one part moves, every part moves; one part still, every part still.

又曰：先在心，後在身，腹鬆淨
，氣斂入骨，神舒體靜，刻刻存
心。切記一動無有不動，一靜無
有不靜。

The mind leads the body. First you must quiet your mind, then the body can be calm. The abdomen is relaxed and sunken. The imagery of the Chinese is that of water that is clear because it is still and all the impurities have sunk to the bottom. When you do this the Chi can circulate throughout the body and penetrate into the bones, making them strong.

Remember, the body always moves as a unit. Don't push with just a hand or arm, push with your entire body, mind, and Spirit. When you are still, be totally still, with no stray motions.

(The mind) leads the Chi flowing back and forth, adhering to the back, then condensing into the spine; strengthen the Spirit of Vitality (Jieng-Shen) internally, and express externally peacefully and easily.

牽動往來氣貼背，而斂入脊骨，
內固精神，外示安逸。

As the mind leads and circulates the Chi it accumulates in the back and penetrates into the spine. As mentioned, the spine is the distributor in the application of Chi to techniques. As you continue to practice and pay attention carefully, the Spirit of Vitality will be strengthened. Be aware of all that is around you, but keep centered on your Dan Tien. When you express your will in an external motion, move efficiently and peacefully.

Step like a cat walks; applying Jing is like drawing silk from a cocoon.

邁步如貓行，運勁如抽絲。

A cat steps carefully and quietly. Touch the ground lightly with your foot before you put your weight forward. When applying Jing, your Yi and Chi should be smooth and continuous, as when you are drawing a thread of silk from a cocoon.

(Throughout your) entire body, your mind is on the Spirit of Vitality (Jieng-Shen), not on the Chi. (If concentrated) on the Chi, then stagnation. A person who concentrates on Chi has no Li (strength); a person who cultivates Chi (develops) pure hardness (power).

全身意在精神，不在氣。在氣則
滯，有氣者無力，養氣者純剛。

Here "Chi" refers to both breath and Chi (intrinsic energy) because breathing is used to control the circulation of Chi. In the beginning of your training you must consciously coordinate your movement, breath, and Chi. However, this coordination must become automatic so that you can concentrate on the Spirit of Vitality. The mind leads the Chi which leads the body. If you have to pay attention to breathing or the movement of your body, you will be clumsy and weak. If your Spirit is clear and your mind alert, and if you have cultivated your Chi, your movements will be quick and strong.

The Chi is like a cartwheel, the waist is like an axle.

氣如車輪，腰似車軸。

When you move, your waist directs the rolling, flowing Chi.

4. SONG OF EIGHT WORDS
八字歌

Wardoff (Peng), Rollback (Lu), Press (Ghi), and Push (An) are rare in this world. Ten martial artists, ten don't know. If able to be light and agile, also strong and hard, (then you gain) Adhere-Connect, Stick-Follow with no doubt. Pluck (Chai), Split (Lie), Elbow-Stroke (Zou), and Shoulder-Stroke (Kau) are even more remarkable. When used, no need to bother your mind. If you gain the secret of the words Adhere-Connect, Stick-Follow, then you will be in the ring and not scattered.

掤攦擠按世界稀，十個藝人十不
知。若能輕靈並堅硬，沾連粘隨
俱無疑。採挒肘靠更出奇，行之
不用費心思。果得沾連黏隨字，
得其環中不支離。

Wardoff, Rollback, Press, and Push are the four basic movements of Tai Chi Chuan. Few people understand them properly. The movements are done with Chi-supported Jing, which allows the power to be either soft or hard. One must avoid external muscular power, called Li, which makes movement stiff, clumsy, and stagnant. You must stay light and agile, avoid meeting force with force, and wait for the right opportunity. If you do the right move at the right time in the proper direction, then your techniques will be powerful. You must also learn "Adhere-Connect, Stick-Follow". This is the technique of remaining lightly attached to the opponent, and following him without break or let up, without resistance or force. This is the only way you can really learn how to take advantage of the opponent's actions. If you master the first four moves, then the second four will come much more easily, and in time you will be able to do them automatically. But again, your actions must be based on the opponent's movements and postures, and this can only come about through "Adhere-Connect, Stick-Follow".

5. THREE IMPORTANT THESES OF TAI CHI CHUAN

太極拳之三要論

A. THE THESIS OF THE MIND COMPREHENDING

心會論

The waist and the spine are the first master.
The throat is the second master.
The heart (mind) is the third master.
The Dan Tien is the first chancellor.
The fingers and palms are the second chancellor.
The foot and sole are the third chancellor.

腰脊為第一主宰。
喉頭為第二主宰。
心地為第三主宰。
丹田為第一賓輔。
指掌為第二賓輔。
足掌為第三賓輔。

In Tai Chi applications, the waist is the source of all movement. It is like the axle of a wheel, directing and controlling the movement and direction. In addition, the Chi from within the spine strengthens the Jing and enables it to reach its maximum. Without the waist and Chi from the spine, you are missing the major center of control and the major source of power. Therefore, the waist and the spine are the first master.

Even when you have control, and Chi from the spine, if you can't use the Chi, then it is in vain. In order to move Chi to the extremities, the Spirit of Vitality must be raised up by coordinating your breathing (exhale when attacking, inhale when yielding), and making the Hen-Ha sound corresponding to the Yin or Yang of the force used. When the Spirit of Vitality is raised up, the Chi is instantly guided to the extremities for application. Therefore, the throat (breathing and sound) is the second master.

In addition to the above two factors, the mind must be calm, steady, and clear. The mind must constantly lead the Chi as it is being used, and it must also be able to sense the opponent's intentions. Thus the mind is the third master.

The above three factors are important for Tai Chi Chuan. However, they are not enough to make the techniques perfect. Unless the Chi is generated from the Dan Tien it will not be strong. It is said "Chi sinks to the Dan Tien". This must be done to keep generating Chi, as well as to increase downward stability.

In addition, you need sensitive feeling in the fingers and palms to listen to and understand the enemy's Jing. This enables you to neutralize and react appropriately.

Finally, if you have mastered all of the above elements but do not have a root, then your postures will not be stable and your Jing will lose its foundation. Therefore, the Dan Tien, fingers and palms, and feet and soles are the three chancellors of Tai Chi technique.

B. THE MARVELOUS APPLICATION OF THE ENTIRE BODY
週身大用論

(You) want your heart (mind) to be natural, and your Yi (thinking) to be calm, then naturally nowhere will not be light and agile.

要心性與意靜，自然無處不輕靈
。

The mastery of the mind over the body is emphasized. Your awareness and perception of things around you must be clear and not distorted by emotions or preconceptions. If your judgements and intentions are calmly arrived at, then your body and Chi will freely and easily follow your will.

(You) want the entire body's Chi to circulate smoothly, (it) must be continuous and non-stop.

要遍體氣流行，一定繼續不能停
。

Good Chi circulation throughout the body is necessary for Tai Chi and for health. Since Chi is linked with awareness and sensing, good Chi circulation is also necessary for the body to be obedient to the mind.

(You) don't ever want to give up your throat (voice); question every talented person in heaven and earth.

要喉頭，永不拋，問盡天下眾英
豪。

The voice here refers firstly to the Hen and Ha sounds made during practice, which help to raise up the Spirit of Vitality and to control and direct energy. Secondly, you must be humble enough to use your voice to ask guidance of those who have achieved the higher levels. There is so much to life and the martial arts that other people's views and experiences are necessary to fill out our own partial understanding.

If (you are) asked: how can one attain this great achievement, (the answer is) outside and inside, fine and coarse, nothing must not be touched upon.

如詢大功因何得，表裡精粗無不到。

You can specialize in one small area of the art and become very good at it, but the only way to achieve real mastery and true understanding is to explore every facet of the art, which includes the postures on the outside and the Chi on the inside. Large and small, fine and coarse, all aspects must be explored.

C. SEVENTEEN KEY THESES
十七關要論

1. Rotate on the feet. 旋之於足。

The root of your body is in your feet. When your body twists and turns, the movement starts in your feet, and goes all the way up to your fingers and your head. Your root must be stable in order to have controlled and accurate motion.

2. Move on the legs. 行之於腿。

Energy is generated by the legs. When you walk, your upper body does very little, and the legs do all the work. When you push or yield, your legs move your upper half, which remains relaxed.

3. Spring on the knees. 蹤之於膝。

Your bent knees provide the springiness to your legs which is crucial to the generation and accumulation of Jing. The strength and flexibility of the sinews of the knees determines to a great extent the strength and effectiveness of the whole body.

4. Lively waist. 活潑於腰。

The waist controls your energy in both offense and defense. Your waist must be flexible and relaxed in order to do this effectively.

5. Agility (Ling) passes through the back. 靈通於背。

The energy that is generated by the legs and directed by the waist then passes through the body. The body, especially the back, must be relaxed in order to move freely and accurately.

6. Shen (Spirit) threads up through the head. 神貫於頂。

"The Tai Chi Chuan Classic" by Wang Dsung-Yueh states that an insubstantial energy should lead the head upward, so that it feels as if it were suspended by a thread from above. This helps the rest of the body to relax and the Spirit of Vitality to rise to the top of the head.

7. Chi should flow and move (in your entire body). 流行於氣。

Cultivate your Chi so that it fills your whole body and circulates through all the channels. This will clear up stagnant Chi which can cause health problems. Doing the Tai Chi sequence stimulates and moves the Chi, and trains it so that it can support Jing.

8. Transport (Chi) to the palms. 運之於掌。

To use Tai Chi Chuan you have to be able to use the mind to transport Chi instantly to any part of the body, particularly to the hands.

9. (It) passes into the fingers. 通之於指。

You must be able to move Chi from your palms into your fingers, for that is where your will expresses itself.

10. (Chi) condenses into the marrow. 斂之於髓。

After many years of practice the Chi will sink into the bones, making them as strong as steel.

11. Approach (the opponent's) Shen (Spirit). 達之於神。

After practicing for a long time, you will be able to reach a level of enlightenment where you can sense your opponent's intentions and Spirit. Then, at your opponent's slightest move, you can move first.

12. Concentrate on the ears. 凝之於耳。

In pushing hands and sparring you must pay careful attention to your opponent. You must be very sensitive to his motion and energy. This is done by touch—through the sensitivity of the skin and also by the eyes. In Tai Chi Chuan this acute paying attention is called "listening".

13. Breathe through the nose. 息之於鼻。

Breathing, which is normally through the nose, should be regular, relaxed, and natural.

14. Exhale and inhale in the lungs. 呼吸於肺。

This means your breathing should be deep, done with the lower abdomen, so the Chi can sink to the Dan Tien. If you can breathe fully and calmly, your mind will become clear, your Chi will settle, and impurities will be cleansed out of your system.

15. To and fro from the mouth. 往來於口。

This refers to the Hen-Ha sounds made as you draw in your opponent and expel him.

16. Let the body return to its original state. 渾噩於身。

After long years of practice your body will regain the health of a little baby, and you will be able to respond to everything around you with the simplicity and naturalness of a child.

17. The entire body emits on the hair. 全體發之於毛。

If your entire body is filled with Chi and all the small channels out to the skin (roots of the hair) are opened, then you will be more sensitive. You will be able to develop your sensing Jings to a very high level, and you will be able to emit Jing anywhere on your body.

6. THE FIVE MENTAL KEYS
TO DILIGENT STUDY
用功五誌

1. **Study wide and deep.**
2. **Investigate, ask.**
3. **Ponder carefully.**
4. **Clearly discriminate.**
5. **Work perseveringly.**

博學　　審問　　慎思　　明辨　　篤行

Tai Chi Chuan has been developed and refined over many centuries. It has many facets and great depth. To truly master the art you must study the solo form including the applications for all the moves, the two-person sequence, weapons, meditation, and Chi Kung. You should push hands with as many people as possible to experience a wide range of body types and temperaments. It is desirable to study with several teachers, because each one has a different viewpoint and emphasis. You must be humble and open to learning from anyone. The more you ask and investigate, the more you will learn. You must carefully ponder everything you hear and see, discriminating good points from bad, evaluating what is true and false, and determining when something is valid or usable and when it is not. Most important of all is to persevere, for you can never approach your goal if you don't take all the steps to get there. It is desirable to have good teachers and helpful to have natural talent, but unless you are willing and able to train diligently, it is all to no avail.

7. SONG OF PUSHING HANDS
打手歌

Be concientious about Wardoff (Peng), Rollback (Lu), Press (Ghi), and Push (An). Up and down follow each other, (then) the opponent (will find it) difficult to enter.

掤擺擠按須認真，上下相隨人難
進。

Wardoff, Rollback, Press, and Push are the four basic moves of Tai Chi pushing hands. You must be serious in your study, and must practice and research these moves extensively to find out just what they are, and how and when they are used. When practicing, you and your opponent should adhere lightly to each other, following the motion back and forth, up and down. Also remember that when you attack high you are vulnerable and must cover low, and vice versa.

Similarly, when the opponent attacks high, counterattack low. If you do this, it will be difficult for the opponent to get in on you.

No matter (if) he uses enormous power to attack me, (I) use four ounces to lead (him aside), deflecting (his) one thousand pounds.

任他巨力來打我，牽動四兩撥千
斤。

Tai Chi Chuan is based on the principle of not meeting force with force. When an opponent attacks with great strength, you lead his attack away from you. The key word here is "lead". You cannot push a large bull around, but if it has a ring through its sensitive nose, you can lead it this way or that with only a light force. When a punch is coming at you with great force, you should adhere lightly to it, and lead it slightly off its course. If you tried to make a major change in the course of his attack, you might get bowled over by his forward momentum, and even if you succeeded, you would need a considerable force.

Guide (his power) to enter into emptiness, then immediately attack; Adhere-Connect, Stick-Follow, do not lose him.

引進落空合即出，沾連黏隨不丟
頂。

Your opponent expects his attack to meet resistance. If instead, you lead his attack past you, he will lose balance in the direction of his motion. This is the time to attack. Adhere-Connect means to attach a hand to him, and to become one with his motion, wherever he moves. Stick-Follow means to stay with him and not let him get away.

8. SONG OF
THE REAL MEANING

真義歌

No shape, no shadow.
Entire body transparent and empty.
Forget your surroundings and be natural.
Like a stone chime suspended from West Mountain.
Tigers roaring, monkeys screeching.
Clear fountain, peaceful water.
Turbulent river, stormy ocean.
With your whole being, develop your life.

無形無象。	全身透空。
忘物自然。	西山懸磬。
虎吼猿鳴。	泉清水靜。
翻江鬧海。	盡性立命。

When practicing Tai Chi Chuan you must let go of everything. Your mind must be clear and centered. No concepts (preconceptions) should cloud your vision, no thoughts should hinder your action. The body must be relaxed and stable so that you can be light and agile. Forget your surroundings and just do what needs to be done. West Mountain is a famous mountain. "Like a stone chime suspended from West Mountain" means your mind must be clear, your head held as if suspended from above, and your body as stable and rooted as a great mountain. Sound is important in Tai Chi Chuan because it is linked to your Chi and the emission of power. Your sound must be as powerful as a tiger's roar and as penetrating as a monkey's screech. If you lift your Spirit (Shen) and guide your Chi throughout your body, your mind will be as clear and pure as a fountain full of spring water. If you practice Tai Chi Chuan for a long time, cultivating your Chi, your Chi will fill your body and circulate peacefully. But, like water, it can move powerfully and quickly so that nothing can stand before it.

This is not something that can be done lightly or casually, for it takes your full attention and effort. When done this way, Tai Chi Chuan fills your whole life, tying in to everything else you do. At this stage the separation between your life and your art disappears, and your efforts are directed at improving yourself as a whole, unified person.

9. THE SECRET OF WITHDRAW AND RELEASE

撒放密訣

First Saying: Deflect
Deflect and open opponent's body and borrow opponent's Li (strength).

一曰擎，擎開彼身借彼力。

Do not meet the opponent's attack head on, or try to block it with force. Let your arm touch the opponent's arm, match his speed and direction, and deflect his attack from its original direction. If the opponent throws a right punch and you deflect it to your right, his right side will be exposed. When the opponent uses strength he will tend to be stiff. If you deflect him properly, his strength and momentum will cause him to lose balance. In this sense you are "borrowing" his strength to defeat him.

Second Saying: Lead
Lead (opponent's power) near (my) body, Jing thereby stored.

二曰引，引到身前勁始蓄。

When you neutralize an opponent's attack, draw him into you somewhat, and accumulate energy in your posture and Chi in your Dan Tien and spine. This is just like a bow accumulating energy when it is drawn, or a coil spring when it is compressed. You should also inhale in order to coordinate the motion with your Chi.

Third Saying: Relax
Relax and expand my Jing, without bends.

三曰鬆，鬆開我勁勿使屈。

The major difference between the Jing used in Tai Chi Ch'uan and the Jing of other styles is that Tai Chi emphasizes Chi support. This makes it possible to develop the Jing to a higher level. The first step of this development is relaxation. You must relax all of your muscles so that the Chi can flow wherever you want it without any hindrance. The Chi will then suffuse the muscles so that they function at peak efficiency.

When you counterattack you relax and emit Jing the way a bow relaxes from a state of tension as it shoots an arrow. Your posture should not have any kinks or awkward bends. Thus it is said: "Relax and expand my Jing, without bends".

When you apply force with your hand, there should be a counterforce into your rear foot to balance it. The line from the hand to the rear foot should be direct, without any "bends" (awkwardness in the posture) to disperse the energy. Thus it is said in Tai Chi Chuan: "Jing is straight and not curved".

Fourth Saying: Release
When (I) release, the waist and the feet must be timed carefully and accurately.

四 曰 放 ， 放 時 腰 脚 認 端 的 。

In order for the released Jing to reach its maximum level, your feet must be firmly rooted in the ground, the Jing must be generated from the legs, and the waist must control and direct it. Timing is critical in order to release your Jing effectively and efficiently. If you do not grasp the right moment to accurately express your Jing in attack or defense, it will be clumsy and inefficient, and you will miss the opportunity and lose the advantage. It is just like shooting at a moving target with a bow and arrow. The timing of the arrow's release and the accuracy of the aim are the keys to hitting the target.

10. TAI CHI CHUAN
FUNDAMENTAL KEY POINTS
太極拳基本要點

1. An insubstantial energy leads the head (upward). 虛領頂勁．

The head should feel like it is suspended from above. This will raise the Spirit of Vitality and let the whole body move lightly and agilely.

2. The eye gazes with concentrated Spirit. 眼神注視．

When a person has concentrated and raised his Spirit, his eyes will be bright and he will be able to pay attention to even the slightest movement of the enemy.

3. Hold the chest in, arc the back. 含胸拔背．

The back between the shoulders has the feeling of being lifted, and the chest is slightly sunken. This lets the chest relax and the lungs move naturally. This is also used to neutralize the opponent's attack and to store energy within the posture.

4. Sink the shoulders, drop the elbows. 沉肩垂肘．

Dropping the shoulders and elbows helps relaxation, and facilitates the transmission of energy into the hands. When the elbows and shoulders are sunken, the Jing can thread through from the waist to the hands so that they can function as one unit. Otherwise the Jing will be broken. Furthermore, sinking the elbows and shoulders will seal major cavities such as the armpit to an enemy's attack. This posture also helps you to neutralize attacks because you are compact and can more easily evade or deflect an attack.

5. Settle the wrists, extend the fingers. 坐腕伸指．

When the hand is extended palm downward, to "settle the wrist" means to drop the wrist slightly, so that the base of the palm is facing forward. This facilitates striking with the palm. Remember to keep the wrist relaxed. "Extend the fingers" means to let the fingers be straight, but not tensed. This should not be forced. Gradually get used to holding the fingers fairly straight so that there is no hindrance to the flow of blood and Chi.

6. Body central and upright. 身體中正．

The body should be straight and erect, not leaning to any side.

7. Pull up the tailbone. 尾閭 收住．

The tailbone should be pulled up slightly to the front in order to keep the pelvis at the proper angle and the lower back straight. When the tip of the tailbone is allowed to move backward, the pelvis tilts and the lower back curves inward. This deprives the lower abdomen of its support and lets the belly bulge forward. A bent lower back also hinders the efficient transmission of energy up and down the spine. Therefore, it is very important to keep the tailbone tucked under.

8. Relax your waist and relax your thighs. 鬆腰鬆胯 ．

The waist controls and directs the application of force. The thighs connect the waist to the knees, which are very important in all movement and in the generation of force by the legs. It is therefore important to keep the waist and thighs relaxed and movable.

9. The knees look relaxed, but are not relaxed.
膝部似鬆非鬆．

In Tai Chi Chuan, the Jing is generated from the legs. In order to do this, the legs must behave like springs to spring out the power. Therefore, the knees must be relaxed. However, the legs are also vital in changing the steps during the fight. When this happens, they must move fast and firm. In order to move fast with a firm root, the knees must be able to change their tension skillfully. Therefore, this statement means that the knees look relaxed but can be tensed whenever necessary.

10. Soles touch the ground. (or Feet flat on the ground.)
足掌貼地．

The feet (or foot) must always be flat on the ground and relaxed, so that your root will be stable. Unless a specific posture calls for it, don't rest your weight on just the heels or the toes, but instead let the weight spread over the whole of the foot. Keep your attention on the center of the foot, a little bit behind the Bubbling Well point. This is where the center of gravity naturally falls.

11. Top and bottom follow each other, the entire body should be harmonious.
上下相隨週身一致．

The entire body must move in a unified, coordinated way. Your upper body movement determines what your legs do, and your legs control your upper body. Arms and legs must move together, especially when pushing.

12. Distinguish insubstantial and substantial. 分清虛實．

The body as a whole, as well as each individual part of the body, has a substantial and an insubstantial aspect. Usually only one leg and one arm should be substantial at a time. Which part of the body is substantial or insubstantial depends upon the opponent's actions. When the opponent is substantial, I become insubstantial where he contacts me and substantial somewhere else, either left or right, up or down. Also, one must clearly judge whether the opponent's attack is substantial or insubstantial. Very often an opponent can change a substantial force into insubstantial, or vice versa. Therefore, I must know my Yin and Yang, and also know my opponent's Yin and Yang. Then I know the enemy, but the enemy doesn't know me. I can control him, but I cannot be controlled.

13. Internal and external are mutually coordinated. Breathe naturally.

內外相合，呼吸自然。

Breathing, Chi, muscular strength and Yi must all act together. Breathing should be relaxed and should match your actions in a comfortable way. If the breathing is tense or jerky, then there is tension in the body, the mind is not still, and the Chi flow is hindered and unable to support the Jing.

14. Use Yi (mind), not Li (strength). 用意不用力。

This means you should use skill, technique, and intelligence to defeat your opponent, and not just overwhelm him with strength. It also means that when you do a technique you should think only of what you are doing—e.g., pushing your opponent, locking an arm, etc. Do not think of Chi, strength, or your body, for this will split your attention and will weaken the technique. When you use Yi (mind) to move, Chi is automatically circulated, but when you use Li you will be more tense and Chi circulation will be hindered.

15. Chi circulates through the whole body; dividing, it moves up and down.

氣遍週身分行上下。

Although Chi is always circulating, it is also moving simultaneously to the Dan Tien where it is stored, and to the spine to be used in techniques. Of these two ways, the movement down the front of the body to the storage area at the Dan Tien is Yin. The movement through the tailbone and up the spine to the hands is Yang. Thus it is said, Chi adheres closely to the bones of the spine and flows upward.

16. Where Yi (the mind) is, Chi is. 意氣相連。

Chi follows the mind, so that wherever you put your attention, Chi accumulates. This is the reason that mental self-discipline is so important.

17. Every form of every posture follows smoothly; no forcing, no opposition, the entire body is comfortable.

式式勢順，不拗不背，週身舒適。

The entire sequence should flow smoothly from beginning to end. There should be no breaks, jerks, or sharp angles. The movements should be natural and comfortable for your body. In each posture, every part of the body contributes either directly or by counterbalancing. No part of the body should be hindering this unified flow.

18. Each form smooth. 式式均勻．

Every form in the sequence should be done smoothly, with Yi, Chi, and the body all unified.

19. Postures should not be too little or too much (i.e., neither insufficient nor excessive). They (the postures) should seek to be centered and upright.

姿勢無過，或不及當求其中正．

Your body should be natural, centered, balanced, and controlled. Your arms and legs should be neither too extended nor drawn in too much. Strive to be efficient.

20. Your applications should be concealed, and not exposed.

用法含而不露．

The opponent should not be able to sense or predict your intentions. Your attack and defense should be concealed and unpredictable in order to confuse your opponent.

21. Attain stillness in motion. 動中求靜．

You should maintain a meditative state while moving, then you will be calm and your mind clear.

22. Attain motion in stillness. 靜中求動．

If you are in a meditative state you will move your Chi and body naturally and correctly without conscious effort.

23. Light, then agile; agile, then move; move, then vary.

輕則靈，靈則動，動則變．

This is Tai Chi Chuan in a nutshell. The first requirement is to clear the mind, relax the body, and circulate the Chi. Then you will be light. If you adhere to your opponent, not resisting and not letting go, then you will be agile. You can then move to attack and defend, but remember to vary your attacks and responses so that your intentions cannot be read by your opponent.

11. SONG OF APPLICATION
功用歌

Light, agile, and alive, seek Dong Jing (to understand Jing); Yin and Yang cooperate mutually without the fault of stagnation; If (you) acquire (the trick), four ounces neutralizes one thousand pounds; Expand and close, stimulate the "drum", the center will be steady.

輕靈活潑求懂勁，陰陽相濟無滯病，若得四兩撥千斤，開合鼓蕩主宰定。

"Alive" here means alert and active. In practice you must pay close attention to your opponent/partner. In time you will be able to interpret his intention from the slightest of motions. Where the opponent is heavy, you are light. When one part of you is light, another part of you is heavy. You and your partner continually follow one another, never resisting, never separating. In this way the motion will continue to flow. In time you will acquire the knack of being light enough to avoid the opponent's attack, and substantial and controlled enough to deflect or attack him. Your postures alternately expand and close up with the circumstances. The drum is the abdomen in the area of the Dan Tien. You stimulate the Chi centered there with sound, attention, breathing and movement. This strengthens the Chi and exercises your control of it. When your attention and actions are thus centered on the Dan Tien, your stance will be stable and your mind calm and clear.

12. FIVE KEY WORDS

五字訣

First Saying: The Hsin (heart, mind) is quiet (calm).
When the heart (mind) is not quiet (calm), then (I am) not concentrated on one (thing). When I lift hands, forward and backward, left and right, (I am) totally without direction (purpose). In the beginning the movements do not follow the mind. Put the heart on recognizing and experiencing. Follow the opponent's movements, follow the curve, then expand. Don't lose (him), don't resist, don't extend or withdraw by yourself. (If the) opponent has Li (power), I also have Li, but my Li is first. (If the) opponent is without power, I also am without power, however my Yi (mind) is still first. One must be careful every movement. Wherever I am in contact, there the heart (mind) must be. One must seek information from not losing and not resisting; if I do that from now on, in one year or in half a year I will then be able to apply this with my body. All of this is using Yi (the mind), not using Jing. If I practice longer and longer, then the opponent is controlled by me, and I am not controlled by the opponent.

一曰心靜。心不靜則不專一，一舉手，前後左右，全無定向。起初舉動，未能由己，要悉心體認，隨人所動，隨屈就伸，不丟不頂，勿自伸縮，彼有力，我亦有力，我力在先，彼無力，我亦無力，我意仍在先。要刻刻留心，挨何處，心須用在何處，須向不丟不頂中討消息；從此做去，一年半載，便能施於身，此全是用意，不是用勁，久之則人為我制，我不為人制矣。

In Tai Chi Chuan, the mind is most important and controls movement. You cannot achieve this control by asserting your will. You must "give up yourself and follow the other". Don't resist, don't lose contact. Your power and mind are first in that you lead the opponent's attack away, rather than push it away. If you always remain lightly attached to the opponent you will gradually learn to sense his intentions. When you can follow automatically, your mind will be quiet and able to control your body and the opponent.

Second Saying: The body is agile.

If the body is stagnant, then (moving) forward and backward can't be at will. Therefore the body must be agile. When you lift your hands you must not have a clumsy appearance. When the opponent's power just touches my skin, my Yi (mind) is already deep into his bones. Two hands support, one Chi threading all through. (If) the left is heavy (attacked), then the left becomes insubstantial, (and) the right is gone (attacks). (If) the right is heavy, then the right becomes insubstantial and the left is gone. Chi is just like a cartwheel. Each part of the body must be mutually coordinated. If there is a place not mutually coordinated, then the body is dispersed and disordered, then you cannot gain power. (If you have) this fault, you must look to the waist and legs. First use your heart (mind) to master your body, following the opponent, not following your own will. Then the body will be able to follow the heart. Now you can follow your own will and also follow the opponent. If you follow your own will, then stagnation. If you follow the opponent, then you are alive. If able to follow the opponent, then the top of your hand has centimeters and inches. Weigh the opponent's Jing, big or small, then you have centimeters and millimeters with no mistakes. Measure the opponent's movement, long or short, then (you will make) no errors, even by a hairsbreadth. Forward and backward, everywhere just match (the opponent). The longer you study, then the finer your technique.

二曰身靈。身滯則進退不能自如，
，故要身靈。舉手不可有呆像已入，
彼之力方礙我手支撐，而右之意貫穿，則
彼骨裡。兩手支撐，而右重則週
左重則左虛，而左已去。氣如車輪，身便求
右虛俱要相隨，其病於腰腿己，
身散亂，便不得使身，從人不從人，從己上厘
之。先認從心，由己仍從人，手分差
後身能從人則活，能從人之大小，毫髮無久
則滯，從人則活，秤彼勁之大小，分彌
便有分寸，權彼來之長短，毫髮無差
不錯，權彼來之長短，處處恰合，工彌久
。前進後退，處處恰合，
而技彌精。

When you are light and agile and practice following for a long time, you can interpret the opponent's intentions at his lightest touch. Your two hands work together as a unit. When the opponent puts pressure on (attacks) your right side, that side becomes insubstantial (yields) and your left side has already attacked. When you can follow the opponent, then you can judge and interpret his actions and respond appropriately. The more you practice, the finer your sensitivity and control will be. It is as if your hand had a ruler or micrometer on it to measure the opponent's actions.

Third Saying: Chi condenses.
When the appearance of Chi is dispersed and diffused, then it is not conserved, and the body can easily be scattered and disordered. In order to make Chi condense into the bones your exhalation and inhalation must flow agilely (smoothly). The entire body is without gap. Inhalation is storage, and exhalation is emitting. That is because inhalation lifts up naturally (the Spirit of Vitality). It can also lift (control) the opponent. (When you) exhale, then (your Chi) can sink naturally. (You) also can release (Jing) out to the opponent. That means use Yi (your mind) to move your Chi, don't use Li (strength).

三曰氣歛。氣勢散漫，便無含蓄，身易散亂，務使氣歛入骨，呼吸通靈，週身罔間，吸為蓄，呼為發，蓋吸則自然提得起，亦拏得人起，呼則自然沉得下，亦放人得出，此是以意運氣，非以力運氣也。

When your Chi is scattered about your body in an undisciplined fashion, your body will be disorganized. You must calm the mind. When you inhale, let the Chi accumulate in the Dan Tien and spine, and raise up the Spirit of Vitality. When you exhale, move the Chi from the spine, to the shoulders, and out to the hands. When you exhale, the Chi is also fully sunk to the tailbone. Breathing must be unhindered and must comfortably match your actions.

Fourth Saying: Jing is integrated.
The entire body's Jing, (when) trained, becomes one family (one unit). Distinguish clearly insubstantial and substantial. Emitting Jing must have root and origin. Jing begins at the foot's root, is controlled by the waist, expressed by the fingers, emitted by the spine and back. (You) must also lift up the entire Spirit of Vitality. When the opponent's Jing is just about to be emitted, but is not yet emitted, my Jing already accepts it in (senses it). Just right, not late, not early. (It is) just like the skin (senses) fire. Like a spring bubbling up from the ground. Forward, backward, not the slightest scattering or confusion. Look for the straight in the curved. Store and then emit. (If you do this) then (you will be) able to follow the (opponent's) hands and act effectively. This is borrowing (the opponent's) Li to strike the opponent, and (using) four ounces to repel a thousand pounds.

四曰勁整。一身之勁，練成一家，分清虛實，發勁要有根源，勁起於腳根，主宰於腰，形於手指，發於脊背，又要提起全副精神，於彼勁將出未發之際，我勁已接入彼勁，恰好不後不先，如皮燃火，如泉湧出，前進後退，無絲毫散亂，曲中求直，蓄而後發，方能隨手奏效，此借力打人，四兩撥千金也。

You must learn how all parts of the body contribute to the technique, what parts are heavy or active, and what parts are light or insubstantial. Jing is rooted in the feet, it originates in (is generated by) the legs, is controlled by the waist, emitted by the spine, and expressed by the hands. Raising the Spirit of Vitality allows you to have a strong root and a clear mind. Timing is crucial for effective technique. You must develop the lightness and sensitivity to respond to the opponent's attack as quickly and unconsciously as the skin responds to fire. At the first touch, or even before the touch, you know his intention and are already neutralizing him. Your movement and response must be continuous and flowing like a spring bubbling up out of the ground. You are continuously moving in curves and circles. This allows you to bend like a bow or coil like a spring and accumulate energy in your posture. You also accumulate Chi in your spine and Dan Tien. When you neutralize you curve or bend, and then you attack in a straight line. If you learn these skills you will be able to defeat your opponent easily and automatically.

Fifth Saying: Spirit condenses.
All in all, (if) the above four items (are) totally acquired, it comes down to condensing Shen (Spirit). When Shen condenses, then one Chi (can be) formed, like a drum. Training Chi belongs to Shen. Chi appears agitated and smooth. The Spirit of Vitality is threaded and concentrated. Opening and closing have numbers (degrees of fineness). Insubstantial and substantial are clearly distinguished: if the left is insubstantial, then the right is substantial; if the right is insubstantial, then the left is substantial. Insubstantial doesn't mean absolutely no Li. The appearance of Chi must have agitation and smoothness; in actuality it does not happen instantly (by magic). The Spirit of Vitality should be emphasized, it must be threaded and concentrated. Li is borrowed from the opponent. Chi is emitted from the spine. How can Chi come from the spine? (When) Chi sinks downward from the two shoulders, condenses into the bones of the spine, concentrates at the waist (Dan Tien), this Chi from the top to the bottom is called closing. From the waist, appearing in the bones of the spine, then spreading to the shoulders, appearing

in the fingers, this Chi from the bottom to the top is called opening. Closing means to draw in, opening means to release. If able to understand opening and closing, then (you) know Yin and Yang. When you understand these steps, then (if you) practice one day, your technique is refined one day. (Then you) gradually approach (the point) where you can not but achieve what you want.

五曰神聚。上四者俱備，總歸神聚，神聚則一氣鼓鑄，煉氣歸神，氣勢騰挪，精神貫注，開合有數，虛實清楚：左虛則右實，右虛則左實，虛非全然無力，氣勢要有騰挪；實非全然占煞，精神要有貫注。力從人借，氣由脊發，胡能氣由脊發？氣向下沉，由兩肩收入脊骨，注於腰間，此氣之由上而下也，謂之合。由腰形於脊骨，布於兩膊，施於手指，此氣之由下而上也，謂之開。合便是收，開便是放；能懂得開合，便知陰陽，到此地步，工用一日，技精一日，漸至從心所欲，罔不如意矣。

Just as you train your Chi to thread through every part of your body, so too must you train your Spirit. Your awareness must reach to every part of your body and even beyond, but yet it must also be focused or concentrated. When your Spirit is concentrated your Mind will be able to move the Chi. It is said "Yi Sou Dan Tien". This means the mind (Yi) is kept on the Dan Tien. The mind will move as you move or do techniques, but it always returns to the abdomen. As you do this you are developing and training your Chi, which is an important part of Spirit. As Chi accumulates it will fill the Dan Tien and the abdomen will be taut like a drum. This is not a rigid tightness. It is the firmness that comes from inflation. Like a drum, Chi has a vibrating and pulsating energy. The Chinese translated here as "agitated" has the sense of motion up and down like a prancing horse or a bubbling well; the word translated here as "smooth" has the sense of smooth motion back and forth. The Spirit of Vitality is an aspect of Shen. It must be lifted up to raise the Spirit as a whole. Shen does not exist in a vacuum. You must develop your techniques, and learn about Yin and Yang. Techniques do not happen by magic—they depend upon a firm grasp of principles, and Jing supported by Chi, all guided by your Spirit. You must understand closing and opening. As you neutralize an attack, you draw him into you, drawing in and borrowing his energy, as well as accumulating the energy of your own body in the Dan Tien. This is called closing, and is done on the inhale. Chi sinks from the shoulders to the Dan Tien down the front of the body. This is Yin and is used to withdraw. At the appropriate time you release the accumulated energy up the spine and out to the hands. This is called opening and is done on the exhale. Chi is raised from the tailbone up the spine to the shoulders and out to the fingers. This is Yang and is used to emit Jing. Again, in all of this, the mind is the master.

13. OLD TAI CHI CHUAN CLASSIC OF CHING CHYAN LON DYNASTY (1736-1796 A.D.)

乾隆舊鈔本歌訣

Follow the neck to thread (the Chi) to the head, the two shoulders relaxed. Condense the strong lower Chi, and support the hips. The stomach sound extends the Jing to strengthen the two fist's (Jing). Five toes grasp the ground, the top bent like a bow.

順項貫頂兩膀鬆，束烈下氣把襠
撐，胃音開勁兩捶爭，五指抓地
上彎弓。

An insubstantial energy lifts the head and straightens the neck. This allows the Chi to flow naturally, and keeps the shoulders relaxed and sunken. The Chi of the lower abdomen condenses into the Dan Tien. The Chi sinks downward into the Dan Tien and into the feet, and at the same time there is force coming up and supporting the hips. This sinking and lifting allows the posture to be stable and flexible. The "Ha" sound, which comes from the "stomach" or abdomen, helps you raise the Spirit of Vitality, coordinate Chi and Jing, and extend energy out to your hands. When your feet "grasp the ground" the root should be firm and alive, but the feet should still remain relaxed. The legs should be bent like a bow. The Chinese word for toes can also mean fingers, and so an alternate meaning for this sentence can be that the hand should be shaped as if it were holding a large ball, and should be bent backward a bit.

Lift and move lightly and agilely and condense the Spirit internally. Don't be broken and then continuous, refine your one Chi. Left and right as appropriate have insubstantial and substantial places. When Yi (mind) is up, this implies down; and give up post-birth strength.

舉動輕靈神內斂，莫教斷續一氣
研，左宜右有虛實處，意上寓下
後天還。

You should be light and agile and should keep your Spirit inside. If you expose your Spirit externally, people can see what you are doing and thinking. Your postures and motion should be fluid and continuous, and all should be one flow of Chi. The different parts of the body are substantial or insubstantial, and this changes constantly with the circumstances. To do this appropriately requires correct timing. When your attention is up, don't forget down. When the opponent attacks down, don't forget up. All of this is not done with post-birth strength (Li), but rather with Chi-supported Jing.

Grasp and hold the Dan Tien to train internal Kung Fu. Hen, Ha, two Chi's are marvellous and infinite. Move open, quiet close, bend and extend following your opponent. Slow respond (slow), fast follow (fast), the principles must be understood thoroughly.

拿住丹田鍊內功，哼哈二氣妙無窮，動分靜合屈伸就，緩應急隨理貫通。

When your attention remains on your Dan Tien you will gradually generate internal energy. When you coordinate this with your breathing and motions, your Kung Fu will be internal and superior to the external variety. The two sounds, Hen and Ha, help you to mobilize and express your energy. When you move you open, or extend your energy. When you close you accumulate energy, but calmly, so the opponent doesn't notice. You bend and extend, contract and expand, yield and adhere, neutralize and attack, all depending upon your opponent. You move slow or fast, following the opponent, and always according to the Tai Chi principles.

Suddenly disappear, suddenly appear. Forward, then expand. A feather cannot be added; be perfect like the Taoist bible. Hand slow, hand fast, all not alike. Four ounces repel a thousand pounds, apply this principle and neutralize well.

忽隱忽現進則長，一羽不加至道藏，手慢手快皆非似，四兩撥千運化良。

As you exchange substantial and insubstantial, you disappear in front of the enemy's attack and reappear elsewhere to attack him. You remain insubstantial, and when you find an opportunity you move forward and "expand", i.e., become substantial. "Forward, then expand" can also mean that when the opponent moves forward you become insubstantial in front of his attack, and attack on the other side. This is just like the Tai Chi diagram, where each side is small where the other side is large, and large where the other side is small. You must be so light, agile, and responsive that a feather cannot touch you without setting you in motion. If you can do this, your art will be as perfect as the Taoist bible. Slow or fast, the situation is always changing, but if you adhere to the principles you will be able to neutralize an attack of a thousand pounds with four ounces.

Peng (Wardoff), Lu (Rollback), Ghi (Press), An (Push) are the four main directions. Chai (Pluck), Lie (Split), Zou (Elbow-Stroke), Kau (Shoulder-Stroke) complete the four diagonal corners. Chyan (Heaven), Kuen (Earth), Jenn (Thunder), Duey (Lake) are the eight trigrams. Forward, backward, look to the left, look to the right, and central equilibrium are the five elements

棚擺擠按四方正，採挒肘靠斜角
成，乾坤震兌乃八卦，進退顧盼
定五行。

Tai Chi Chuan is said to be comprised of thirteen postures. These are the eight basic moves and the five directions. These are coordinated with the eight trigrams (the author lists only four, assuming the reader is already quite familiar with them) and the five elements.

Chyan (Heaven) .... Peng (Wardoff)
Kuen (Earth) .... Lu (Rollback)
Kann (Water) .... Ghi (Press)
Lii (Fire) .... An (Push)
Shiunn (Wind) .... Chai (Pluck)
Jenn (Thunder) .... Lie (Split)
Duey (Lake) .... Zou (Elbow-Stroke)
Genn (Mountain) .... Kau (Shoulder-Stroke)

Jinn Bu (Forward) .... Gin (Metal)
Twe Bu (Backward) .... Moo (Wood)
Sou Gu (Left) .... Sui (Water)
Yu Pan (Right) .... For (Fire)
Sung Dien (Center) .... Tu (Earth)

Extremely soft means hardness. That means extremely insubstantial and agile. When you transport (Chi) it is like drawing silk from a cocoon. Everywhere clear. Open and expanding, tight and compact, one right after the other, should be threaded together tightly. Wait for the opportunity, then move as a cat moves.

極柔即剛極虛靈，運若抽絲處處
明，開展緊湊乃縝密，待機而動
如貓行。

In Tai Chi, you achieve hardness through softness. You remain light and agile, avoiding the opponent's attack, and waiting for the opportunity when you can mobilize all your forces and attack with certainty. Your motion is smooth, continuous and unbroken so that you can mobilize and transport your Chi effectively. When you are experienced at moving Chi throughout your body, you will be able to clearly sense where the energy is. When you are opening and closing, expanding and contracting in response to your opponent's moves, your postures should mesh together seamlessly so that there is no opportunity for him to attack. You adhere and stick, neutralize and follow, always paying careful attention. When the opportunity to attack presents itself, you attack instantly.

14. SONG OF COMPREHENSION AND APPLICATION

體用歌

Tai Chi Chuan, thirteen postures, it's marvelous, (because there are) two Chi's, discriminated as Yin and Yang.

太極拳，十三式，妙在二氣分陰
陽。

Tai Chi Chuan, because it includes thirteen movements and directions in its fighting strategy, is also called the thirteen postures. This extraordinary training and fighting strategy is made up of two Chi's—Yin and Yang. All the movements, breathing, Chi circulation, and techniques are based on Yin and Yang principles and derive into insubstantial and substantial fighting strategies.

Neutralization generates a thousand million (techniques), all belonging to one (principle). All belongs to one. Tai Chi Chuan has two poles, four faces, it is infinite.

化生千億歸抱一，歸抱一，太極
拳兩儀四象渾無邊。

From Yin and Yang (insubstantial and substantial) fighting strategies, the principle of neutralization is generated. From the principle of neutralization, numerous techniques are created. Though the techniques are many, there is only one principle. From Tai Chi's two poles—Yin and Yang—are generated four faces; the four faces generate eight trigrams, the eight trigrams generate sixty-four hexagrams, and the hexagrams generate everything else. The four faces are extreme Yin, extreme Yang, deficient Yin and deficient Yang. The Chinese translated here as "infinite" is literally "blurred no sides". This has the feeling of being on a foggy river where everything is indistinct and the shores cannot be seen.

If you follow the wind, how can your head be suspended? I have one guiding sentence. Today I want to tell it to the people who can comprehend. (If) the Bubbling Well (Yongquan cavity) has no root, the waist has no master, (then) you can try hard to learn until you almost die, you will still not succeed.

御風何似頂頭懸，我有一轉語，
今為知者吐，湧泉無根，腰無主
，力學垂死終無補。

If you sway and move around like a kite in the wind, you cannot cultivate the feeling of being suspended from above. You must keep the body straight and erect, with an insubstantial energy lifting the head and giving you the feeling of being suspended from above. At the same time you must sink your Chi to the soles of the feet into the Bubbling Well cavities. Having a good root is absolutely essential for getting force out to the hands, or to any part of the body for any of the techniques. A good root is also necessary for effective use of the waist. If there is no root and waist control, all your practice is in vain and your techniques are useless.

When comprehension and application mutually support one another—is there any other trick to do this? (No), because marvelous Chi can approach the hands.

體用相兼豈有他，浩然氣能行乎手。

A Tai Chi practitioner must learn the principles and techniques first, and then he should ponder and comprehend the deeper meaning of the theory. Only after that can he apply all the theory and techniques. After he has gained enough experience in applying the techniques, he should go back to the theory and ponder again, and then apply it to the techniques and so on. Comprehension and application mutually support each other, and will help one become a high level Tai Chi artist. If one practices this way his Chi will be able to reach his hands. This will not only benefit his health, but will also be useful in martial applications.

Peng (Wardoff), Lu (Rollback), Ghi (Press), An (Push), Chai (Pluck), Lie (Split), Zou (Elbow-Stroke), Kau (Shoulder-Stroke), and Jinn (Forward), Twe (Backward), Gu (Left), Pan (Right), and Dien (Center). Don't neutralize, automatically neutralize; (don't) yield, automatically yield.

掤攦擠按採挒肘，靠及進退顧盼定，不化自化走自走。

For all thirteen postures, one should follow the rule of natural response. Yielding and neutralizing should not be big, conscious moves. They should be natural and automatic. Don't try to yield. Stay calm and centered and let it happen automatically. Just stick to the enemy, follow, and automatically neutralize.

(When you) wish the foot to go forward, you must push off from the rear (foot). Your body is like moving clouds. (When you) strike with the hands, why use hands? The entire body is hands, but the hands are not your hands. However (you) must be careful to protect what should be protected at all times.

足欲向前先挫後，身似行雲打手安用手，渾身是手手非手，但須方寸隨時守所守。

When you wish to move, push off the rear foot. Move lightly like a cloud. When you strike don't use the force of the arms. Instead use the force of the whole body, generated from the legs and controlled by the waist. It may not be necessary to use the hands at all. Instead you may use any part of the body in contact with the opponent. However, when you do this you must remember to do whatever is necessary to protect yourself.

15. SONG OF THE THIRTEEN POSTURES

十三勢歌

All the thirteen postures (of Tai Chi Chuan) must not be treated lightly. The meaning of life originates at the waist.

十三總勢莫輕視，命意源頭在腰際。

The thirteen postures are the foundation of Tai Chi Chuan. The waist is important because it governs all of your movements, and because Chi is generated and stored in the Dan Tien.

(When you) vary and exchange insubstantial and substantial (you) must take care that Chi (circulates) in the entire body without the slightest stagnation.

變換虛實須留意，氣遍身軀不少滯。

When you move your body, you are changing and exchanging substantial and insubstantial and transporting Chi to various parts of your body. It is important that the whole body is relaxed and the mind is clear so that the Chi can move through the whole body without hindrance. When Chi moves easily there is health, when Chi stagnates there is illness.

Touch (find) the movement in the stillness, (although there is) stillness even in movement. Vary (your) response to the enemy and show the marvelous technique.

靜中觸動動猶靜，應敵變化示神奇。

Tai Chi has been called meditation in motion. While moving, the mind is still centered and quiet as in sitting meditation. At the same time, while in this meditative state one is still actively circulating Chi. When attacked, remain in the meditative state, calm and aware. When the principles have been learned and internalized, you can respond naturally and comfortably to the opponent's moves. Tai Chi is the art of change. As you follow the opponent's actions, your response subtly changes and varies with the situation.

Pay attention to every posture and gauge its purpose, (then you will) gain (the art) without wasting your time and energy.

勢勢存心揆用意，得來全不費功夫。

The care and seriousness you put into your study determines the degree of success you will have. Every posture has its nature and purpose, and must be researched and studied before it can be really understood.

In every movement the heart (mind) remains on the waist, the abdomen is relaxed and clear, and Chi rises up.

刻刻留心在腰間，腹內鬆淨氣騰然。

In all the postures the principle is the same: the mind must remain on the Dan Tien (Yi Sou Dan Tien). The abdomen must be relaxed and the mind calm and clear so that the Chi will rise up and circulate throughout the body.

The tailbone is central and upright, the Spirit is threaded through the head. The entire body is light and easy (relaxed), the top of the head is suspended.

尾閭中正神貫頂，滿身輕利頂頭懸。

The lower vertebrae must be erect and the back straight, and an insubstantial energy must lift the head upward.

Pay attention carefully in (your) research, bent-extended, open-closed follow their freedom.

仔細留心向推求，屈伸開合聽自由。

Bent-extended, open-closed are the tricks of pushing hands. Bend to neutralize the enemy's power, at the same time close to store your Jing, and then open and extend to emit your Jing. All these techniques must be natural and freely follow your opponent's intention, then you can Adhere-Connect, Stick-Follow and defeat your opponent. If you do not research these tricks with all your heart, you will not gain the key to Tai Chi Chuan.

To enter the door and be led along the way, one needs oral instruction; practice without ceasing, the way is through self-study.

入門引路須口授，功夫無息法自修。

To learn Tai Chi well a teacher is needed. There are so many subtleties that it is very easy to get something wrong or emphasize the wrong things. It is said "a slight error can cause a thousand mile divergence". Traditionally in the martial arts there were two kinds of students—the outer and the inner. The outer students were often accepted for their money or to test their seriousness. They were taught only the forms and a minimum of applications and principles. Once a student was judged worthy he was taken into the temple and shown the inner secrets of the style. Today it is often much easier to learn the secrets of a martial art because so much has been published. However, having a good teacher in the flesh is still almost a necessity. Once one has been shown the way, the only thing remaining is to practice unceasingly and to continually research on one's own.

If asked, what is the standard (criteria) of its (thirteen postures) application, (the answer is) Yi (mind) and Chi are the master, and the bones and muscles are the chancellor.

若 問 體 用 何 為 準 ， 意 氣 君 來 骨 肉 臣 。

The criteria for judging whether the postures are applied correctly is: are the mind and Chi directing the movement? All movement is done with Jing supported by Chi and directed by Yi (mind). If the movement is done only with bones and muscles, it is considered Li, or muscular strength, and is incorrect.

Investigate in detail what the ultimate meaning is: to increase the age, extend the years, and achieve never-aging youthfulness.

詳 推 用 意 終 何 在 ， 益 壽 延 年 不 老 春 。

You must remember that the ultimate purpose of Tai Chi is to maintain a healthy body and a youthful mind.

The song, the song, one hundred and forty (words), every word is real and true, no meaning is left behind. If not approached from this (song), your time and energy are wasted in vain, and you will sigh in regret.

歌 兮 歌 兮 百 四 十 ， 字 字 真 切 意 無 遺 。 若 不 向 此 推 求 去 ， 枉 費 功 夫 貽 歎 息 。

Whether you study the art for health or self-defense, you must follow the words of this song or your efforts will be wasted.

APPENDIX B
GLOSSARY

An: Push. A technique for pushing or striking the opponent. It is one of the Four Directions of the eight basic Tai Chi fighting techniques, which correspond to the Eight Trigrams (Ba Kua).

Ba Kua: the Eight Trigrams. The Yi Ching, a book of philosophy, lists eight basic principles, which are derived from Yin and Yang, and which in turn give rise to other variations. These eight principles are each represented by three broken and/or straight lines known as trigrams (See Yi Ching). In Tai Chi Chuan the trigrams correspond to the basic techniques Peng, Lu, Ghi, An, Chai, Lie, Zou, and Kau.

Ba Kua Chang: Eight Trigrams Palm. One of the internal Chinese martial styles, based on the Ba Kua theory. It emphasizes the application of palm techniques and circular movements. Ba Kua Chang was created by Tung Hai-Chuan in the nineteenth century.

Ba Tuan Gin: Eight Pieces of Brocade. A style of Chi Kung training, said to be created by Marshal Yeuh Fei in the Sung Dynasty (960-1279 A.D.). Originally called Shih Er Tuan Gin (twelve pieces of brocade), it was later shortened to eight forms.

Bi Chi: Seal the Breath. One of the four major categories of Chin Na techniques, it specializes in sealing (obstructing) the opponent's breath or a blood vessel, causing unconsciousness or death.

Chai: Pluck. A technique for unbalancing the opponent or pulling him into an exposed position. One of the Four Corners of the eight basic Tai Chi fighting techniques.

Chian Gin Juey: Thousand Pound Sinking. A popular training in Chinese martial arts, used to train the root and the stability of the postures. Refers to the practitioner imagining sinking into the ground as if he weighed a thousand pounds.

Chang Chuan: Long Fist or Long Sequence. When it means Long Fist, it is a northern Shaolin Chinese martial style which specializes in kicking techniques. When it means Long Sequence, it refers to Tai Chi Chuan and implies that the Tai Chi sequence is long and flowing like a river.

Chang San-Feng: Said to be the creator of Tai Chi Chuan in the Sung Dynasty (960-1279 A.D.), however, there is no certain documentary proof of this.

Chen Chang-Shen: The fouteenth generation master of Chen style Tai Chi Chuan, who taught the art to Yang Lu-Shann.

Cheng Man-Ching: A famous Yang style Tai Chi master from Taiwan, who taught in the United States during the 1960s. He taught a shortened version of the form (which is very popular here and in Taiwan) and stressed relaxation and the health aspect.

Chen Jar Gou: The name of the village of the Chen family, where Chen Style Tai Chi Chuan originated.

Chen Yen-Lin: A famous Chinese Yang Style master in the 1940s. At that time he wrote a book on Tai Chi Chuan which is still considered one of the best. Born in 1906, he is still alive and living in Shanghai, China.

Chi: The "intrinsic energy" which circulates in all living things.

Chi Li (or Li Chi): Chi supported muscular power. When you concentrate your mind (Yi) and keep the muscles relaxed, the Chi flow will increase and invigorate the muscles.

Chi Kung: A type of Kung Fu training which specializes in building up the Chi circulation in the body for health and/or martial purposes.

Chiang Fa: The Tai Chi master who passed the art of Tai Chi Chuan to the Chen family.

Chin Woo Association: A Chinese martial art organization, founded in 1909 by Huo Yuen-Jar in Shanghai.

Ching: The main Chi (energy) channels. In the human body there are twelve pairs of these channels, which are related to the internal organs.

Ching Ling: Lightness and agility. These words are often used to describe the motion of monkeys—responsive, controlled, and able to move quickly.

Chin Na: literally Grasp and Control. An aspect of Chinese martial art training, Chin Na specializes in controlling the enemy through "misplacing the joint", "dividing the muscle", "sealing the breath", and "cavity press".

Chuan: Fist. This term in Chinese martial arts is also used to denote a Kung Fu style, e.g. Shaolin Chuan or Tai Chi Chuan, or a sequence, for example, Lien Bu Chuan and Gung Li Chuan.

Chung: Layering. The same character, when pronounced as Jong, means weight or heaviness.

Chyan: One of the Eight Trigrams (Ba Kua). Corresponds to Heaven.

Da Chou Tien: Grand Circulation. A Chi Kung training in which the Chi is led to circulate throughout the entire body.

Da Lu: Large Rollback. Rollback is one of the eight basic Tai Chi fighting techniques, and is a method of leading the opponent's attack past you. There are two versions—large and small rollback. Da Lu also refers to a two-person pushing hands exercise which concentrates on using the four "corners" (Chai, Lie, Zou, Kau), as well as the four "directions"(Peng, Lu, Ghi, An).

Da Mo's Yi Gin Ching: Da Mo was an Indian prince who went to China to preach Buddhism around 527 A.D. His book "Yi Gin Ching" (Muscle Change Classic) describes methods for generating and circulating Chi in the body to improve the health. This training was later found to be useful for increasing the power of martial techniques.

Dan Tien: Field of Elixir. There are three Dan Tiens in the body: between the eyebrows, the solar plexus area, and the lower abdomen. Tai Chi is primarily interested in the lower Dan Tien. It is considered the resevoir of Chi, and is located approximately one and one-half inches below the navel and about a third of the way toward the spine. In acupuncture this point is known as Qihai (Sea of Chi).

Dsao Gu: Beware of the Left. One of the five fundamental strategic movements which correspond to the Five Elements.

Dsung Dien: Central Equilibrium. One of the five basic strategic movements.

Du Mei: Governing Vessel. One of the eight Chi vessels which, along with the twelve channels, are the major Chi pathways in the human body. Du Mei runs from the tailbone, along the spine, to the roof of the mouth.

Duey: One of the Eight Trigrams (Ba Kua). Corresponds to Lake.

For: Fire. One of the Five Elements (Wu Hsing).

Genn: One of the eight trigrams (Ba Kua). Corresponds to Mountain.

Ghi: Press. One of the Four Directions of the eight basic Tai Chi fighting techniques. Usually done with one hand on the other forearm, it often pushes the opponent at an angle to his line of motion.

Gin: Metal. One of the Five Elements (Wu Hsing).

Gin Chung Tsao: Golden Bell Cover. A Kung Fu training which enables a person to be struck without injury.

Gung Sou: Arc Hands. Also known as "Universal Post", it is a standing meditation form of Chi Kung training, in which Chi is built up in the shoulders and then circulated to the limbs and internal organs.

Ha: One of the two sounds used in Tai Chi Chuan and other Chinese martial styles. The Ha sound is positive (Yang) and is used to raise the Spirit of Vitality, enabling power to reach its maximum.

Hen: The other sound used in Tai Chi. The Hen sound is purely negative (Yin) when done during the inhale. When done this way it condenses the Yi and Chi into the marrow. When done on the exhale, Hen is negative with some positive. This allows you to attack while conserving some energy.

Hou Tien Far: Post-Heaven Techniques. A Kung Fu style which existed hundreds of years before Tai Chi Chuan and was said to embody the same principles.

Hsin: Heart. In Chinese it often means mind. It refers to an intention, idea or thought which has not been expressed.

Hsin—Yi: Heart—Mind. Hsin has the sense of "mind", and Yi has the sense of "intention". When used together they refer to the desire to do something specific.

Hsing Yi C~~hdsfds Shdsf Mind Fist. O~~ of the internal Chinese martial styles. It is ~~...~~ (Wu Hsing), as well as motions c~~...~~ was created by Marshal Yueh Fei during the Sung Dynasty.

Jenn: One of the eight trigrams (Ba Kua). Corresponds to Thunder.

Jieng: Essence. What is left after something has been refined and purified. In Chinese medicine, Jieng can mean semen, but it generally refers to the basic substance of the body which the Chi and Spirit enliven.

Jieng-Shen: Essence of the Spirit; Spirit of Vitality. A person with a strong Jieng-Shen is active, vigorous, and concentrated.

Jing: Power; flow of energy. In Chinese martial arts there are many types of Jing, but they all deal with the flow of energy. These range from sensing Jings (sensing the enemy's power), to neutralizing Jings (neutralizing or deflecting the enemy's power), to emitting Jings (emitting power in a smooth pulse). In general, the higher the level of Jing, the more Chi and the less Li (muscular strength) is used.

Jing Kung: A type of Kung Fu which specializes in training Chi to support Jing so that the Jing can reach its maximum.

Jinn Bu: Step Forward. One of the five basic strategic movements of Tai Chi.

Jong: Weight or heaviness. The same Chinese character, when pronounced as Chung, means layering.

Juan—Hsin: Juan means concentrated; Hsin means heart or mind. Juan—Hsin means concentrated mind.

Kann: One of the eight trigrams (Ba Kua). Corresponds to Water.

Kau: Shoulder—Stroke. A technique of using the shoulder to strike or throw the opponent. One of the "four corners" of the eight basic Tai Chi fighting techniques.

Kon Chi: Air.

Kuen: One of the eight trigrams (Ba Kua). Corresponds to Earth.

Kung Fu: literally energy and time. Anything which takes time and energy to master is called Kung Fu. Nowaday, it commonly means Chinese martial arts.

Kuoshu: National Technique. The name for Chinese martial arts used by Chiang Kai-Shek since 1926, and still used in Taiwan. Mainland China uses the term Wushu.

Li: Muscular power, strength.

Lii: One of the eight trigrams (Ba Kua). Corresponds to Fire.

Lie: Rend. The use of two opposing forces to lock or unbalance the opponent. One of the "four corners" of the eight basic Tai Chi fighting techniques.

Lu: Rollback. A technique for leading the opponent's attack past you. One of the Four Directions of the eight basic Tai Chi fighting techniques.

Liu Ho Ba Fa: Six Combinations and Eight Methods. One of the internal Chinese martial styles. Said to have been created by Chen Bou during the Sung Dynasty.

Lou: Branches. The numerous tiny Chi channels which extend from the major channels (Ching) and allow the Chi to reach from the skin to the marrow.

Mei: Vessels. The eight auxillary Chi channels which are not associated with internal organs.

Moo: Wood. One of the five basic elements (Wu Hsing).

Nanking Central Kuoshu Institute: A Chinese martial arts institute, founded by the Chinese government in 1926 to promote the martial arts.

Nei Dan: Internal Elixir. Chi Kung training in which the Chi is generated at the Dan Tien, then circulated throughout the entire body.

Nei Jar: Internal Family. Refers to the internal Chinese martial styles, the most famous of which are Tai Chi Chuan, Hsing Yi, and Ba Kua. The external styles are known as Wai Jar (External Family).

Nei Jing: Internal Power. The Jing or power in which Chi from the Dan Tien is used to support the muscles. This is characterized by relatively relaxed muscles. When the muscles predominate and local Chi is used to support them, it is called Wai Jing (external Jing).

Nei Jing Li: Internal Jing Li. Same as Nei Jing. Called Li because no matter how much Chi you use to generate the power, you must still use the muscles to some degree. For the same reason, Wai Jing is also sometimes called Wai Jing Li.

Nei Kung: Internal Kung Fu. This is another name for Chi Kung.

Pai Huo: White Crane. A style of southern Shaolin Kung Fu which imitates the fighting techniques of the crane.

Peng: Ward-off. A technique for bouncing the opponent's force back in the direction it came from. One of the "four directions" of the eight basic Tai Chi fighting techniques.

Ren Mei: Conception Vessel. One of the eight auxillary Chi channels (Mei) in the human body. It runs from the base of the body up the front of the body and ends in the tongue.

Roan Jing: Soft Jing. In this Jing the Chi predominates and muscle usage is reduced to the minimum.

Roan Ying Jing: Soft Hard Jing. When this Jing is generated, the muscles are relaxed as much as possible to allow the Chi to flow. Right before the Jing reaches the target, they are then suddenly tightened to avoid injuring the hands, and also to focus the Jing to the spot being attacked.

San Bao: Three Treasures—Jieng (essence), Chi (internal energy), and Shen (Spirit). The Chinese people believe that if these three things are properly cultivated and guarded, they will have a long and healthy life.

San Shih Chi Shih: Thirty-Seven Postures. According to historical records, one of the predecessors of Tai Chi Chuan.

Shao Chou Tien: Small Circulation. Nei Dan Chi Kung training where Chi is generated at the Dan Tien, and then moved in a circle through the Conception and Governing Vessels.

Shao Jeou Tien: Small Nine Heaven. According to the historical records, one of the predecessors of Tai Chi Chuan.

Shaolin: The name of a Buddihist Temple, built in 377 A.D., which later became a Chinese martial arts training center.

Shao Lu: Small Rollback. Another name for Rollback.

Shen: Spirit. The consciousness within which the mind and thought function.

Shih Er Chuang: Twelve Postures. A style of Chi Kung training.

Shiunn: One of the eight trigrams (Ba Kua). Corresponds to Wind.

Shuang: Double or Pair.

Shuang Jong: Double Weighting. The fault of not distinguishing between substantial and insubstantial.

Sui: Water. One of the five basic elements (Wu Hsing).

Tai Chi: Supreme Ultimate. The state in which things are differentiated into opposites, known as Yin and Yang.

Tai Chi Chuan: Grand Ultimate Fist. (Pronounced Tie Jee Chuen)

Tiea Bu Shan: Iron Shirt. Kung Fu training which enables a person to endure a strike or blow without injury. Similar to Golden Bell Cover.

Tien Hsueh: Cavity Press. A high level technique of Chinese Kung Fu in which certain acupuncture points are struck or grasped in order to injure or kill the opponent.

Tu: Earth. One of the five basic elements (Wu Hsing).

Tou Tien: Supporting the Heavens. A form of Chi Kung training used to train the strength and endurance of the legs, and also build up Chi in the spine.

Twe Bu: Step Backward. One of the five basic strategic movements of Tai Chi.

Wa Sou: Tile Hand. This is the typical open-hand form used in Tai Chi Chuan.

Wai Dan: External Elixir. A kind of Chi Kung training in which the Chi is generated in local areas of the body (especially limbs) and circulated to the other parts of the body.

Wai Jing: External Power. The type of Jing where the muscles predominate and only local Chi is used to support the muscles. See also Nei Jing.

Wu Chi: Literally No Extremity. This is the state of undifferentiated emptiness before a beginning. As soon as there is a beginning or a movement, there is differentiation and opposites, and this is called Tai Chi.

Wu Chin Si: Five Animal Sport. A Chi Kung exercise which imitates the movements of five animals: tiger, deer, monkey, bear, and bird.

Wu Dan: A Mountain located to the South of Chun Hsien, in Hubei Province, China. It is believed that a number of Taoist martial arts such as Tai Chi and Wu Dan were created in this area.

Wushu: Martial Technique. In the beginning, Chinese martial arts were called Wu Yi (Martial Arts), and the techniques of Wu Yi were called Wushu (martial techniques). In 1926, the name was changed to Kuoshu but was changed back to Wushu in 1949. It is still called Kuoshu in Taiwan.

Yang: The positive pole of Tai Chi (Grand Ultimate), the other pole being Yin (Negative). Chinese people believe that everything follows from the interaction of Yin and Yang.

Yang Chen-Fu: A very famous Tai Chi master. (1883-1935).

Yang Chien-Huo (1842-1917): A very famous Tai Chi master; the father of Yang Chen-Fu .

Yang Lu-Shann (1799-1872): The first generation master of Yang Style Tai Chi Chuan. He learned his Tai Chi Chuan from Chen Chang-Shen.

Yi: Mind. It is commonly expressed as Hsin-Yi. Hsin is an idea and Yi is the expression of this idea. Therefore, Yi can be translated as Mind by itself.

Yi Ching: The Book of Changes. One of the most ancient philosophic writings in existence, this classic has affected Chinese culture and tradition for thousands of years. See also Ba Kua.

Yin: The Negative pole of Tai Chi (Grand Ultimate). See also Yang.

Ying Jing: Hard Jing. A type of Jing in which the muscles predominate in the expression of power. In this Jing the muscles are relatively stiff and Chi from the local area is used in support.

Yu Pan: Look to the Right. One of the five basic Tai Chi strategic movements.

Zou: Elbow-Stroke. The technique of striking with the elbow. One of the "four corners" of the eight basic Tai Chi fighting techniques.

APPENDIX C
CHINESE TERMS AND TRANSLATIONS

ABOUT THE AUTHOR & PREFACE

Yang Jwing-Ming
Taiwan
Wushu
Kung Fu
Shaolin
Pai Huo
Cheng Gin-Gsao
Chin Na
Tai Chi Chuan
Kao Tao
Taipei
Tamkang College
Taipei Hsien
Chang Chuan
Li Mao-Ching
Kuoshu
Chi Kung
Lien Bu Chuan
Gung Li Chuan
Yi Lu Mei Fu
Shaw Fu Ien
Shih Tzu Tan
Chi
Jing

CHAPTER 1

Ba Kua
Hsing I
Liu Ho Ba Fa
Nei Kung
Nei Jar
Wu Chin Si
Ba Tuan Gin
Da Mo's Yi Gin Ching
Shih Er Chuang
Chang San-Feng
Sung Wei Dsung
Liang Dynasty
Han Goong-Yueh

Chen Ling-Shih
Chen Bi
Tang Dynasty
Sheu Hsuan-Pin
Li Tao-Tzu
Ien Li-Hen
San Shih Chi Shih
Hou Tien Far
Shao Jeou Tien
Nan Lei Gi Wang Jeng Nan Moo Tzu Min
Sung Dynasty   南雷集王征南墓誌銘
Wu Dan
Wei Dsung
Yuen
Gin
Ming
Ming Shih Fan Gi Chwan
Lieu Dong Yi County
Chuan-Yi
Jiun-Bao
Chang Lar-Tar
Hung Wu
Ming Tai Tzu
Ming Lan Yin Chi Shou Lei Kou
Shuan-Shuan   明郎瑛七修類稿
Tien Suen
Ming Ying Dsung
Ton Wei Sien Far Jinn Zen
Fon Yi-Yuen   通微顯化真人
Wang Dsung
Sanshi
Chen Ton-Jou
Wen County
Chang Soun-Shi
Hai Yen
Yeh Gi-Mei
Shyh Ming
Wang Dsung-Yueh
San You
Chiang Fa

-268-

河北 溝	Hebei
陳家府溝	Chen Jar Gou
懷慶府南	Hwai Ching County
河南	Henan
陳長興	Chen Chang-Shen
陳有本雲	Chen You-Ban
耕雲	Ken-Yun
陳懷遠	Chen Hwai-Yuen
陳華梅	Chen Hwa-Mei
楊露禪	Yang Lu-Shann
李伯魁	Li Bao-Kuai
十三勢老架	Shih San Shih Lao Jiah
楊班侯	Yang Ban-Huo
楊健侯	Yang Chien-Huo
楊少侯	Yang Shao-Huo
楊澄甫	Yang Chen-Fu
吳全佑	Wu Chun-Yu
吳派	Wu Style
陳清洋	Chen Ching-Pin
趙堡派	Tsao Bao Style
武禹讓	Wuu Yu-Larn
武派	Wuu Style
李亦畬	Li Yi-Yu
李派	Li Style
郝為楨	Heh Wei-Jinn
郝派	Heh Style
孫祿堂	Sun Lu-Tan
孫派	Sun Style
福魁	Fu-Kuai
祿纏	Lu-Chan
永年縣	Youn Nien Hsien
廣平府	Kuan Pin County
哼	Hen
哈	Ha
楊拳	Yang Chuan
綿拳	Mei Chuan
化拳	Far Chuan
北京	Peking
清	Ching
楊無敵	Yang Wu Di
楊錡	Yang Chyi
楊鈺	Yang Yuh
楊鑑	Yang Jiann
廣平	Kuan Pin
吳鑑泉	Wu Chien-Chun
兆鵬	Jaw-Peng
鏡湖	Gien-Fu
兆熊	Jaw-Shyong
兆元	Jaw-Yuen
兆清	Jaw-Ching
夢祥	Mum-Shiang

楊振聲	Yang Jen-Shen
南京中央國術館	Nanking Central Kuoshu Institute
振銘	Jeng-Min
振基	Jeng-Gi
振鐸	Jeng-Zer
振國	Jeng-Kuo
無極	Wu Chi
陰	Yin
陽	Yang
掤	Peng
擺	Lu
擠	Ghi
按	An
採	Chai
挒	Lie
肘	Zou
靠	Kau
進步	Jinn Bu
退步	Twe Bu
左顧	Dsao Gu
右盼	Yu Pan
中定	Dsung Dien
乾	Chyan
坤	Kuen
坎	Kann
離	Lii
巽	Shiunn
震	Jenn
兌	Duey
艮	Genn
金	Gin
木	Moo
水	Sui
火	For
土	Tu
易經	Yi Ching
外丹	Wai Dan
內丹	Nei Dan

CHAPTER 2

意	Yi
空氣	Kon Chi
經	Ching
脈	Mei
奇經八脈	Chyi Ching Ba Mei
督脈	Du Mei
任脈	Ren Mei
絡	Lou
丹田	Dan Tien
小週天	Shao Chou Tien

大週天	Da Chou Tien		勁敵	Jing Tee
心	Hsin		氣力	Chi Li (Li Chi)
專心	Juan-Hsin		硬勁	Ying Jing
心意	Hsin-Yi		軟硬勁	Roan Ying Jing
陳炎林	Chen Yen-Lin		軟勁	Roan Jing
以意引氣	Yii Yi Yin Chi		外勁	Wai Jing
金鐘罩	Gin Chung Tsao		內勁	Nei Jing
鐵布衫	Tiea Bu Shan		覺勁	Jywe Jing
一指禪	Yi Jyy Chan		形勁	Hsing Jing
金鋼指	Gin Garn Jyy		攻勁	Gong Jing
點穴	Tien Hsueh		發勁	Fa Jing
手太陰肺	Hand Taiyin Lung		守勁	Shoou Jing
手厥陰心包	Hand Jueyin Pericardium		化勁	Huah Jing
手陽明大腸	Hand Yangming Large Intestine		純陽勁	Chwen Yang Jing
手少陽三焦	Hand Shaoyang Triple Burner		純攻勁	Chwen Gong Jing
手少陰心	Hand Shaoyin Heart		陽中帶陰勁	Yang Jong Dai Yin Jing
手太陽小腸	Hand Taiyang Small Intestine		攻中帶守勁	Gong Jong Dai Shoou Jing
豹扑勁	Bao Pu Jing		純陰勁	Chwen Yin Jing
鴨嘴勁	Ya Tzoei Jing		純守勁	Chwen Shoou Jing
鶴嘴勁	Heh Tzoei Jing		陰中帶陽勁	Yin Jong Dai Yang Jing
通天勁	Ton Tien Jing		守中帶攻勁	Shoou Jong Dai Gong Jing
龍衝舉勁	Long Shyan Ju Jing		非攻非守勁	Fei Gong Fei Shoou Jing
劍訣開氣勁	Jen Jyue Kai Chi Jing		近	Gin
蛇頭勁	Sher Tou Jing		遠	Yeuan
平指勁	Pin Jyy Jing		長	Chang
八卦掌	Ba Kua Chang		短	Doan
鷹爪勁	Ien Jao Jing		聽勁	Tien Jing
鶴爪勁	Heh Jao Jing		沾勁	Tsan Jing
虎爪勁	Fu Jao Jing		黏勁	Nien Jing
螳手	Tan Lang Sou		借勁	Jieh Jing
佛手	For Sou		懂勁	Dong Jing
	Wai lien gin gu pie, nei lien yi kou chi	擦皮虛臨勁	Tsa Pi Shiu Lin Jing
拱手	Gung Sou 外鍊筋骨皮，內鍊一口氣		掤勁	Peng Jing
托天	Tou Tien		鑽勁	Tzuann Jing
會陰	Huiyin		斷勁	Duan Jing
力	Li		橫勁	Hen Jing
神	Shen		掛勁	Kua Jing
精	Jieng		轉勁	Joan Jing
精神	Jieng-Shen		長勁	Charng Jing
三寶	San Bao		沉勁	Chen Jing
湧泉	Yongquan		閉氣	Bi Chi
瓦手	Wa Sou		寸勁	Tsuenn Jing
			分勁	Fen Jing
			冷勁	Leenz Jing
			提勁	Tyi Jing
			擠勁	Ghi Jing

CHAPTER 3

花拳繡腿	Far chuan shiou twe		膺窗	Yingchuang
練拳不練功，到老一場空	Lien chuan bu lien kung, tao lao yi tsang kong	乳根	Rugen
勁弓	Jing Gung		鳩尾	Jiuwei
勁風	Jing Fong		天宗	Tianzong
			採勁	Chai Jing

勁	Zou Jing		血海	Xuehai
肘靠	Tsen Zou Kau		伏兔	Femur-Futu
正側肘靠	Tseh Zou Kau		踢勁	Ti Jing
拿勁	Na Jing		蹬勁	Deng Jing
曲池	Quchi		中脘勁	Jong Chiau Jing
少海	Shaohai		中切勁	Jong Chie Jing
小海	Xiaohai		外擺勁	Wai Bai Jing
搓挫勁	Tsuo Jing		内擺勁	Nei Bai Jing
送勁	Sung Jing		旋風腿	Shain Fon Twe
擺勁	Lu Jing		滿招損,謙受益.	Maan jau soen,chian show yi
大擺	Da Lu			
小擺	Shao Lu			
引勁	Yinn Jing			
走勁	Dsou Jing			
頂抗勁	Dien Kan Jing		**APPENDIX**	
截勁	Gieh Jing			
合勁	Her Jing		輕	Ching
捲勁	Jeuan Jing		靈	Ling
纏絲勁	Chan Szu Jing		重	Jong
撅勁	Jiue Jing		重	Chung
按勁	An Jing		双	Shuang
挒勁	Lie Jing		双重	Shuang Jong
靠勁	Kau Jing		内勁力	Nei Jing Li
鄭曼青	Cheng Man-Ching		海底	Haidi
開勁	Kai Jing		尾閭	Wyelu
辰勁	Jann Jing		意守丹田	Yi Sou Dan Dien
撥勁	Bo Jing		精武門	Chin Woo Association
摺叠勁	Jer Dye Jing			
抖擻勁	Dou Sou Jing			
頂勁	Ding Jing			
盤勁	Pan Jing			
千斤墜	Chian Gin Juey			
凌空勁	Lin Korn Jing			
腿勁	Twe Jing			
一分長,一分利	Yi fen charng, yi fen li			
條口	Tiaokou			
中都	Zhongdu			
解溪	Jiexi			
太冲	Taichong			
足不過膝	Tzwu bu guoh shi			
踩勁	Tsae Jing			
踹勁	Chuay Jing			
低切勁	Di Chie Jing			
低跪勁	Di Chiau Jing			
上頂	Sarn Ding			
蹓腿	Lieu Twe			
低掃勁	Di Shaou Jing			
中脘	Zhongwan			
章門	Zhangmen			
下陰門	Shayin			
箕門	Jimen			

VIDEOTAPES PUBLISHED BY YANG'S MARTIAL ARTS ACADEMY (YMAA)

YANG STYLE TAI CHI CHUAN AND ITS APPLICATIONS

This one hour professionally-made split-screen color tape covers fundamental stances and breathing exercises, and the complete (128 posture) Yang style solo form, including breath coordination. The martial applications of each posture are shown in slow motion and regular speed. All the solo forms and applications are performed by Dr. Yang Jwing-Ming. A textbook, Dr. Yang's *YANG STYLE TAI CHI CHUAN,* is available from Unique Publications. The tape is available in **VHS, BETA,** and **PAL.**

CONTENTS:
1. Fundamental Stances
2. Fundamental Breathing Drills
3. Yang Style Solo Tai Chi Chuan (with low stances and large postures)
4. Martial Applications of Tai Chi Chuan.

NORTHERN SHAOLIN LONG FIST KUNG FU LIEN BU CHUAN AND ITS APPLICATIONS

This forty-five minute, professionally-made, split-screen color tape covers fundamental stances and basic training of Lien Bu Chuan, which was the first basic barehand sequence taught at both the Chin Woo Association and the Nanking Central Kuoshu Institute. This tape was designed for the beginning martial artist who wishes to study by himself, as well as for the experienced practitioner to use as a reference tape. The primary and hidden martial applications of each posture are shown in slow motion and regular speed. All the solo forms and applications are performed by Dr. Yang Jwing-Ming. A textbook, Dr. Yang's *SHAOLIN LONG FIST KUNG FU*, is available from Unique Publications. The tape is available in **VHS, BETA**, and **PAL.**

CONTENTS:
1. Fundamental Stances
2. Basic Training
3. Learning Lien Bu Chuan
4. Lien Bu Chuan - Slow Speed
5. Lien Bu Chuan - Regular Speed
6. Martial Applications of Lien Bu Chuan

NORTHERN SHAOLIN LONG FIST KUNG FU
GUNG LI CHUAN AND ITS APPLICATIONS

This forty-five minute, professionally-made, split-screen color tape covers fundamental stances and basic training of Gung Li Chuan. Gung Li Chuan was the second basic barehand sequence taught at the Chin Woo Association and the Nanking Central Kuoshu Institute. This tape was designed for the beginning martial artist who wishes to study by himself, as well as for the experienced practitioner to use as a reference work. The primary and hidden martial applications of each posture are shown in slow motion and regular speed. A textbook, Dr. Yang's *SHAOLIN LONG FIST KUNG FU,* is available from Unique Publications. The tape is available in **VHS, BETA,** and **PAL.**

CONTENTS:
1. Fundamental Stances
2. Basic Training
3. Learning Gung Li Chuan
4. Gung Li Chuan - Slow Speed
5. Gung Li Chuan - Regular Speed
6. Martial Applications of Gung Li Chuan

BOOKS PUBLISHED BY YANG'S MARTIAL ARTS ACADEMY (YMAA)

CHI KUNG - HEALTH AND MARTIAL ARTS

Chi Kung is the science of energy circulation within the body. For thousands of years Chinese scientists, philosophers, and physicians have researched the circulation of Chi (energy). This book presents several methods of external-internal (Wai Dan) energy generation and circulation training, including the one used by the monks in the Shaolin temple. The internal-internal (Nei Dan) meditation training used in internal martial arts such as Tai Chi Chuan is explained in detail. This book will help both the beginning as well as the experienced martial artist increase his power and effectiveness. Anyone who invests the time and effort to practice these exercises can increase his or her health and vitality.

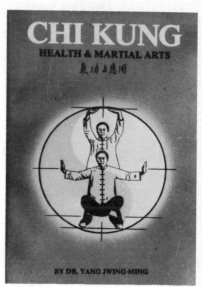

CONTENTS:
CHAPTER 1: INTRODUCTION
  1-1. General Introduction
  1-2. Historical Survey
  1-3. General Principles
  1-4. Popular Martial Styles of Chi Kung Training
CHAPTER 2: WAI DAN
  2-1. Introduction
  2-2. Theory of Wai Dan
  2-3. Da Mo's "Yi Gin Ching"
  2-4. Other Wai Dan Exercises
CHAPTER 3: NEI DAN
  3-1. Introduction
  3-2. Principles of Nei Dan
  3-3. Nei Dan Practice
  3-4. Chi Enhancement and Transport
  3-5. Massage and Exercises after Meditation
CHAPTER 4: CHI KUNG AND HEALTH
  4-1. Introduction
  4-2. Chinese Diagnosis
  4-3. Acupuncture
  4-4. Massage and Rubbing
  4-5. Miscellaneous Chi Kung Exercises
CHAPTER 5: MARTIAL ARTS APPLICATIONS
  5-1. Introduction
  5-2. Cavity Press
  5-3. Sealing the Vein and Sealing the Breath
  5-4. Golden Bell Cover or Iron Shirt
CHAPTER 6: CONCLUSION
APPENDIX A: CHINESE POETRY
  A-1. A Poem by Lu Yu About Da Mo
  A-2. Tai Shih Ching
APPENDIX B: TRANSLATION OF CHINESE TERMS

NORTHERN SHAOLIN SWORD

This volume presents the history of the Chinese sword, fundamental training principles and exercises, and three famous northern Shaolin sword sequences. The applications of each form are included. This book can be used for self-instruction by those with a foundation in martial arts.

CONTENTS:

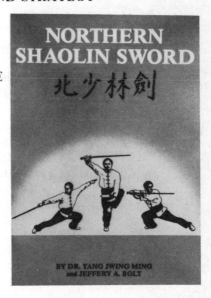

NORTHERN SHAOLIN SWORD
北少林劍

BY DR. YANG JWING MING
and JEFFERY A. BOLT

NEXT SCHEDULED PUBLICATION
(DATE: MARCH, 1986)

ADVANCED YANG STYLE TAI CHI CHUAN
VOLUME 2
MARTIAL APPLICATIONS

The first volume of this series introduced the theory and principles of Tai Chi Chuan and Tai Chi's Jing (power) training. This volume focuses on the discussion and analysis of the martial applications. Tai Chi students who have learned the form and started pushing hands will find these books a gold mine of information which will give depth and realism to their training.

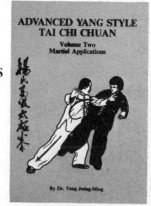

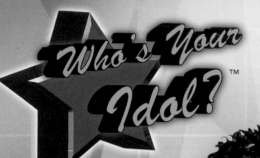

Who's Your Idol?™

FANTASIA
BARRINO

Liz Sonneborn

rosen publishing's
rosen central®

New York

Published in 2008 by The Rosen Publishing Group, Inc.
29 East 21st Street, New York, NY 10010

Library of Congress Cataloging-in-Publication Data

Sonneborn, Liz.
Who's your idol?: Fantasia Barrino / Liz Sonneborn.—1st ed.
    p.cm.
Includes bibliographical references (p. 46) and index.
ISBN-13: 978-1-4042-1369-2 (library binding)
1. Fantasia, 1984—Juvenile literature. 2. Singers—United States—
Biography—Juvenile literature. I. Title.
ML3930.F26S66 2008
782.421643092   dc22
(B)
                                                   2007027124

Manufactured in the United States of America

Unless otherwise attributed, all quoted material comes from *Life Is Not a Fairy Tale* by Fantasia.

On the cover: Fantasia Barrino delivered a powerhouse performance at the Kodak Theater during the finale of season three of *American Idol*.

Contents

Introduction

On April 14, 2004, millions of Americans gathered around their television sets. For many, this was a weekly ritual. Every Tuesday night, they settled in to get their fix of *American Idol*, the singing competition that had become the country's number-one show.

Two singers already had been crowned "Idols." In Season One, there was Kelly Clarkson, a husky-voiced pop singer from Texas. In Season Two, there was Ruben Studdard, a portly soul artist from Alabama. Season Three was in its fifth episode, since the selection of the twelve finalists. With eight contestants still in the game, who would win was anyone's guess. Many viewers thought the season's competitors were the best yet, with several standouts deserving of the Idol title.

The theme of the show was songs from movies. The first half was a mixed bag. Contestants George Huff and Diana

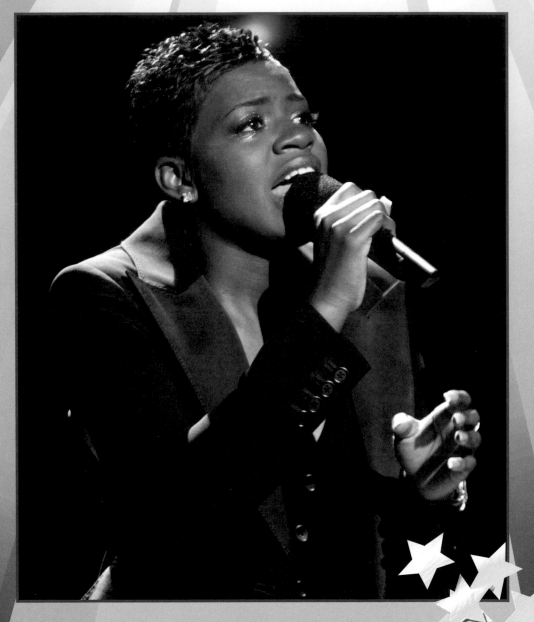

"Summertime" from *Porgy and Bess* immediately became Fantasia's signature song after she performed it on *American Idol*. Her hit recording of the song was later nominated for a Grammy Award.

DeGarmo delivered lackluster performances, while Jon Peter Lewis and Jennifer Hudson wowed the judges with their songs.

Next up was the evening's fifth contestant, Fantasia Barrino. Host Ryan Seacrest announced she would sing "Summertime," from *Porgy and Bess*. The camera then closed in on the stage, showing a small figure seated on the floor. *Idol* viewers were used to animated performances, with singers dancing and gesturing, hoping to rouse the audience and win their approval. Clearly, Fantasia had something else in mind. She stayed put on center stage, content to express herself with nothing but her voice.

She wore an elegant dress and glittering earrings that dangled like chandeliers. Her glamorous appearance seemed at odds with the character she was portraying with the song. In *Porgy and Bess*, "Summertime" is sung by Clara, a poor young woman trying to comfort her crying child. Fantasia delivered a passionate performance, showing an intimate understanding of the emotions expressed in the beautiful lullaby.

In truth, despite her gown and jewelry, Fantasia was not that different from Clara. She, too, was a young mother struggling to care for her daughter. In her charged performance, Fantasia seemed to recall her own experiences of singing to her child. At the end, her voice soared as she promised that nothing would ever harm her little one.

As Fantasia raised herself from the floor, the audience rose to its feet. The theater filled with applause. Randy Jackson, the first judge to speak, joined in the standing ovation and declared

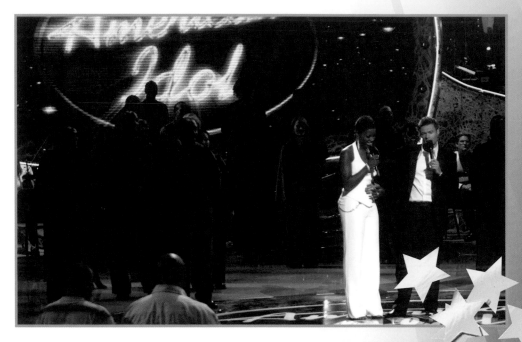

In the season finale, *Idol* host Ryan Seacrest bantered with Fantasia after her performance of the song "I Believe," backed by a gospel choir.

that Fantasia's performance was the best ever on any season of *American Idol*. Even the ever-cranky Simon Cowell could not think of anything negative to say. He told her that her singing was magical. Then, he added with a wink that she had never put her lips to better use, prompting an embarrassed giggle from the performer.

Even as she laughed, Fantasia wiped a tear from her cheek. She'd been crying since she stopped singing. Seacrest saw her tears and put his arm around her. The host was clearly confused,

finding it hard to believe that she would still be crying after the judges' enthusiastic praise. Fantasia gave a simple explanation: She had truly felt the words she was singing.

Throughout the *Idol* competition and since, Fantasia has displayed an emotional connection to her songs. But that is not what makes her an incredible performer. Her greatest talent is that she makes her audience feel her songs with just as much passion as she does.

1 A LITTLE GIRL WITH A BIG VOICE

Fantasia's story began on June 30, 1984, when she was born in High Point, North Carolina. Her grandmother Addie Collins came up with her unusual name. Collins was inspired by a brand of fine crystal and gifts that advertised a line called "Fantasia."

High Point was a small city known mostly for its furniture stores. Homeowners from across the United States went there to take advantage of the deals they offered. Most people who lived in High Point were not as well-off as these visitors. Outside of the furniture stores, there were few good jobs in the city.

Fantasia's mother, Diane, worked for low wages in hospitals and daycare centers. Her father, Joseph, made a little more as a truck driver, a job that often

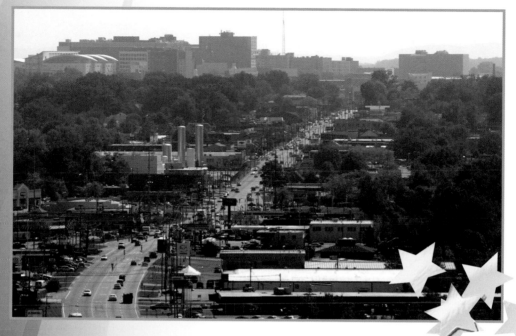

The city of High Point, North Carolina, is best known today as Fantasia's hometown.

took him away from home. Even with both parents working full time, the Barrino family struggled to get by. At the end of the month, they often did not have enough money to pay their bills. Sometimes, they did not have money even for food.

Family, Faith, and Music

While growing up poor, Fantasia was sustained by three things: family, faith, and music. Aunts, uncles, and cousins surrounded her. They often would come by the house at

511 Montlieu Avenue where she lived with her parents and three brothers, Rico, Joseph ("Tiny"), and Xavier. Aside from company, these relatives provided support for one another. Whenever anyone fell on hard times, someone in the family would step up, offering a meal or whatever cash he or she had.

Of all her relatives, Fantasia was closest to her grandmother Addie. Addie had had a difficult life. Her husband had left her with three young daughters to raise on her own. After praying for help, she decided God wanted her to start her own church. Her Mercy Outreach church grew slowly. At first, it attracted just a handful of worshippers. But in time, hundreds gathered there each Sunday to hear Addie preach. Another draw was the beautiful gospel singing of young Fantasia and her family. She later remembered, "Everyone wanted to be blessed by our voices."

The Barrino house was filled with music. Fantasia once recalled, "It was the place where everyone in the neighborhood would gather to sing. Family members and neighbors would come over and sing. People who *couldn't* sing would come over to our house to sing."

The Barrino Family

Her parents certainly were among those who *could* sing. In fact, they were good enough to earn money performing at churches and weddings. Fantasia loved hearing them sing duets. One of her favorites was the song "Inseparable," which they often sang at wedding receptions.

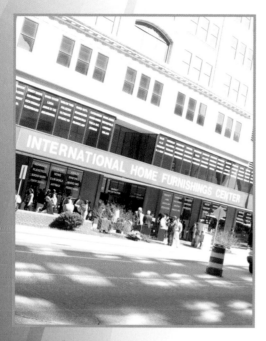

People from across the country visit High Point to hunt for bargains in its many furniture stores and outlets.

Practicing in front of the bathroom mirror, she and her brother Rico began to mimic their parents' act, even down to their facial expressions and gestures. One day, their parents caught their little show. Instead of being mad, they were astounded at how good Fantasia and Rico were.

At the next wedding performance, Joseph Barrino announced to the crowd that a new pair of singers was taking the stage. To five-year-old Fantasia's shock, he pointed at her and Rico. She said, "The first note that I hit made the bathroom scene come to life for me and I was no longer nervous. The further along in the song we got, the more I could feel the audience's reaction."

The crowd loved the song and Joseph got an idea. He decided to start a gospel group featuring him, Diane, and the children. Billed as "The Barrino Family," they traveled throughout the South, playing at churches, revivals, and fairgrounds. Their audiences were always enthusiastic, but the act never earned them much. Most of the time, the family slept in their van while they toured. Sometimes, they had so little money for food that,

as Fantasia explained, "we would eat Vienna sausages and chips and call it a night." Despite the difficulties of life on the road, Fantasia "never complained because I was doin' what I wanted to do—sing."

At one point, the Barrinos attracted the attention of a record label. Excited by the chance to make a record, Joseph quickly signed a contract. They eventually recorded two CDs that received airplay on Southern gospel stations. But because of the terms of the contract, they earned little from their recordings.

Losing Her Way

Disappointed and restless, Fantasia's older brothers Rico and Tiny left the group. Both started their own bands, playing R & B instead of gospel. By the time she was twelve, Fantasia also was losing interest in the family singing group. She was growing bored with a social life that revolved around church. As she later recalled, "My heart was empty and seeking somethin' to do. I cried a lot because I could feel God's spirit pulling me toward Him and boredom pulling me toward trouble. *Trouble won.*"

As a girl, Fantasia was uncomfortable with her looks. Skinny with large lips, she was teased on the schoolyard. In her teenage years, she decided to imitate the popular girls, experimenting with makeup, clothes, and hairstyles. With her new look, Fantasia began attracting plenty of male attention. At fourteen, she had her first boyfriend, who she called "B." in her autobiography, *Life Is Not a Fairy Tale*.

For as long as she could remember, Fantasia's mother had warned her against becoming too involved with boys at a young age. Both she and Fantasia's grandmother had children when they were still teenagers. Diane wanted something different for Fantasia. She told her daughter she needed to grow up herself before taking on the responsibility of raising a family. Fantasia, though, was convinced she was in love with B. She ignored her mother and tuned out her teachers. All she cared about was the next time she would see her boyfriend.

From Bad to Worse

While Fantasia was seeing B., another boy began flirting with her. Since she already had a boyfriend, she did not think much about the attention he was paying her. But what seemed like an innocent flirtation turned into a disaster. The boy trapped and raped her in the school auditorium.

After the rape, Fantasia wandered home and collapsed on her bed. She did not get up for two days. Her mother knew something was wrong. Finally, Fantasia confessed to her mother, who insisted that she go to the police. After the boy was arrested, Fantasia was threatened and harassed by his friends. It was more than she could take. Unable to face a trial, she dropped the charges. And unable to deal with her tormentors, she dropped out of school in the ninth grade.

The experience left Fantasia feeling hopeless. She moved in with an older friend, who had an apartment in the projects.

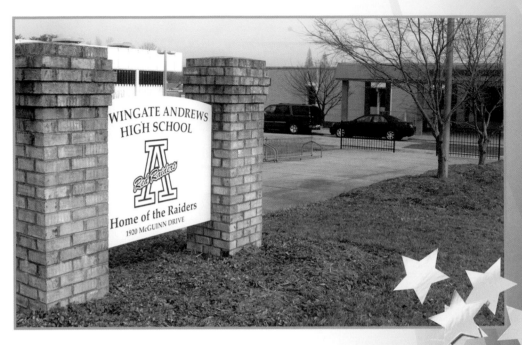

Unhappy at high school, Fantasia dropped out of T. Wingate Andrews High School in the ninth grade.

She began hanging out with a rougher crowd. She spent her evenings at clubs, drinking and smoking, even though it was bad for her voice.

Soon, Fantasia discovered she was pregnant. She was so terrified of what her mother and grandmother would say that she had her brother Tiny tell them. They both began to weep. Fantasia told B. herself. He said the baby was not his and refused to talk to her. The rest of the town, though, was only too eager to

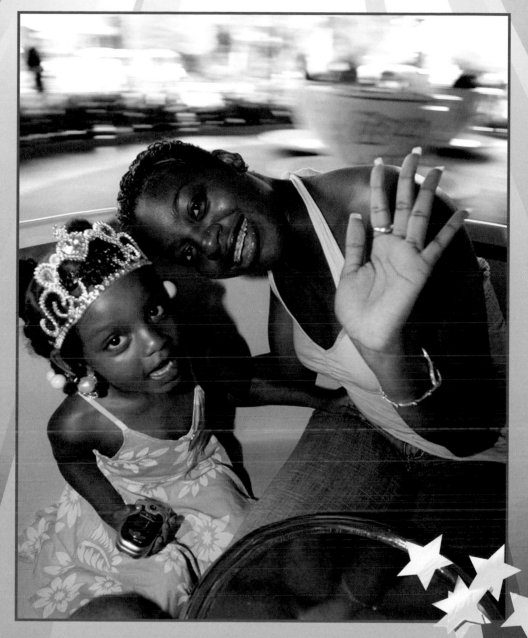

Fantasia celebrated the fourth birthday of her beloved daughter, Zion, with a trip to Walt Disney's Magic Kingdom.

talk about Fantasia. Their gossip made her more depressed and desperate.

"This Ain't Fantasia!"

On August 8, 2001, Fantasia gave birth to a daughter. She named her Zion, after the place in the Bible where the disciples of Jesus prayed. By then, B. had reentered her life. He moved in with her and Zion, all three living off of government welfare and pocket money Fantasia earned by singing.

Fantasia later said she was caught up in "the fantasy of being a real family." But that fantasy did not last. When she managed to stash away $100, B. insisted she give it to him and hit her when she refused. She fought back but ultimately gave him the money. Her apartment went dark and cold when she could not pay the electric bill. Fantasia even had to steal to get milk and diapers for her baby. "I was beginning to feel hopeless," she has explained. "I no longer wanted to wake up in the same life that I went to sleep in."

Another fight with B. proved to be the last straw. In an argument over money, he hit her so hard that she passed out. At her mother's urging, she called the police and B. was arrested. Moving back in with her family, Fantasia spied her black eye and cut lip in a mirror. "I looked at myself and said out loud, 'This ain't Fantasia!'" she said. "This life ain't for me! I ain't supposed to be like this." She then looked at Zion and realized things were going to have to change.

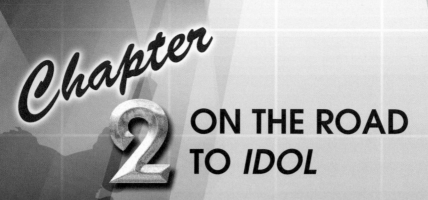

Chapter 2

ON THE ROAD TO *IDOL*

With B. gone for good, Fantasia wanted to get her life back on track. She started going to church again and became determined to get a high school education. On her own, she began studying for the General Educational Development (GED) test.

Fantasia also started seeing a new man, whom she called J. B. in her book. He was as kind and giving as B. was angry and violent. J. B. gave Fantasia both the financial and emotional support she needed. With his help, she focused on solving a problem she used to be too embarrassed to admit: She could not read very well. Fantasia worked hard to improve her reading skills, driven by one special goal—she wanted to be able to read bedtime stories to her daughter, Zion.

Ready to Audition

J. B. encouraged Fantasia to make the most of her singing talent. One day, he brought her a pile of information about the upcoming August 2003 auditions for Season Three of *American Idol*. One of the auditions was being held in Atlanta, Georgia, only a four-hour car ride from High Point, North Carolina.

Fantasia had never watched *American Idol*, but she had friends who did. Like J. B., they all told her she should try out for it.

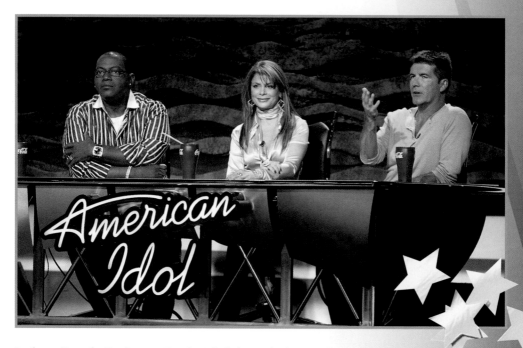

Judges Randy Jackson, Paula Abdul, and Simon Cowell were enthusiastic about Fantasia's singing even at her first audition for them.

Fantasia began to think they were right. She realized "(t)he only thing that was needed was that you sing, and that I could do, without any fear. For once, I could do something without any help from anyone."

Fantasia's family, though, was eager to give her whatever help they could. Her older brother Rico agreed to drive her to Atlanta. Her mother volunteered to watch Zion while Fantasia was away. Her grandmother gave her gas money, and her father offered her cash to buy meals along the way. A cousin agreed to put up Rico and Fantasia at his apartment in Atlanta.

Fantasia spent the two weeks before the audition practicing and then practicing some more. For the first time in a long while, she was excited about her life.

In Atlanta

Finally, the time had come. Fantasia and Rico headed off to the Georgia Dome, a sports arena where *Idol* auditions were being held. As their car pulled into the parking lot, Fantasia was stunned. There were people everywhere. About 7,000 would-be contestants were milling around, all as hopeful as she that they could become the next "Idol."

Fantasia waited nervously until it was her turn to audition. For a producer of the show, she sang a spirited version of Stevie Wonder's "Signed, Sealed, Delivered." The producer calmly told her she was going on to the next round. Fantasia had hoped for more feedback, but she was thrilled that she was still in the running. The next day, she auditioned a second

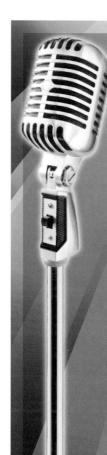

Locked Out

Fantasia's journey in the *American Idol* competition nearly ended before it had begun. After her first audition in Atlanta, she and Rico left the Georgia Dome and spent the evening trying to relax at their cousin's apartment. Refreshed, they showed up at the arena the next morning. In a moment, they realized something was wrong. The doors were closed, and about 100 contestants were outside, crying and yelling at security guards. The arena was so crowded that guards were not letting anyone else in.

Rico and Fantasia went back to her cousin's. In tears, she called her mother and said she was coming home. A few minutes after Fantasia had hung up, the phone rang. It was her father, and he was mad. He demanded she get back to the Georgia Dome and find a way to get in. A little stunned, Fantasia stopped crying long enough to choke out, "Yes, sir." Back at the arena, she spotted a security guard she had spoken to the day before. He helped her sneak in and make her next audition on time.

time, singing Roberta Flack's "Killing Me Softly" for another producer. Again, she passed the tryout.

Two weeks later, Fantasia was back in Atlanta for the next round of competition. In her first tryout, she sang Creedance Clearwater Revival's "Proud Mary." The song got her the most enthusiastic response yet. The producer declared, "Fantasia, you are beautiful. I love your name. You are the one."

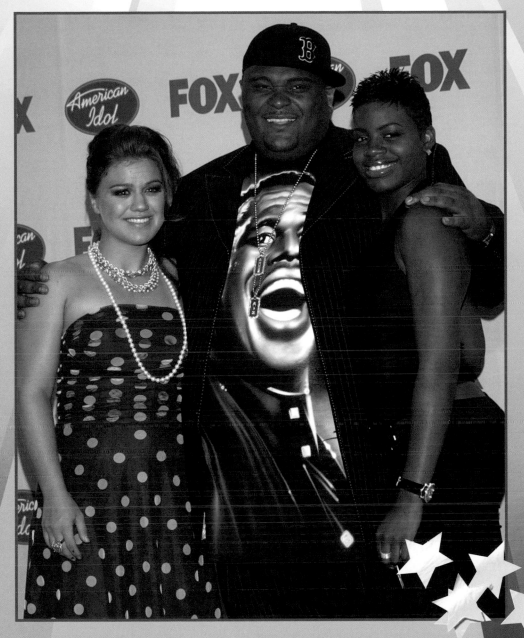

Backstage at *American Idol*, Fantasia got to know the first two *Idol* winners, Kelly Clarkson and Ruben Studdard.

Next up was the most important audition of all. Fantasia was led into a room with the show's three celebrity judges: Randy Jackson, Paula Abdul, and Simon Cowell. When they asked her why she should be the next "Idol," she said, "My name is Fantasia Barrino. I have a two-year-old daughter; her name is Zion. My lips are big, but my talent is bigger." She began to sing and proved her point. After Fantasia's soulful rendition of Marvin Gaye's "I Heard It Through the Grapevine," Cowell told her that she was going to Hollywood.

"*Idol* Boot Camp"

Out of 42,000 hopefuls, Fantasia was one of 117 contestants to continue on in the competition. She headed to California for what the producers called "*Idol* Boot Camp." Every day, competitors had to perform a song in a different style. And every day, a few were sent home. Some flubbed their lyrics. Others missed a note. Still others just lacked the star quality the producers were looking for.

Fantasia knew she could be voted off any minute. Even so, her confidence was growing. She had always listened to a wide range of music and already knew plenty of songs by heart. No matter what challenge the producers threw at her, she could muster up a good performance, flavored with her own flair.

Nevertheless, the stress of the competition left Fantasia feeling anxious and drained. Other competitors spent nights out partying. But Fantasia always stayed in, practicing and

concentrating on the next day's contest. She realized something else set her apart from the others. If they did not win, they had jobs to go back to and plans for the future. For Fantasia, though, competing on *Idol* seemed like her one last chance to do something with her life.

The Final Twelve

By the end of boot camp, Fantasia and thirty-one other contestants were still standing. They were divided into four groups. Each group would perform on the show, and viewers would choose two as finalists. (The rest of the twelve contestants would be chosen in a special "wild card" show.)

Fantasia was in Group One. On February 10, 2004, she made her television debut. Belting out Bonnie Raitt's "Something to Talk About," she scored an immediate hit. But it was clear she had strong competition. In fact, Randy Jackson called that night's singers the best group of eight he had ever heard. In the end, though, only Fantasia—along with a sixteen-year-old named Diana DeGarmo—won enough viewer votes to continue.

While the rest of the twelve were chosen, Fantasia got to go home. She was thrilled to see Zion and the rest of her family and friends. But everywhere she went, she had a production assistant from *Idol* following and filming her. Fantasia thought all the focus on her home life was a little strange. After all, it was a singing competition. She wondered why anything else about her should matter.

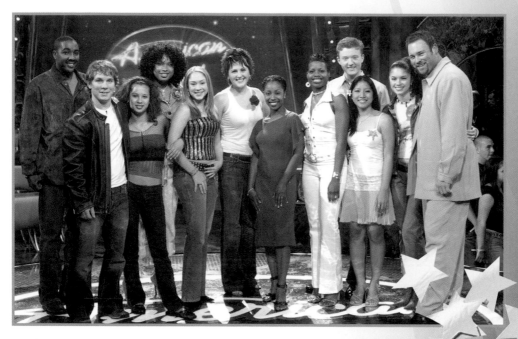

The final twelve contestants of *Idol's* third season were a
talented bunch. In addition to Fantasia, early standouts included
Jennifer Hudson, La Toya London, Diana DeGarmo, and George Huff.

As it turned out, plenty of people seemed interested in her
personal life. On the *American Idol* Web site, some fans began
saying unkind things about Fantasia. They claimed that as a
single mother, she was a bad role model for girls and therefore
did not deserve to be an "Idol." Some said she should hide
Zion from the cameras, so no one would know about her past.
Their comments were deeply hurtful to Fantasia, but she
refused to quit. She decided that, no matter what her critics
said, she was staying with the competition as long as she could.

3

SINGING TO WIN

In the first *American Idol* show featuring the final twelve contestants, Fantasia hit the ground running. Her crowd-pleasing rendition of "Signed, Sealed, Delivered" received high praise even from Simon Cowell, whose sarcastic remarks had cut many would-be "Idols" down to size. But Randy Jackson gave Fantasia the best compliment. He compared her to Aretha Franklin, her own musical idol.

From the start of Season Three, Fantasia looked like a winner. But, based on that first show, she was far from a shoe-in. John Stevens emerged as an appealing young crooner, while George Huff showed a talent for classy soul. The other women, however, were especially formidable. There was Jasmine Trias, a beautiful Hawaiian with a lilting sound, and Diana DeGarmo, the sweet sixteen-year-old who delivered powerhouse vocals. Jennifer Hudson and La Toya London were even

more of a threat. Like Fantasia, both were African American women with strong voices and a preference for R & B. Fantasia knew she would have to work hard to distinguish herself in this talented group.

Impressing the Crowd

In the next few shows, Fantasia continued to wow the viewers and the judges. The top-eleven show had a country theme, a musical genre Fantasia knew little about. Even so, her version of Willie Nelson's "Always on My Mind" was well-received, although Cowell complained her black gown made her look old.

In the top-ten show, Fantasia was on more familiar ground with Motown Night. She delivered a blistering rendition of "I Heard It Through the Grapevine," commanding

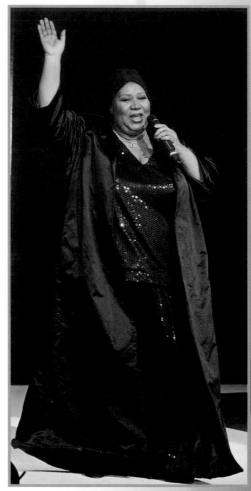

When Fantasia was growing up, her favorite singer was R & B great Aretha Franklin. In 2007, Fantasia had the honor of singing for her idol during a televised tribute to Franklin.

the stage and interacting with the band like a seasoned pro. Veteran Motown performer and guest judge Nick Ashford gushed that she should change her name from Fantasia to Fantastic. On the top-nine show, devoted to the music of Elton John, Fantasia continued her streak. Showing her range, she put a soulful twist on the ballad "Something About the Way You Look Tonight."

With the top-eight show, Fantasia faced a dilemma. The theme was movie music, and she had no idea what to sing. A vocal coach tried to help. He began playing different possibilities on a piano. None seemed right.

Then he began playing "Summertime," a classic by George and Ira Gershwin that Fantasia had never heard before. She loved the music but responded even more to the lyrics. The rousing song, lovingly sung by a mother to her baby, seemed perfect. With so many people gossiping about her past, she wanted to sing about something that was really important in her life—her love for Zion.

Her performance of "Summertime" was a huge hit. Among *Idol* fans, it is considered one of the show's greatest moments. DeGarmo, London, Hudson, Huff—all had plenty of fans. However, at the end of the top-eight show, for many viewers, Fantasia seemed a sure thing to take it all.

A Close Call

On the top-seven show, featuring the hits of Barry Manilow, Fantasia threw herself into a spirited version of "It's a Miracle."

Her performance showcased her training as a church singer. She shouted for the audience to stand up, urging everyone to feel the music completely, body and soul.

The judges were ecstatic. Convinced she would become a big star, Manilow told Fantasia she should open her concerts with the song. Cowell once again said Fantasia had an exciting quality that made her more than just a great singer. Host Ryan Seacrest then appeared on stage, carrying little Zion, so she could share in her mother's triumph. Cooing over her girl, Fantasia told the audience that Zion was the real miracle.

The next night, the results show revealed how viewers had voted. When Seacrest announced the bottom three performers, there was an audible gasp from the audience. London, Hudson, and Fantasia were on the chopping block. The crowd was stunned to realize that one of the contest's best performers would be going home. In the end, London and Fantasia squeaked through, while Hudson was sent packing.

The judges were upset by the decision. Even Seacrest seemed disturbed. As he signed off, he urged viewers to vote for their favorites, clearly convinced that Hudson lost because her fans, assuming she was safe, had not bothered to vote.

Facing the Judges

On the top-six show, Fantasia put in her two cents on the controversy. Bounding onstage, she shouted out Jennifer's name, dedicating her song to her former rival. Her performance of Gloria Estefan's "Get on Your Feet," however, got mixed

reviews. Abdul and guest judge Estefan praised her efforts, but Jackson complained that her pitch was off. Even worse was Cowell's critique. He said she sounded like Donald Duck.

Fantasia had a good week with the Big Band theme of the top-five show. She won special praise for her quiet performance of Woody Herman's "What Are You Doing the Rest of Your Life?" which she dedicated to Zion. She stumbled on the top-four show, though, when the judges did not like the disco songs she chose. On the results night, Fantasia found herself in the bottom two. But once again, she was declared safe. London had to say good-bye, and Fantasia was one step closer to the *Idol* crown.

Down to Two

By that time, one of Fantasia's biggest fans was Clive Davis, the top-three show's guest judge. Davis was a legendary record producer. He had worked with many of the music industry's greatest artists, including Dionne Warwick, Whitney Houston, and Aretha Franklin.

Before the show, Davis came backstage to introduce himself to the final three competitors. He shook hands with DeGarmo and Trias. Then he came over to Fantasia. Instead of shaking her hand, he looked in her eyes and said, "I want you to go out there and sing like you ain't never sang before." He smiled wide every time Fantasia performed, letting her know he was on her side.

The viewers voted off Trias, leaving Fantasia and DeGarmo to fight it out for the top spot. Many of Fantasia's fans were certain

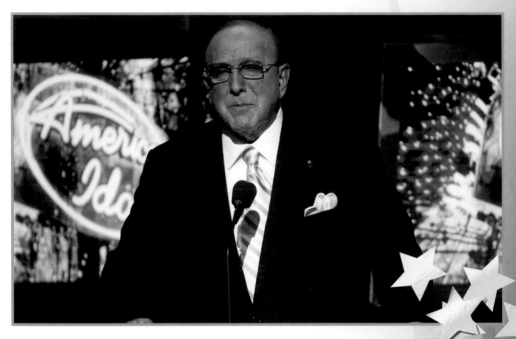

Music industry legend Clive Davis was blown away by Fantasia's voice when he appeared as a guest on *American Idol*. He went on to produce her first two albums.

she would win. Fantasia, though, was not so sure. In an interview before the final show, she noted that DeGarmo was popular with the youngest *Idol* fans. They were more likely to vote over and over than Fantasia's older audience.

A Finale to Remember

On May 25, 2004, Fantasia took the *Idol* stage for the top-two show. Both she and DeGarmo would sing three songs, including "I Believe," which the winner would record as her first single.

For Fantasia, the night started badly. Her rendition of "All My Life" left the judges' cold. Cowell said she was lucky that she was going to have another chance to sing, implying that she would lose if the competition were based on her first effort alone.

For her second song, Fantasia went back to an old favorite, "Summertime." Her moving performance was enough to bring Cowell back into her camp. He declared she was the best singer ever to appear on *Idol*. But the most exciting moment of the evening was her interpretation of "I Believe." Earlier in the show, DeGarmo won praise for her powerful performance. But Fantasia took the song to another level. Backed by a choir of thirty, she drew on her gospel background to bring out all the emotion in its inspirational message.

"The American Idol for 2004 Is . . ."

The next night, millions of Americans tuned in to the final results show. It featured the reunion of the twelve finalists and filmed footage from Fantasia and DeGarmo's hometowns. But viewers had to wait until the end of the show for what they wanted to see most—the announcement of who would become the newest "American Idol."

Alone onstage with Seacrest, Fantasia and DeGarmo put their arms around one another. Behind them was a giant screen that would soon flash a picture of the contest winner. Seacrest talked a little about the season. He also revealed that a record 65 million votes had been cast on the final performances.

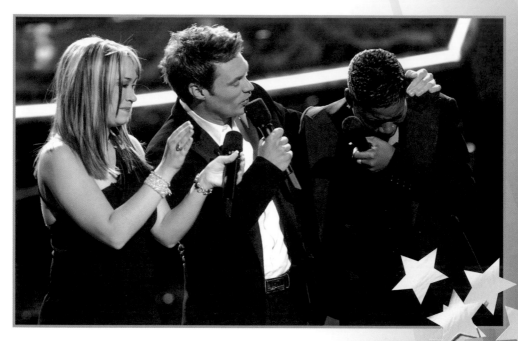

Fantasia was overwhelmed when Ryan Seacrest announced live on air that she had become the third American Idol.

Fantasia was so nervous that she could barely listen: "(H)is lips were moving, but I couldn't understand a word he was sayin'. I opened my eyes a little bit at a time, thinking that Diana DeGarmo would be on the screen. Instead I looked up to see 'Tasia. Ryan was saying my name: 'The "American Idol" for 2004 is Fantasia Barrino.'"

4 THE FANTASIA PHENOMENON

After her win, Fantasia was thrown into a whirlwind. She and the other top-ten contestants spent the summer on the *American Idol* tour, stopping at fifty-two cities in North America. The hectic schedule was exhausting, but adjusting to her sudden fame was more difficult. Everywhere they went, their bus was greeted by fans eager to get a look at their favorite singers. For Fantasia, the attention was a little scary. "I wasn't worried they would hurt me," she explained. "I was worried they would be disappointed when they saw me in person . . . What if they had made a mistake by voting for me?"

Despite her worries, the tour was a big success. Once competitors, the singers now worked together to put on the best show they could. Fantasia made a point of ensuring that everyone got his or her

chance to shine. When they began to tour, Fantasia, as the "Idol" winner, sang more songs than anyone else. But she insisted on giving some of her solos to other singers so they, too, could have their moment in the spotlight.

In the Studio

On days off, the other singers played tourist in the cities they visited or just relaxed in their hotel rooms. Fantasia, however, had to jump on a plane and head to Los Angeles. Anytime she was not onstage or traveling, she was working in a recording studio there.

Her single of "I Believe" hit record stores in July. Within a week, it had sold more than 142,000 copies, earning it the top spot on *Billboard* magazine's Hot 100. It also made history. Fantasia became the first artist ever to debut at number one with her first record.

In November 2004, Fantasia's first CD, *Free Yourself*, was released. The album went platinum, eventually selling more than 1.7 million copies. It included four songs that made the *Billboard* charts. The CD earned four Grammy nominations— Best R & B Album, Best R & B Song ("Free Yourself"), Best Female R & B performance ("Free Yourself"), and Best Traditional R & B Performance ("Summertime").

Telling Her Story

Fantasia's career headed in a new direction in September 2005 with the release of her memoir, *Life Is Not a Fairy Tale*. In the

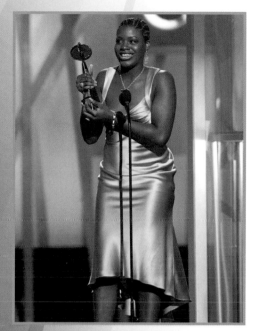

Fantasia was all smiles when she accepted the award for "I Believe," the top-selling single of 2004, at the Billboard Music Awards.

book, she recounts the many struggles she had experienced before *Idol*—from her rape in high school to her teenage pregnancy to her struggles with poor reading skills. Brutally honest, Fantasia's story struck a chord with the public and became a surprise best seller.

After the release of her book, Fantasia set out on the road again, touring with rap artist Kanye West. When the tour ended, she was presented with a new challenge. The Lifetime cable network wanted to make a television movie out of *Life Is Not a Fairy Tale*. Fantasia had appeared in cameos on several TV shows, including *All of Us* and *American Dreams*, on which she portrayed Aretha Franklin. But other than those brief spots, she had never acted before. Even so, Lifetime took a chance and hired her to play herself in the movie.

Premiering on August 18, 2006, *Fairy Tale* was a hit. On its first telecast, it drew 6.6 million viewers, making it the second-highest-rated television movie in Lifetime's history. Both viewers and reviewers were impressed by Fantasia's emotional

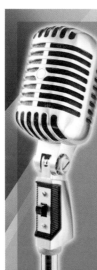

Advice from Fantasia

In her autobiography, *Life Is Not a Fairy Tale*, Fantasia offers fans advice based on lessons she has learned in her own life.

On grabbing opportunities: "When a door is opened for you, you have to step up your game . . . Anyone with talent and hunger can succeed when given the chance."

On loving yourself: "Good love in your life doesn't have to come in the form of a man. The best love in your life is your self-love."

On children: "Cherish the relationship with your children; it's the only lifelong relationship you will have."

On learning from others: "Listen and learn. You don't know everything, even when you think you do."

On respect: "Know that you are a child of God and treat everyone with the same respect that you want because they are children of God, too."

On dreams: "Having dreams are the first part of making things happen . . . If you are not dreamin' big, then you are just sleepin' on life."

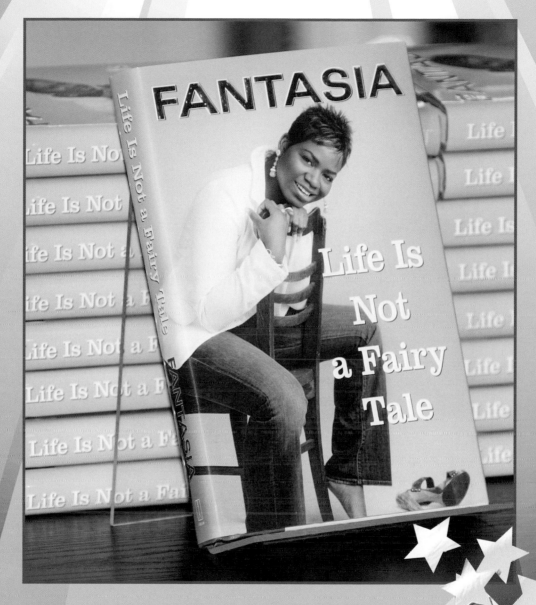

Fantasia's autobiography became a surprise best seller and inspired a successful television movie, in which Fantasia played herself.

performance. The *New York Post* declared, "(S)he does a terrific job in the title role—a performance that marks this movie as another personal triumph for her, on par with writing a best-selling book and winning 'Idol.'"

For Fantasia, the movie represented something even bigger: a complete break from her former life. In the biography on her Web site, she said, "I was able to let go of the past with the Lifetime movie, and now I'm on a whole different level."

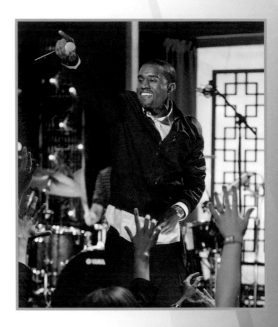

In 2005, Fantasia joined rap artist Kanye West on his "Touch the Sky" tour.

Bold and Daring

Fantasia's new attitude was evident on her second self-titled CD, which was released in December 2006. She had regretted that *Free Yourself* showed only one side of her. As she explained to *Entertainment Weekly*, "I didn't have enough songs on *Free Yourself* for the DJs. All of the songs were slow ballads."

On *Fantasia*, she purposely cultivated a more daring sound. The album included several hits such as "Hood Boy"

and "When I See U." It also allowed her to collaborate with some of the biggest names in R & B and rap music, including Babyface, Big Boi, and her close friend Missy Elliott.

Even as her career continued to blaze white hot, Fantasia faced one big disappointment. She was invited to audition for the pivotal role of Effie in the film version of the musical *Dreamgirls*. In the end, though, she lost the part to fellow *Idol* alum Jennifer Hudson, who went on to win the Best Supporting Actress Oscar in February 2007 for her performance. Fantasia told *Entertainment Weekly*, "I was a little hurt. I had stayed up late reading that script, trying to get Effie in my spirit. I worked so hard. But it wasn't for me."

A New Stage

Soon, though, another great part came along for Fantasia. She was approached by Oprah Winfrey and Quincy Jones, producers of the Broadway musical *The Color Purple*. Based on the Pulitzer Prize-winning novel by Alice Walker, the show had opened more than a year earlier. They invited Fantasia to take over the lead role of Celie, beginning in April 2007. Given her biography, Fantasia seemed a natural to play Celie, a poor woman who, through the power of love, overcomes abuse and adversity. Winfrey and Jones were so confident Fantasia could handle the part that they did not even ask her to audition.

Fantasia, however, was a little hesitant. After all, she had never been to a Broadway show, much less performed in one.

But after seeing the musical, she was eager to take the part. As she told Winfrey on her television talk show, "It's such a powerful role . . . And I'm ready. I've got so much to let out, and I feel like I can take all of that and put it out there on the stage."

In the first week, ticket sales for her Broadway debut soared to $1.2 million, setting a record for the theater. The reviews for her performance were even more impressive. The Associated Press said she gave the production "new heart, soul, and star

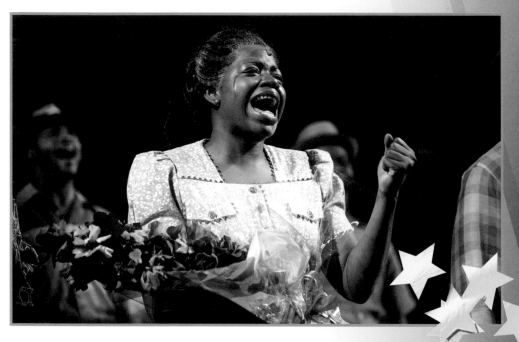

For her performance as Celie in *The Color Purple*, Fantasia won the prestigious Theater World Award. The award honors outstanding Broadway debuts.

power," while *Newsday* called her performance a "phenomenal stage debut." The *New York Times* declared, "Fantasia exudes a sweetness, simplicity, and honesty that gives it a core of authentic feeling."

In just three years since becoming an "American Idol," Fantasia had made an amazing journey. Once a poor teenage mother ready to surrender her hopes and dreams, Fantasia had transformed herself into a television celebrity, a beloved singer, a best-selling author, and a Broadway star. More than ever, she is willing to take on any and all new challenges that come her way. As Fantasia exclaims on her Web site, "(H)ey, I'm gonna ride this train till the wheels fall off!"

Glossary

ballad A slow, romantic song.

boot camp A place that provides a short, intense period of training in a specific field.

cameo A small part, often in a single scene in a television show.

critique A critical discussion of a performance or piece of art.

debut A performer's first public appearance.

General Educational Development (GED) test A test that dropouts can take to demonstrate that they have mastered a body of knowledge equivalent to a high school education.

gospel A style of African American religious music that combines elements of old spirituals with folk and jazz music.

Grammy One of many music awards in various categories given annually by the National Academy of Recording Arts and Sciences.

Motown A record company originally based in Detroit, Michigan, that pioneered a popular style of R & B music in the 1960s and 1970s.

platinum record A single or an album that has sold more than one million copies.

producer A person who supervises the creation of an artistic production such as a television show or a CD.

projects Informal term for government-financed housing.

R & B Meaning "rhythm and blues," a style of music combining blues and jazz and associated with African American performers.

rendition A particular performance of a song.

For More Information

Fox Broadcasting Co.
P.O. Box 900
Beverly Hills, CA 90213
(310) 369-1000
Web site: http://www.fox.com
   Fox is the network that broadcasts the television program *American Idol*.

J Records
745 Fifth Avenue, 6th Floor
New York, NY 10151
(646) 840-5600
Web site: http://www.jrecords.com
   This American record label produces and distributes Fantasia Barrino's recordings.

Web Sites

Due to the changing nature of Internet links, Rosen Publishing has developed an online list of Web sites related to the topic of this book. This site is updated regularly. Please use this link to access the list:

http://www.rosenlinks.com/wyi/faba

For Further Reading

Carroll, Jillian. *Aretha Franklin.* Chicago, IL: Raintree, 2004.

Cowell, Simon. *I Don't Mean to Be Rude, But...: Backstage Gossip from American Idol & the Secrets That Can Make You a Star.* New York, NY: Broadway Books, 2003.

Fantasia. *Life Is Not a Fairy Tale.* New York, NY: Fireside, 2005.

Fonseca, Nicholas. "Fantasia Voyage." *Entertainment Weekly.* December 15, 2006, pp. 23–27.

Handyside, Christopher. *Soul and R & B.* Chicago, IL: Heinemann Library, 2006.

Hoffmann, Frank W. *Rhythm and Blues, Rap, and Hip-Hop.* New York, NY: Facts On File, 2006.

Rich, Jason. *American Idol Season 3: All Access.* Roseville, CA: Prima Games, 2004.

Bibliography

American Idol Web Site. Retrieved May 3, 2007 (http://www. americanidol.com).

Fantasia. *Life Is Not a Fairy Tale.* New York, NY: Fireside, 2005.

Fantasia's Official Web Site. Retrieved May 5, 2007 (http:// www.fantasiabarrinoofficial.com).

Fonseca, Nicholas. "Fantasia Voyage." *Entertainment Weekly.* December 15, 2006, pp. 23–27.

Rich, Jason. *American Idol Season 3: All Access.* Roseville, CA: Prima Games, 2004.

Index

About the Author

Liz Sonneborn is a writer living in Brooklyn, New York. A graduate of Swarthmore College, she has written more than sixty books for children and adults, including *A to Z of American Women in the Performing Arts* and the *New York Public Library's Amazing Native American History*, winner of a 2000 Parent's Choice Award.

Usually a casual *American Idol* fan, Sonneborn was drawn completely into Season Three, mostly because of Fantasia and her outsized talent. "I was eager to work on this book because I like Fantasia and wanted to know more about her," she explained. "What I learned really earned my respect. I went to a high school in the South that was right across the street from a housing project. Many of the kids I knew were like Fantasia as a teenager, poor and hopeless. It was a hard life. Knowing about that firsthand only makes me admire Fantasia's success all the more."

Photo Credits

Cover, pp. 1, 5, 7, 16, 19, 22, 27, 33, 36, 38, 39, 41 © Getty Images; pp. 10, 15 The High Point Enterprise; p. 12 High Point Market Authority; pp. 21, 37 www.istockphoto.com; p. 25 © AP/WideWorld Photos; p. 31 © Getty Images for Fox.

Designer: Tahara Anderson; **Editor:** Kathy Kuhtz Campbell; **Photo Researcher:** Marty Levick